Statistics in the Health Sciences

Series Editors
K. Dietz, M. Gail, K. Krickeberg, B. Singer

Springer
New York
Berlin
Heidelberg
Barcelona
Budapest
Hong Kong
London
Milan
Paris
Tokyo

Statistics in the Health Sciences

David G. Kleinbaum

SURVIVAL ANALYSIS

A Self-Learning Text

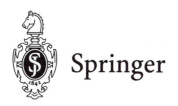 Springer

David G. Kleinbaum
Department of Epidemiology
Emory University
Atlanta, GA 30333
USA

Series Editors
K. Dietz
Institut für Medizinische Biometrie
Universität Tübingen
West Bahnhotstrasse 55
7400 Tübingen
Germany

M. Gail
National Cancer Institute
Rockville, MD 20892
USA

K. Krickeberg
3 Rue de L'Estrapade
75005 Paris
France

B. Singer
Office of Population Research
Princeton University
Princeton, NJ 08544
USA

Library of Congress Cataloging-in-Publication Data
Kleinbaum, David G.
    Survival Analysis: a self-learning text / David G. Kleinbaum.
      p.   cm. — (Statistics in the health sciences)
    Includes bibliographical references and index.
    ISBN 0-387-94543-1 (hardcover: alk. paper)
    1. Survival analysis (Biometry)   I. Title   II. Series: Springer
series in statistics. Statistics in the health sciences.
    R853.S7K543 1995
    610′.72—dc20   95-18632

Printed on acid-free paper.

Production managed by Steven Pisano; manufacturing supervised by Jeffrey Taub.
Typeset by Impressions, Inc., Madison, WI.
Printed and bound by Edwards Brothers, Inc., Ann Arbor, MI.
Printed in the United States of America.

9 8 7 6 5 4 3 2 1

ISBN 0-387-94543-1 Springer-Verlag New York Berlin Heidelberg   SPIN 10490574

To my mother,
Janet Leventhal Kleinbaum Cohen

Preface

This text on survival analysis methods contains the following chapters:

1 Introduction to Survival Analysis
2 Kaplan–Meier Survival Curves and the Log–Rank Test
3 The Cox Proportional Hazards Model and Its Characteristics
4 Evaluating the Proportional Hazards Assumption
5 The Stratified Cox Procedure
6 Extension of the Cox Proportional Hazards Model for Time-Dependent Variables

Each chapter contains a presentation of its topic in "lecture-book" format together with objectives, an outline, key formulae, practice exercises, and a test. The "lecture-book" has a sequence of illustrations and formulae in the left column of each page and a script in the right column. This format allows you to read the script in conjunction with the illustrations and formulae that highlight the main points, formulae, or examples being presented.

The reader may also purchase directly from the author audio cassette tapes of each chapter. The use of the audiotape with the illustrations and formulae, ignoring the script, is intended to be similar to a lecture. Tapes may be obtained by writing or calling the author at the following address: Department of Epidemiology, Rollins School of Public Health, Emory University, 1518 Clifton Rd. N.E., Atlanta, GA 30322; phone (404) 727–9667.

Suggestions for Use

This text is intended for self-study. The text may be used to supplement material covered in a course, to review previously learned material, or to provide the primary learning material in a self-instructional course or self-planned learning activity. A more individualized learning program may be particularly suitable to a working professional who does not have the time to participate in a regularly scheduled course. If you purchase the audiotapes, you may consider using the tapes without the script, although, if used this way, the learner will have difficulty visualizing any formulae or calculations being explained on the tape. Such use, however, may be beneficial for review of previously studied material. (You may be able to glance at the pictures while driving and listening to the tape, particularly if stuck in traffic, but the author assumes no responsibility for the consequences!)

In working with any chapter, the learner is encouraged first to read the abbreviated outline and the objectives and then work through the presentation, by using either the script or the audiotape with the picture sequence. After finishing the presentation, the user is encouraged to read the detailed outline for a summary of the presentation, review the key formulae and other important information, work through the practice exercises, and, finally, complete the test to check what has been learned.

Recommended Preparation

The ideal preparation for this text on survival analysis is a course on quantitative methods in epidemiology and a course in applied multiple regression. Also, knowledge of logistic regression, modeling strategies, and maximum likelihood techniques is crucial for the material on the Cox model described in modules 3–6 of this series.

Recommended references on these subjects, with suggested chapter readings, are:

Kleinbaum D., Kupper L., and Morgenstern, H., *Epidemiologic Research: Principles and Quantitative Methods*, Van Nostrand Reinhold Publishers, New York, 1982, Chaps. 20–24.

Kleinbaum, D., Kupper, L., and Muller, K., *Applied Regression Analysis and Other Multivariable Methods*, Second Edition, Duxbury Press, Boston, 1987, Chaps. 1–16, 20.

Kleinbaum, D., *Logistic Regression: A Self-Learning Test*, Springer-Verlag Publishers, New York, 1994.

A first course on the principles of epidemiologic research would be helpful, since all modules in this series are written from the perspective of epidemiologic research. In particular, the learner should be familiar with the basic characteristics of epidemiologic study designs (follow-up, case control, and cross sectional), and should have some idea of the frequently encountered problem of controlling or adjusting for variables.

As for mathematics prerequisites, the reader should be familiar with natural logarithms and their relationship to exponentials (powers of e), and, more generally, should be able to read mathematical notation and formulae.

Acknowledgments

I wish to thank John Capelhorn at Sydney University's Department of Public Health for carefully reading the manuscript, and for providing meaningful criticism, support, and continued friendship. I also wish to thank Chris Nardo for his contribution to the computer aspects of this text, particularly the appendix on computer programs for survival analysis. I thank Holly Hill for reviewing portions of the manuscript, for computer assistance, and for her friendship. I thank G. David Williamson at the Centers for Disease Control and Prevention for arranging institutional support for this project. I thank Phil Rhodes at the Centers for Disease Control and Prevention for reviewing the manuscript and providing many thoughtful comments. I also thank the faculty of the Rollins School fo Public Health at Emory University and John Boring, in particular, for providing a wonderful working environment and colleagueship during the latter stages of this project.

Finally, I thank Edna Kleinbaum, my wife, whose love, support, companionship, and sense of humor has made my life so joyful during the past two and a half years.

Contents

Chapter 5   **The Stratified Cox Procedure   171**

Chapter 6   **Extension of the Cox Proportional Hazards Model for Time-Dependent Variables   211**

Appendix A: Computer Programs for Survival Analysis   255

Appendix B: Datasets   291

Test Answers   305

References   319

Index   321

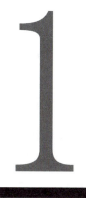

1 Introduction to Survival Analysis

Introduction

This introduction to survival analysis gives a descriptive overview of the data analytic approach called **survival analysis.** This approach includes the type of problem addressed by survival analysis, the outcome variable considered, the need to take into account "censored data," what a survival function and a hazard function represent, basic data layouts for a survival analysis, the goals of survival analysis, and some examples of survival analysis.

Because this chapter is primarily descriptive in content, no prerequisite mathematical, statistical, or epidemiologic concepts are absolutely necessary. A first course on the principles of epidemiologic research would be helpful. It would also be helpful if the reader has had some experience reading mathematical notation and formulae.

Abbreviated Outline

The outline below gives the user a preview of the material to be covered by the presentation. A detailed outline for review purposes follows the presentation.

Objectives   Upon completing the module, the learner should be able to:

1. Recognize or describe the type of problem addressed by a survival analysis.
2. Define what is meant by censored data.
3. Define or recognize right-censored data.
4. Give three reasons why data may be censored.
5. Define, recognize, or interpret a survivor function.
6. Define, recognize, or interpret a hazard function.
7. Describe the relationship between a survivor function and a hazard function.
8. State three goals of a survival analysis.
9. Identify or recognize the basic data layout for the computer; in particular, put a given set of survival data into this layout.
10. Identify or recognize the basic data layout, or components thereof, for understanding modeling theory; in particular, put a given set of survival data into this layout.
11. Interpret or compare examples of survivor curves or hazard functions.
12. Given a problem situation, state the goal of a survival analysis in terms of describing how explanatory variables relate to survival time.
13. Compute or interpret average survival and/or average hazard measures from a set of survival data.
14. Define or interpret the hazard ratio defined from comparing two groups of survival data.

Presentation

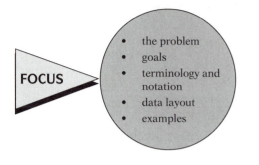

- the problem
- goals
- terminology and notation
- data layout
- examples

This presentation gives a general introduction to survival analysis, a popular data analysis approach for certain kinds of epidemiologic and other data. Here we focus on the problem addressed by survival analysis, the goals of a survival analysis, key notation and terminology, the basic data layout, and some examples.

I. What Is Survival Analysis?

Outcome variable: **Time until an event occurs**

We begin by describing the type of analytic problem addressed by survival analysis. Generally, survival analysis is a collection of statistical procedures for data analysis for which the outcome variable of interest is *time until an event occurs.*

Start follow-up   TIME   Event

By **time,** we mean years, months, weeks, or days from the beginning of follow-up of an individual until an event occurs; alternatively, time can refer to the **age** of an individual when an event occurs.

Event: death
disease
relapse
recovery

By **event,** we mean death, disease incidence, relapse from remission, recovery (e.g., return to work) or any designated experience of interest that may happen to an individual.

Assume 1 event

> 1 event   Competing risk

Although more than one event may be considered in the same analysis, we will assume that only one event is of designated interest. When more than one event is considered (e.g., death from any of several causes), the statistical problem is generally characterized as a **competing risk** problem, which is beyond the scope of this presentation.

Time ≡ survival time

Event ≡ failure

In a survival analysis, we usually refer to the time variable as **survival time,** because it gives the time that an individual has "survived" over some follow-up period. We also typically refer to the event as a **failure,** because the kind of event of interest usually is death, disease incidence, or some other negative individual experience. However, survival time may be "time to return to work after an elective surgical procedure," in which case failure is a positive event.

EXAMPLE

1. Leukemia patients/time in remission (weeks)
2. Disease-free cohort/time until heart disease (years)
3. Elderly (60+) population/time until death (years)
4. Parolees (recidivism study)/time until rearrest (weeks)
5. Heart transplants/time until death (months)

Five examples of survival analysis problems are briefly mentioned here. The first is a study that follows leukemia patients in remission over several weeks to see how long they stay in remission. The second example follows a disease-free cohort of individuals over several years to see who develops heart disease. A third example considers a 13-year follow-up of an elderly population (60+ years) to see how long subjects remain alive. A fourth example follows newly released parolees for several weeks to see whether they get rearrested. (This type of problem is called a recidivism study.) The fifth example traces how long patients survive after receiving a heart transplant.

All of the above examples are survival analysis problems because the outcome variable is time until an event occurs. In the first example, involving leukemia patients, the event of interest (i.e., failure) is "going out of remission," and the outcome is "time in weeks until a person goes out of remission." In the second example, the event is "developing heart disease," and the outcome is "time in years until a person develops heart disease." In the third example, the event is "death" and the outcome is "time in years to death." Example four, a sociological rather than a medical study, considers the event of recidivism (i.e., getting rearrested), and the outcome is time in weeks until rearrested. Finally, the fifth example considers the event "death," with the outcome being "time until death (in months from receiving a transplant)."

We will return to some of these examples later in this presentation and in later presentations.

II. Censored Data

Censoring: don't know survival time exactly

Most survival analyses must consider a key analytical problem called **censoring.** In essence, censoring occurs when we have some information about individual survival time, but **we don't know the survival time exactly.**

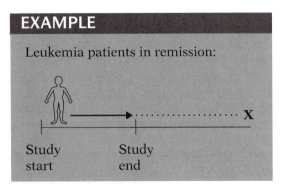

EXAMPLE

Leukemia patients in remission:

Why censor?

1. study ends—no event
2. lost
3. withdraws

As a simple example of censoring, consider leukemia patients followed until they go out of remission, shown here as **X.** If for a given patient, the study ends while the patient is still in remission (i.e., doesn't get the event), then that patient's survival time is considered censored. We know that, for this person, the survival time is at least as long as the period that the person has been followed, but if the person goes out of remission after the study ends, we do not know the complete survival time.

There are generally three reasons why censoring may occur:

(1) a person does not experience the event before **the study ends;**
(2) a person is **lost to follow-up** during the study period;
(3) a person **withdraws from the study** because of death (if death is not the event of interest) or some other reason (e.g., adverse drug reaction).

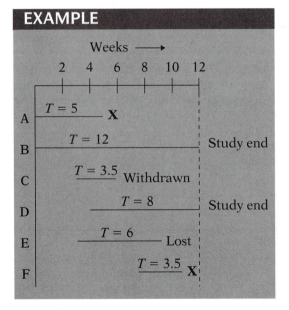

EXAMPLE

These situations are graphically illustrated here. The graph describes the experience of several persons followed over time. An **X** denotes a person who got the event.

Person A, for example, is followed from the start of the study until getting the event at week 5; his survival time is 5 weeks and is *not* censored.

Person B also is observed at the start of the study but is followed to the end of the 12-week study period without getting the event; the survival time here is censored because we can say only that it is *at least* 12 weeks.

Person C enters the study between the second and third week and is followed until he/she withdraws from the study at 6 weeks; this person's survival time is censored after 3.5 weeks.

Person D enters at week 4 and is followed for the remainder of the study without getting the event; this person's censored time is 8 weeks.

Person E enters the study at week 3 and is followed until week 9, when he is lost to follow-up; his censored time is 6 weeks.

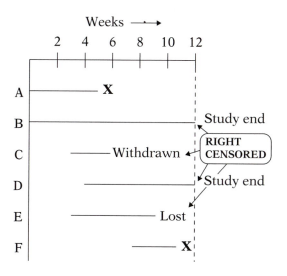

X ➡ Event occurs

Person F enters at week 8 and is followed until getting the event at week 11.5. As with person A, there is no censoring here; the survival time is 3.5 weeks.

SUMMARY
Event: A, F
Censored: B, C, D, E

In **summary,** of the six persons observed, two get the event (persons A and F) and four are censored (B, C, D, and E).

Person	Survival time	Failed (1); censored (0)
A	5	1
B	12	0
C	3.5	0
D	8	0
E	6	0
F	3.5	1

A table of the survival time data for the six persons in the graph is now presented. For each person, we have given the corresponding survival time up to the event's occurring or up to censorship. We have indicated in the last column whether this time was censored or not (with 1 denoting failed and 0 denoting censored). For example, the data for person C is a survival time of 3.5 and a censorship indicator of 0, whereas for person F the survival time is 3.5 and the censorship indicator is 1. This table is a simplified illustration of the type of data to be analyzed in a survival analysis.

Notice in our example that for each of the four persons censored, we know that the person's exact survival time becomes incomplete at the **right** side of the follow-up period, occurring when the study ends or when the person is lost to follow-up or is withdrawn. We generally refer to this kind of data as **right-censored.** For these data, the complete survival time interval, which we don't really know, has been cut off (i.e., censored) at the right side. Although data can also be **left-censored,** most survival data is right-censored. In the remainder of this text, we will consider right-censored data only.

Left-censored data:

Left censored   Observed survival time

················· ————————**X**

↑   ↑

HIV exposure HIV + test

Left-censored data can occur when a person's survival time becomes incomplete at the left side of the follow-up period for that person. For example, if we are following persons with HIV infection, we may start follow-up when a subject first tests positive for the HIV virus, but we may not know exactly the time of first exposure to the virus. Thus, the survival time is censored on the left side, because there is unknown follow-up time from the time of first exposure up to the time of first positive HIV test.

III. Terminology and Notation

T = survival time $(T \geq 0)$

       ◄———— random variable

t = specific value for T

We are now ready to introduce basic mathematical terminology and notation for survival analysis. First, we denote by a **capital T** the random variable for a person's survival time. Since T denotes time, its possible values include all nonnegative numbers; that is, T can be any number equal to or greater than zero.

EXAMPLE

Survives > 5 years?

$T > t = 5$

Next, we denote by a **small letter t** any specific value of interest for the random variable capital T. For example, if we are interested in evaluating whether a person survives for more than 5 years after undergoing cancer therapy, **small t** equals 5; we then ask whether capital T exceeds 5.

$\delta = (0, 1)$ random variable

$$= \begin{cases} 1 \text{ if failure} \\ 0 \text{ if censored} \end{cases}$$

- study ends
- lost
- withdraws

Finally, we let the Greek letter delta (δ) denote a (0,1) random variable indicating either failure or censorship. That is, $\delta = 1$ for failure if the event occurs during the study period, or $\delta = 0$ if the survival time is censored by the end of the study period. Note that if a person does not fail, that is, does not get the event during the study period, censorship is the **only** remaining possibility for that person's survival time. That is, $\delta = 0$ if and only if one of the following happens: a person survives until the study ends, a person is lost to follow-up, or a person withdraws during the study period.

$S(t)$ = survivor function
$h(t)$ = hazard function

We next introduce and describe two quantitative terms considered in any survival analysis. These are the **survivor function,** denoted by $S(t)$, and the **hazard function,** denoted by $h(t)$.

$S(t) = P(T > t)$

t	$S(t)$
1	$S(1) = P(T > 1)$
2	$S(2) = P(T > 2)$
3	$S(3) = P(T > 3)$
·	·
·	·
·	·

Theoretical $S(t)$:

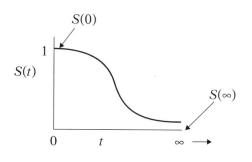

$\hat{S}(t)$ in practice:

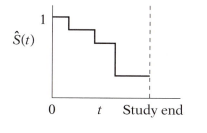

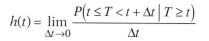

$$h(t) = \lim_{\Delta t \to 0} \frac{P\left(t \leq T < t + \Delta t \mid T \geq t\right)}{\Delta t}$$

The survivor function $S(t)$ gives the probability that a person survives longer than some specified time **t:** that is, $S(t)$ gives the probability that the random variable T exceeds the specified time t.

The survivor function is fundamental to a survival analysis, because obtaining survival probabilities for different values of t provides crucial summary information from survival data.

Theoretically, as t ranges from 0 up to infinity, the survivor function can be graphed as a smooth curve. As illustrated by the graph here, where t identifies the X-axis, all survivor functions have the following characteristics:

- they are nonincreasing; that is, they head downward as to increases;
- at time $t = 0$, $S(t) = S(0) = 1$; that is, at the start of the study, since no one has gotten the event yet, the probability of surviving past time 0 is one;
- at time t = ∞, $S(t) = S(\infty) = 0$; that is, theoretically, if the study period increased without limit, eventually nobody would survive, so the survivor curve must eventually fall to zero.

Note that these are **theoretical** properties of survivor curves.

In practice, when using actual data, we usually obtain graphs that are **step functions,** as illustrated here, rather than smooth curves. Moreover, because the study period is never infinite in length, it is possible that not everyone studied gets the event; the estimated survivor function, denoted by a caret over the S in the graph, thus does not go all the way down to zero at the end of the study.

The hazard function, denoted by **$h(t)$,** is given by the formula: $h(t)$ equals the limit, as Δt approaches zero, of a probability statement about survival, divided by Δt, where Δt denotes a small interval of time. This mathematical formula is difficult to explain in practical terms.

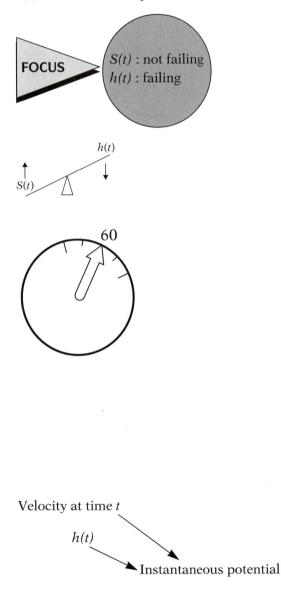

$h(t)$ = instantaneous potential

$S(t)$: not failing
$h(t)$: failing

Before getting into the specifics of the formula, we give a conceptual interpretation. **The hazard function $h(t)$ gives the instantaneous potential per unit time for the event to occur, given that the individual has survived up to time t.** Note that, in contrast to the survivor function, which focuses on *not* failing, the hazard function focuses on failing, that is, on the event occurring. Thus, in some sense, the hazard function can be considered as giving the negative side of the information given by the survivor function. That is, the higher $S(t)$ is for a given t, the smaller is $h(t)$, and vice versa.

To get an idea of what we mean by instantaneous potential, consider the concept of velocity. If, for example, you are driving in your car and you see that your speedometer is registering 60 mph, what does this reading mean? It means that if in the next hour, you continue to drive this way, with the speedometer exactly on 60, you would cover 60 miles. This reading gives the **potential,** at the moment you have looked at your speedometer, for how many miles you will travel in the next hour. However, because you may slow down or speed up or even stop during the next hour, the 60-mph speedometer reading does not tell you the number of miles you *really* will cover in the next hour. The speedometer tells you only how fast you are going *at a given moment;* that is, the instrument gives your instantaneous potential or velocity.

Velocity at time t

$h(t)$

Instantaneous potential

Similar to the idea of velocity, a hazard function $h(t)$ gives the instantaneous potential at time t for getting an event, like death or some disease of interest, given survival up to time t. The given part, that is, surviving up to time t, is analogous to recognizing in the velocity example that the speedometer reading at a point in time inherently assumes that you have already traveled some distance (i.e., survived) up to the time of the reading.

Given

$$h(t) = \lim_{\Delta t \to 0} \frac{P\left(t \le T < t + \Delta t \mid T \ge t\right)}{\Delta t}$$

Conditional probabilities: $P(A \mid B)$

1.2. $P(t \le T < t + \Delta t \mid T \ge t)$

Hazard function $\equiv$ conditional failure **rate**

$$\lim_{\Delta t \to 0} \frac{P\left(t \le T < t + \Delta t \mid T \ge t\right)}{\Delta t}$$

Probability per unit time

Rate: 0 to ∞

$P = P(t \le T < t + \Delta t \mid T \ge t)$

P	Δt	$P/_{\Delta t}$ = rate
$\dfrac{1}{3}$	$\dfrac{1}{2}$ day	$\dfrac{1/3}{1/2} = 0.67/\text{day}$
$\dfrac{1}{3}$	$\dfrac{1}{14}$ week	$\dfrac{1/3}{1/14} = 4.67/\text{week}$

In mathematical terms, the given part of the formula for the hazard function is found in the probability statement—the numerator to the right of the limit sign. This statement is a conditional probability because it is of the form, P of A, given B, where the P denotes probability and where the long vertical line separating A from B denotes "given." In the hazard formula, the conditional probability gives the probability that the event will occur in the time interval between t and $t + \Delta t$, given that the survival time, T, is greater than or equal to t. Because of the given sign here, the hazard function is sometimes called a **conditional failure rate.**

We now explain why the hazard is a **rate** rather than a probability. Note that in the hazard function formula, the expression to the right of the limit sign gives the ratio of two quantities. The numerator is the conditional probability we just discussed. The denominator is Δt, which denotes a small time interval. By this division, we obtain a probability per unit time, which is no longer a probability but a rate. In particular, the scale for this ratio is not 0 to 1, as for a probability, but rather ranges between 0 and infinity, and depends on whether time is measured in days, weeks, months, or years, etc.

For example, if the probability, denoted here by P, is 1/3, and the time interval is one-half a day, then the probability divided by the time interval is 1/3 divided by 1/2, which equals 0.67 per day. As another example, suppose, for the same probability of 1/3, that the time interval is considered in weeks, so that 1/2 day equals 1/14 of a week. Then the probability divided by the time interval becomes 1/3 over 1/14, which equals 14/3, or 4.67 per week. The point is simply that the expression P divided by Δt at the right of the limit sign **does not give a probability. The value obtained will give a different number depending on the units of time used, and may even give a number larger than one.**

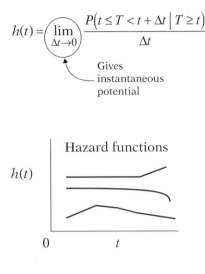

$$h(t) = \left(\lim_{\Delta t \to 0} \right) \frac{P\left(t \le T < t + \Delta t \mid T \ge t\right)}{\Delta t}$$

Gives
instantaneous
potential

When we take the limit of the right-side expression as the time interval approaches zero, we are essentially getting an expression for the instantaneous probability of failing at time t per unit time. Another way of saying this is that the conditional failure rate or hazard function $h(t)$ gives the instantaneous **potential** for failing at time t per unit time, given survival up to time t.

As with a survivor function, the hazard function $h(t)$ can be graphed as t ranges over various values. The graph at the left illustrates three different hazards. In contrast to a survivor function, the graph of $h(t)$ does not have to start at 1 and go down to zero, but rather can start anywhere and go up and down in any direction over time. In particular, for a specified value of t, the hazard $h(t)$ has the following characteristics:

- it is always nonnegative, that is, equal to or greater than zero;
- it has no upper bound.

These two features follow from the ratio expression in the formula for $h(t)$, because both the probability in the numerator and the Δt in the denominator are nonnegative, and since Δt can range between 0 and ∞.

Hazard functions

$h(t)$

0   t

- $h(t) \ge 0$
- $h(t)$ has no upper bound

EXAMPLE

Constant hazard
(**exponential model**)

$h(t)$ for healthy
persons

λ

t

Now we show some graphs of different types of hazard functions. The first graph given shows a constant hazard for a study of healthy persons. In this graph, no matter what value of t is specified, $h(t)$ equals the same value—in this example, λ. Note that for a person who continues to be healthy throughout the study period, his/her instantaneous potential for becoming ill at any time during the period remains constant no matter what time is picked. When the hazard function is constant, we say that the survival model is **exponential.** This term follows from the relationship between the survivor function and the hazard function. We will return to this relationship later.

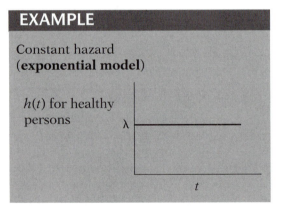

EXAMPLE (continued)

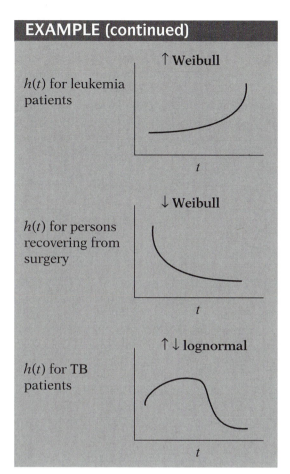

$h(t)$ for leukemia patients

$h(t)$ for persons recovering from surgery

$h(t)$ for TB patients

The second hazard function illustrated shows a graph that is increasing. This kind of graph is called an **increasing Weibull** model. Such a graph might be expected for leukemia patients not responding to treatment, where the event of interest is death. As survival time increases for such a patient, and as the prognosis accordingly worsens, the patient's potential for dying of the disease also increases.

The third hazard function illustrated shows a graph that is decreasing. This kind of graph is called a **decreasing Weibull.** Such a graph might be expected when the event is death in persons who are recovering from surgery, because the potential for dying after surgery usually decreases as the time after surgery increases.

The fourth hazard function given shows a graph that is first increasing and then decreasing. This type of graph is called a **lognormal survival** model. We can expect such a graph for tuberculosis patients, since their potential for dying increases early in the disease and decreases later.

$S(t)$: directly describes survival

$h(t)$: • insight about conditional failure rates
   • identify specific model form
   • math model for survival analysis

Of the two functions we have considered, $S(t)$ and $h(t)$, the survivor function is more naturally appealing for analysis of survival data, simply because $S(t)$ directly describes the survival experience of a study cohort.

However, the hazard function is also of interest for the following reasons:

• it provides insight about conditional failure rates;
• it may be used to identify a specific model form, such as an exponential, a Weibull, or a lognormal curve that fits one's data;
• it is the vehicle by which mathematical modeling of survival data is carried out; that is, the survival model is usually written in terms of the hazard function.

Relationship of *S(t)* and *h(t)*:

If you know one, you can determine the other.

> ## EXAMPLE
>
> $h(t) = \lambda$ if and only if $S(t) = e^{-\lambda t}$

General formulae:

$$S(t) = \exp\left[-\int_0^t h(u)\,du\right]$$

$$h(t) = -\left[\frac{dS(t)\big/dt}{S(t)}\right]$$

Formulae not important:

$S(t)$ 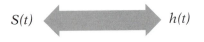 $h(t)$

Regardless of which function $S(t)$ or $h(t)$ one prefers, **there is a clearly defined relationship between the two.** In fact, if one knows the form of $S(t)$, one can derive the corresponding $h(t)$, and vice versa. For example, if the hazard function is constant—i.e., $h(t) = \lambda$, for some specific value λ—then it can be shown that the corresponding survival function is given by the following formula: $S(t)$ equals **e** to the power minus λ times t.

More generally, the relationship between $S(t)$ and $h(t)$ can be expressed equivalently in either of two calculus formulae shown here.

The first of these formulae describes how the survivor function $S(t)$ can be written in terms of an integral involving the hazard function. The formula says that $S(t)$ equals the exponential of the negative integral of the hazard function between integration limits of 0 and t.

The second formula describes how the hazard function $h(t)$ can be written in terms of a derivative involving the survivor function. This formula says that $h(t)$ equals minus the derivative of $S(t)$ with respect to t divided by $S(t)$.

The actual formulae are not important, because in any actual data analysis a computer program can make the numerical transformation from $S(t)$ to $h(t)$, or vice versa, without the user ever having to use either formula. The point here is simply that if you know either $S(t)$ or $h(t)$, you can get the other directly.

SUMMARY

T = survival time random variable
t = specific value of T
δ = (0,1) variable for failure/censorship
$S(t)$ = survivor function
$h(t)$ = hazard function

At this point, we have completed our discussion of key terminology and notation. **The key notation is *T* for the survival time variable, *t* for a specified value of *T*, and δ for the dichotomous variable indicating event occurrence or censorship. The key terms are the survivor function *S(t)* and the hazard function *h(t)*,** which are in essence opposed concepts, in that the survivor function focuses on surviving whereas the hazard function focuses on failing, given survival up to a certain time point.

IV. Goals of Survival Analysis

We now state the basic goals of survival analyses.

Goal 1: To estimate and interpret survivor and/or hazard functions from survival data.

Goal 2: To compare survivor and/or hazard functions.

Goal 3: To assess the relationship of explanatory variables to survival time.

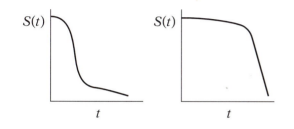

Regarding the first goal, consider, for example, the two survivor functions pictured at the left, which give very different interpretations. The function farther on the left shows a quick drop in survival probabilities early in follow-up but a leveling off thereafter. The function on the right, in contrast, shows a very slow decrease in survival probabilities early in follow-up but a sharp decrease later on.

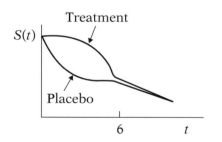

Goal 3: Use math modeling, e.g., Cox
proportional hazards

We compare survivor functions for a treatment group and a placebo group by graphing these functions on the same axis. Note that up to 6 weeks, the graph for the treatment group lies above that for the placebo group, but thereafter the two graphs are at about the same level. This dual graph indicates that up to 6 weeks the treatment is more effective than the placebo but has about the same effect thereafter.

Goal 3 usually requires using some form of mathematical modeling, for example, the Cox proportional hazards approach, which will be the subject of subsequent modules.

V. Basic Data Layout for Computer

Data layouts:
- for computer use
- for understanding

We previously considered some examples of survival analysis problems and a simple data set involving six persons. We now consider the general data layout for a survival analysis. We will provide two types of data layouts, one giving the form appropriate for computer use, and the other giving the form that helps us understand how a survival analysis works.

For computer:

We start by providing, in the table shown here, the basic data layout for the computer. Assume that we have a data set consisting of n persons. The first column of the table identifies each person from 1, starting at the top, to n, at the bottom.

Indiv. #	t	δ	X_1	X_2	$\cdots$	X_p
1	t_1	δ_1	X_{11}	X_{12}	$\cdots$	X_{1p}
2	t_2	δ_2	X_{21}	X_{22}	$\cdots$	X_{2p}
$\vdots$						$\vdots$
5	$t_5 = 3$ got event					
$\vdots$						$\vdots$
8	$t_8 = 3$ censored					
$\vdots$						$\vdots$
n	t_n	δ_n	X_{n1}	X_{n2}	$\cdots$	X_{np}

The remaining columns after the first one provide survival time and other information for each person. The second column gives the survival time information, which is denoted t_1 for individual 1, t_2 for individual 2, and so on, up to t_n for individual n. Each of these t's gives the observed survival time regardless of whether the person got the event or is censored. For example, if person 5 got the event at 3 weeks of follow-up, then $t_5 = 3$; on the other hand, if person 8 was censored at 3 weeks, without getting the event, then $t_8 = 3$ also.

To distinguish persons who get the event from those who are censored, we turn to the third column, which gives the information for δ, the dichotomous variable that indicates censorship status.

Thus, δ_1 is 1 if person 1 gets the event or is 0 if person 1 is censored; δ_2 is 1 or 0 similarly, and so on, up through δ_n. In the example just considered, person 5, who failed at 3 weeks, has a δ of 1; that is, δ_5 equals 1. In contrast, person 8, who was censored at 3 weeks, has a δ of 0; that is, δ_8 equals 0.

Note that if all of the δ_j in this column are added up, their sum will be the total number of failures in the data set. This total will be some number equal to or less than n, because not every one may fail.

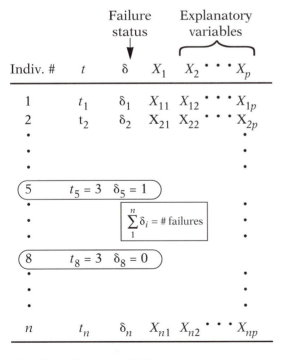

$$X_i = \text{Age, } E, \text{ or Age} \times \text{Race}$$

The remainder of the information in the table gives values for explanatory variables of interest. An explanatory variable, X_i, is any variable like age or exposure status, E, or a product term like age $\times$ race that the investigator wishes to consider to predict survival time. These variables are listed at the top of the table as X_1, X_2, and so on, up to X_p. Below each variable are the values observed for that variable on each person in the data set.

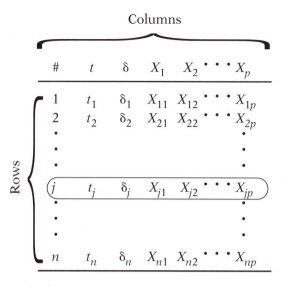

Columns

#	t	δ	X_1	X_2	$\cdots$	X_p
1	t_1	δ_1	X_{11}	X_{12}	$\cdots$	X_{1p}
2	t_2	δ_2	X_{21}	X_{22}	$\cdots$	X_{2p}
$\cdot$						$\cdot$
$\cdot$						$\cdot$
$\cdot$						$\cdot$
j	t_j	δ_j	X_{j1}	X_{j2}	$\cdots$	X_{jp}
$\cdot$						$\cdot$
$\cdot$						$\cdot$
$\cdot$						$\cdot$
n	t_n	δ_n	X_{n1}	X_{n2}	$\cdots$	X_{np}

Rows

For example, in the column corresponding to X_1 are the values observed on this variable for all n persons. These values are denoted as X_{11}, X_{21}, and so on, up to X_{n1}; the first subscript indicates the person number, and the second subscript, a one in each case here, indicates the variable number. Similarly, the column corresponding to variable X_2 gives the values observed on X_2 for all n persons. This notation continues for the other X variables up through X_p.

We have thus described the basic data layout by columns. Alternatively, we can look at the table line by line, that is, by rows. For each line or row, we have the information obtained on a given individual. Thus, for individual j, the observed information is given by the values t_j, δ_j, X_{j1}, X_{j2}, etc., up to X_{jp}. This is how the information is read into the computer, that is, line by line, until all persons are included for analysis.

As an example of this data layout, consider the following set of data for two groups of leukemia patients: one group of 21 persons has received a certain treatment; the other group of 21 persons has received a placebo. The data come from Freireich et al., *Blood*, 1963.

As presented here, the data are not yet in tabular form for the computer, as we will see shortly. The values given for each group consist of time in weeks a patient is in remission, up to the point of the patient's either going out of remission or being censored. Here, going out of remission is a failure. A person is censored if he or she remains in remission until the end of the study, is lost to follow-up, or withdraws before the end of the study. The censored data here are denoted by a plus sign next to the survival time.

EXAMPLE

The data: Remission times (in weeks) for two groups of leukemia patients

Group 1 (Treatment) $n = 21$	Group 2 (Treatment) $n = 21$
6, 6, 6, 7, 10,	1, 1, 2, 2, 3,
13, 16, 22, 23,	4, 4, 5, 5,
6+, 9+, 10+, 11+,	8, 8, 8, 8,
17+, 19+, 20+,	11, 11, 12, 12,
25+, 32+, 32+,	15, 17, 22, 23
34+, 35+	

+ denotes censored

→ In remission at study end

→ Lost to follow-up

→ Withdraws

EXAMPLE (continued)

Group 1 (Treatment) n = 21	Group 2 (Treatment) n = 21
6, 6, 6, 7, 10,	1, 1, 2, 2, 3,
13, 16, 22, 23,	4, 4, 5, 5,
6+, 9+, 10+, 11+,	8, 8, 8, 8,
17+, 19+, 20+,	11, 11, 12, 12,
25+, 32+, 32+,	15, 17, 22, 23
34+, 35+	

	# failed	# censored	Total
Group 1	9	12	21
Group 2	21	0	21

	Indiv. (#)	t (weeks)	δ (failed or censored)	X (Group)
	1	6	1	1
	2	6	1	1
	3	6	1	1
	4	7	1	1
	5	10	1	1
	6	13	1	1
	7	16	1	1
	8	22	1	1
GROUP	9	23	1	1
1	10	6	0	1
	11	9	0	1
	12	10	0	1
	13	11	0	1
	⑭	17	0	1
	15	19	0	1
	16	20	0	1
	17	25	0	1
	18	32	0	1
	19	32	0	1

Here are the data again:

Notice that the first three persons in group 1 went out of remission at 6 weeks; the next six persons also went out of remission, but at failure times ranging from 7 to 23. All of the remaining persons in group 1 with pluses next to their survival times are censored. For example, on line three the first person who has a plus sign next to a 6 is censored at six weeks. The remaining persons in group one are also censored, but at times ranging from 9 to 35 weeks.

Thus, of the 21 persons in group 1, nine failed during the study period, whereas the last 12 were censored. Notice also that none of the data in group 2 is censored; that is, all 21 persons in this group went out of remission during the study period.

We now put this data in tabular form for the computer, as shown at the left. The list starts with the 21 persons in group 1 (listed 1–21) and follows (on the next page) with the 21 persons in group 2 (listed 22–42). Our n for the composite group is 42.

The *second* column of the table gives the survival times in weeks for all 42 persons. The *third* column indicates failure or censorship for each person. Finally, the *fourth* column lists the values of the only explanatory variable we have considered so far, namely, group status, with 1 denoting treatment and 0 denoting placebo.

If we pick out any individual and read across the table, we obtain the line of data for that person that gets entered in the computer. For example, person #3 has a survival time of 6 weeks, and because $\delta = 1$, which means that this person failed, that is, went out of remission, the X value is 1 because person #3 is in group 1. As a second example, person #14, who has a survival time of 17 weeks, was censored at this time because $\delta = 0$. The X value is again 1 because person #14 is also in group 1.

EXAMPLE (continued)

	Indiv. #	t (weeks)	δ (failed or censored)	X (Group)
	20	34	0	1
	21	35	0	1
	22	1	1	0
	23	1	1	0
	24	2	1	0
	25	2	1	0
	26	3	1	0
	27	4	1	0
GROUP	28	4	1	0
2	29	5	1	0
	30	5	1	0
	31	8	1	0
	㉜	8	1	0
	33	8	1	0
	34	8	1	0
	35	11	1	0
	36	11	1	0
	37	12	1	0
	38	12	1	0
	39	15	1	0
	40	17	1	0

As one more example, this time from group 2, person #32 survived 8 weeks and then failed, because $\delta = 1$; the X value is 0 because person #32 is in group 2.

VI. Basic Data Layout for Understanding Analysis

For analysis:

Ordered failure $(t_{(j)})$	# of failures (m_j)	# censored in $(t_{(j)}, t_{(j+1)})$ (q_j)	Risk set $R(t_{(j)})$
$t_{(0)} = 0$	$m_0 = 0$	q_0	$R(t_{(0)})$
$t_{(1)}$	m_1	q_1	$R(t_{(1)})$
$t_{(2)}$	m_2	q_2	$R(t_{(2)})$
•	•	•	•
•	•	•	•
•	•	•	•
$t_{(k)}$	m_k	q_k	$R(t_{(k)})$

We are now ready to look at another data layout, which is shown at the left. This layout helps provide some understanding of how a survival analysis actually works and, in particular, how survivor curves are derived.

The first column in this table gives ordered failure times. These are denoted by t's with subscripts within parentheses, starting t_0, t_1, and so on, up to t_k by $t_{(0)}$, $t_{(1)}$ and so on, up to $t_{(k)}$. Note that the parentheses surrounding the subscripts distinguish ordered failure times from the survival times previously given in the computer layout.

$\{t_1, t_2, \ldots, t_n\}$

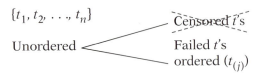

Unordered

Censored t's

Failed t's
ordered $(t_{(j)})$

k = # of distinct times at which subjects
failed ($k \leq n$)

To get ordered failure times from survival times, we must first remove from the list of unordered survival times all those times that are censored; we are thus working only with those times at which people failed. We then order the remaining failure times from smallest to largest, and count ties only once. The value k gives the number of distinct times at which subjects failed.

For example, using the remission data for group 1, we find that nine of the 21 persons failed, including three persons each at 6 weeks and one person each at 7, 10, 13, 16, 22, and 23 weeks. These nine failures have $k = 7$ distinct survival times, because three persons had survival time 6 and we only count one of these 6's as distinct. The first ordered failure time for this group, denoted as $t_{(1)}$, is 6; the second ordered failure time $t_{(2)}$, is 7, and so on up to the seventh ordered failure time of 23.

EXAMPLE

Remission Data: Group 1
($n = 21$, 9 failures, $k = 7$)

$t_{(j)}$	m_j	q_j	$R(t_{(j)})$
$t_{(0)} = 0$	0	0	21 persons survive $\geq$ 0 wks
$t_{(1)} = 6$	③	1	21 persons survive $\geq$ 6 wks
$t_{(2)} = 7$	1	1	17 persons survive $\geq$ 7 wks
$t_{(3)} = 10$	1	2	15 persons survive $\geq$ 10 wks
$t_{(4)} = 13$	1	0	12 persons survive $\geq$ 13 wks
$t_{(5)} = 16$	1	3	11 persons survive $\geq$ 16 wks
$t_{(6)} = 22$	1	0	7 persons survive $\geq$ 22 wks
$t_{(7)} = 23$	1	5	6 persons survive $\geq$ 23 wks
Totals	9	12	

Remission Data: Group 2
($n = 21$, 21 failures, $k = 12$)

$t_{(j)}$	m_j	q_j	$R(t_{(j)})$
$t_{(0)} = 0$	0	0	21 persons survive $\geq$ 0 wks
$t_{(1)} = 1$	2	0	21 persons survive $\geq$ 1 wk
$t_{(2)} = 2$	2	0	19 persons survive $\geq$ 2 wks
$t_{(3)} = 3$	1	0	17 persons survive $\geq$ 3 wks
$t_{(4)} = 4$	2	0	16 persons survive $\geq$ 4 wks
$t_{(5)} = 5$	2	0	14 persons survive $\geq$ 5 wks
$t_{(6)} = 8$	4	0	12 persons survive $\geq$ 8 wks
$t_{(7)} = 11$	2	0	8 persons survive $\geq$ 11 wks
$t_{(8)} = 12$	2	0	6 persons survive $\geq$ 12 wks
$t_{(9)} = 15$	1	0	4 persons survive $\geq$ 15 wks
$t_{(10)} = 17$	1	0	3 persons survive $\geq$ 17 wks
$t_{(11)} = 22$	1	0	2 persons survive $\geq$ 22 wks
$t_{(12)} = 23$	1	0	1 person survive $\geq$ 23 wks
Totals	21	0	

(Ties)

Turning to group 2, shown at the left, we find that although all 21 persons in this group failed, there are several ties. For example, two persons had a survival time of 1 week; two more had a survival time of 2 weeks; and so on. In all, we find that there were $k = 12$ distinct survival times out of the 21 failures. These times are listed in the first column for group 2.

Note that for both groups we inserted a row of data giving information at time 0. We will explain this insertion when we get to the third column in the table.

The *second column* in the data layout gives frequency counts, denoted by m_j, of those persons who failed at each distinct failure time. When there are no ties at a certain failure time, then $m_j = 1$. Notice that in group 1, shown at the bottom left, there were three ties at 6 weeks but no ties thereafter. In group 2, there were ties at 1, 2, 4, 5, 8, 11, and 12 weeks. In any case, the sum of all the m_j's in this column gives the total number of failures in the group tabulated. This sum is 9 for group 1 and 21 for group 2.

EXAMPLE (continued)

q_j = censored in $(t_{(j)}, t_{(j+1)})$

Remission Data: Group 1

$t_{(j)}$	m_j	q_j	$R(t_{(j)})$
$t_{(0)} = 0$	0	0	21 persons survive ≥ 0 wks
$t_{(1)} = 6$	3	1	21 persons survive ≥ 6 wks
$t_{(2)} = 7$ ties	1	1	17 persons survive ≥ 7 wks
$t_{(3)} = 10$	1	2	15 persons survive ≥ 10 wks
$t_{(4)} = 13$	1	0	12 persons survive ≥ 13 wks
$t_{(5)} = 16$	1	3	11 persons survive ≥ 16 wks
$t_{(6)} = 22$	1	0	7 persons survive ≥ 22 wks
$t_{(7)} = 23$	1	5	6 persons survive ≥ 23 wks
Totals	9	12	

Remission Data: Group 1

#	t(weeks)	δ	X(group)
1	6	1	1
2	6	1	1
3	6	1	1
4	7	1	1
5	10	1	1
6	13	1	1
7	16	1	1
8	22	1	1
9	23	1	1
10	6	0	1
11	9	0	1
12	10	0	1
13	11	0	1
14	17	0	1
15	19	0	1
16	20	0	1
17	25	0	1
18	32	0	1
19	32	0	1
20	34	0	1
21	35	0	1

The *third column* gives frequency counts, denoted by q_j, of those persons censored in the time interval starting with failure time $t_{(j)}$ up to the next failure time denoted $t_{(j+1)}$. Technically, because of the way we have defined this interval in the table, we include those persons censored at the beginning of the interval but not at its end.

For example, the remission data, for group 1 includes 5 nonzero q_j's: $q_1 = 1$, $q_2 = 1$, $q_3 = 2$, $q_5 = 3$, $q_7 = 5$. Adding these values gives us the total number of censored observations for group 1, which is 12. Moreover, if we add the total number of q's (12) to the total number of m's (9), we get the total number of subjects in group 1, which is 21.

We now focus on group 1 to look a little closer at the q's. At the left, we list the unordered group 1 information followed (on the next page) by the ordered failure time information. We will go back and forth between these two tables (and pages) as we discuss the q's. Notice that in the table here, one person, listed as #10, was censored at week 6. Consequently, in the table at the top of the next page, we have $q_1 = 1$, which is listed on the second line corresponding to the ordered failure time t_1 in parentheses, which equals 6.

The next q is a little trickier; it is derived from the person who was listed as #11 in the table here and was censored at week 9. Correspondingly, in the table at the top of the next page, we have $q_2 = 1$ because this one person was censored within the time interval that starts at the second ordered failure time, 7 weeks, and ends at the third ordered failure time, 10 weeks. We have *not* counted here person #12, who was censored at week 10, because this person's censored time is exactly at the end of the interval. We count this person in the following interval.

EXAMPLE (continued)

Group 1 using ordered failure times

$t_{(j)}$	m_j	q_j	$R(t_{(j)})$
$t_{(0)} = 0$	0	0	21 persons survive $\geq$ 0 wks
$t_{(1)} = 6$	3	[1]	21 persons survive $\geq$ 6 wks
$t_{(2)} = 7$	1	(1)	17 persons survive $\geq$ 7 wks
$t_{(3)} = 10$	1	(2)	15 persons survive $\geq$ 10 wks
$t_{(4)} = 13$	1	0	12 persons survive $\geq$ 13 wks
$t_{(5)} = 16$	1	3	11 persons survive $\geq$ 16 wks
$t_{(6)} = 22$	1	0	7 persons survive $\geq$ 22 wks
$t_{(7)} = 23$	1	5	6 persons survive $\geq$ 23 wks
Totals	9	12	

We now consider, from the table of unordered failure times, person #12 who was censored at 10 weeks, and person #13, who was censored at 11 weeks. Turning to the table of ordered failure times here, we see that these two times are within the third ordered time interval, which starts and includes the 10-week point and ends just before the 13th week. As for the remaining q's, we will let you figure them out for practice.

One last point about the q information. We inserted a row at the top of the data for each group corresponding to time 0. This insertion allows for the possibility that persons may be censored after the start of the study but before the first failure. In other words, it is possible that q_0 may be nonzero. For the two groups of this example, however, no one was censored before the first failure time.

EXAMPLE

Risk Set: $R(t_{(j)})$ is the set of individuals for whom $T \geq t_{(j)}$.

Remission Data: Group 1

$t_{(j)}$	m_j	q_j	$R(t_{(j)})$
$t_{(0)} = $ (0)	0	0	(21 persons survive $\geq$ 0 wks)
$t_{(1)} = $ (6)	3	1	(21 persons survive $\geq$ 6 wks)
$t_{(2)} = 7$	1	1	17 persons survive $\geq$ 7 wks
$t_{(3)} = 10$	1	2	15 persons survive $\geq$ 10 wks
$t_{(4)} = 13$	1	0	12 persons survive $\geq$ 13 wks
$t_{(5)} = 16$	1	3	11 persons survive $\geq$ 16 wks
$t_{(6)} = 22$	1	0	7 persons survive $\geq$ 22 wks
$t_{(7)} = 23$	1	5	6 persons survive $\geq$ 23 wks
Totals	9	12	

The last column in the table gives the **"risk set."** The risk set is not a numerical value or count but rather a collection of individuals. By definition, the risk set $R(t_{(j)})$ is the collection of individuals who have survived at least to time $t_{(j)}$; that is, each person in $R(t_{(j)})$ has a survival time that is $t_{(j)}$ or longer, regardless of whether the person has failed or is censored.

For example, we see that at the start of the study everyone in group 1 survived at least 0 weeks, so the risk set at time 0 consists of the entire group of 21 persons. The risk set at 6 weeks for group 1 also consists of all 21 persons, because all 21 persons survived at least as long as 6 weeks. These 21 persons include the 3 persons who failed at 6 weeks, because they survived and were still at risk just up to this point.

EXAMPLE (continued)

$t_{(j)}$	m_j	q_j	$R(t_{(j)})$
$t_{(0)} = 0$	0	0	21 persons survive $\geq$ 0 wks
$t_{(1)} = 6$	3	1	21 persons survive $\geq$ 6 wks
$t_{(2)} = 7$	1	1	17 persons survive $\geq$ 7 wks
$t_{(3)} = 10$	1	2	15 persons survive $\geq$ 10 wks
$t_{(4)} = 13$	1	0	12 persons survive $\geq$ 13 wks
$t_{(5)} = 16$	1	3	11 persons survive $\geq$ 16 wks
$t_{(6)} = 22$	1	0	7 persons survive $\geq$ 22 wks
$t_{(7)} = 23$	1	5	6 persons survive $\geq$ 23 wks
Totals	9	12	

$t_{(j)}$	m_j	q_j	$R(t_{(j)})$
$t_{(0)} = 0$	0	0	21 persons survive $\geq$ 0 wks
$t_{(1)} = 6$	3	1	21 persons survive $\geq$ 6 wks
$t_{(2)} = 7$	1	1	17 persons survive $\geq$ 7 wks
$t_{(3)} = 10$	1	2	15 persons survive $\geq$ 10 wks
$t_{(4)} = 13$	1	0	12 persons survive $\geq$ 13 wks
$t_{(5)} = 16$	1	3	11 persons survive $\geq$ 16 wks
$t_{(6)} = 22$	1	0	7 persons survive $\geq$ 22 wks
$t_{(7)} = 23$	1	5	6 persons survive $\geq$ 23 wks
Totals	9	12	

How we work with censored data:

Use all informaton up to time of censorship; don't throw away information.

Now let's look at the risk set at 7 weeks. This set consists of seventeen persons in group 1 that survived at least 7 weeks. We omit everyone in the $\times$-ed area. Of the original 21 persons, we therefore have excluded the three persons who failed at 6 weeks and the one person who was censored at 6 weeks. These four persons did not survive at least 7 weeks. Although the censored person may have survived longer than 7 weeks, we must exclude him or her from the risk set at 7 weeks because we have information on this person only up to 6 weeks.

To derive the other risk sets, we must exclude all persons who either failed or were censored before the start of the time interval being considered. For example, to obtain the risk set at 13 weeks for group 1, we must exclude the five persons who failed before, but not including, 13 weeks and the four persons who were censored before, but not including, 13 weeks. Subtracting these nine persons from 21, leaves twelve persons in group 1 still at risk for getting the event at 13 weeks. Thus, the risk set consists of these twelve persons.

The importance of the table of ordered failure times is that we can work with censored observations in analyzing survival data. Even though censored observations are incomplete, in that we don't know a person's survival time exactly, we can still make use of the information we have on a censored person up to the time we lose track of him or her. Rather than simply throw away the information on a censored person, we use all the information we have.

EXAMPLE

$t_{(j)}$	m_j	q_j		$R(t_{(j)})$
6	3	1	✓	21 persons
7	1	1	✓	17 persons
10	1	2	✓	15 persons
13	1	0	✓	12 persons
16	1	③	✓	11 persons
22	1	0		7 persons
23	1	5		6 persons

For example, for the three persons in group 1 who were censored between the 16th and 20th weeks, there are at least 16 weeks of survival information on each that we don't want to lose. These three persons are contained in all risk sets up to the 16th week; that is, they are each at risk for getting the event up to 16 weeks. Any survival probabilities determined before, and including, 16 weeks should make use of data on these three persons as well as data on other persons at risk during the first 16 weeks.

Having introduced the basic terminology and data layouts to this point, we now consider some data analysis issues and some additional applications.

VII. Descriptive Measures of Survival Experience

EXAMPLE

Remission times (in weeks) for two groups of leukemia patients

Group 1 (Treatment) $n = 21$	Group 2 (Placebo) $n = 21$
6, 6, 6, 7, 10,	1, 1, 2, 2, 3,
13, 16, 22, 23,	4, 4, 5, 5,
6+, 9+, 10+, 11+,	8, 8, 8, 8,
17+, 19+, 20+,	11, 11, 12, 12,
25+, 32+, 32+,	15, 17, 22, 23
34+, 35+	
$\overline{T}_1$ (ignoring + 's) 17.1	$\overline{T}_2 = 8.6$
$\overline{h}_1 = \dfrac{9}{359} = .025$	$\overline{h}_2 = \dfrac{21}{182} = .115$

$$\text{Average hazard rate } (\overline{h}) = \frac{\#\text{ failures}}{\sum\limits_{i=1}^{n} t_i}$$

We first return to the remission data, again shown in untabulated form. Inspecting the survival times given for each group, we can see that most of the treatment group's times are longer than most of the placebo group's times. If we ignore the plus signs denoting censorship and simply average the survival times for each group we get an average, denoted by T "bar," of **17.1** weeks survival for the treatment group and **8.6** weeks for the placebo group. Because several of the treatment group's times are censored, this means that group 1's true average is even larger than what we have calculated. Thus, it appears from the data (without our doing any mathematical analysis) that, regarding survival, the treatment is more effective than the placebo.

As an alternative to the simple averages that we have computed for each group, another descriptive measure of each group is the **average hazard rate,** denoted as h "bar." This rate is defined by dividing the total number of failures by the sum of the observed survival times. For group 1, h "bar" is 9/359, which equals **.025.** For group 2, h "bar" is 21/182, which equals .115.

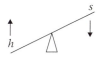

As previously described, the hazard rate indicates failure potential rather than survival probability. Thus, the higher the hazard rate, the lower is the group's probability of surviving.

In our example, the average hazard for the treatment group is smaller than the average hazard for the placebo group.

Placebo hazard > treatment hazard:
  suggests that treatment is more effective than placebo

Thus, using average hazard rates, we again see that the treatment group appears to be doing better overall than the placebo group; that is, the treatment group is less prone to fail than the placebo group.

Descriptive measures ($\overline{T}$ and $\overline{h}$) give **overall** comparison; they do not give comparison over time.

The descriptive measures we have used so far—the ordinary average and the hazard rate average—provide overall comparisons of the treatment group with the placebo group. These measures don't compare the two groups at different points in time of follow-up. Such a comparison is provided by a graph of survivor curves.

Here we present the **estimated survivor curves** for the treatment and placebo groups. The method used to get these curves is called the Kaplan–Meier method, which is described in Chapter 2. When estimated, these curves are actually step functions that allow us to compare the treatment and placebo groups over time. The graph shows that the survivor function for the treatment group consistently lies above that for the placebo group; this difference indicates that the treatment appears effective at all points of follow-up. Notice, however, that the two functions are somewhat closer together in the first few weeks of follow-up, but thereafter are quite spread apart. This widening gap suggests that the treatment is more effective later during follow-up than it is early on.

EXAMPLE

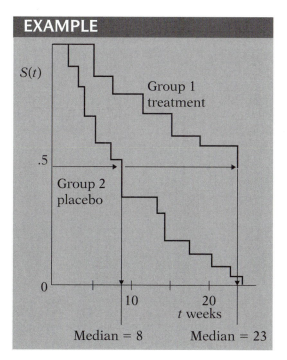

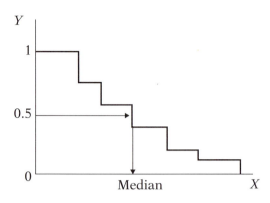

Median (treatment) = 23 weeks

Median (placebo) = 8 weeks

Also notice from the graph that one can obtain the median survival time for each group. Graphically, the median is obtained by proceeding horizontally from the 0.5 point on the Y-axis until the survivor curve is reached, as marked by an arrow, and then proceeding vertically downward until the X-axis is crossed at the median survival time.

For the treatment group, the median is 23 weeks, as indicated at the right-hand corner of the top graph. For the placebo group, the median is 8 weeks. Comparison of the two medians reinforces our previous observation that the treatment is more effective overall than the placebo.

VIII. Example: Extended Remission Data

Before proceeding to another data set, we consider the remission example data (Freireich et al., *Blood*, 1963) in an **extended form.** The table at the left gives the remission survival times for the two groups with additional information about white blood cell count for each person studied. In particular, each person's log white blood cell count is given next to that person's survival time. The epidemiologic reason for adding log WBC to the data set is that this variable is usually considered an important predictor of survival in leukemia patients; the higher the WBC, the worse the prognosis. Thus, any comparison of the effects of two treatment groups needs to adjust for the possible **confounding effect** of such a variable.

Group 1		Group 2	
t (weeks)	log WBC	t (weeks)	log WBC
6	2.31	1	2.80
6	4.06	1	5.00
6	3.28	2	4.91
7	4.43	2	4.48
10	2.96	3	4.01
13	2.88	4	4.36
16	3.60	4	2.42
22	2.32	5	3.49
23	2.57	5	3.97
6+	3.20	8	3.52
9+	2.80	8	3.05
10+	2.70	8	2.32
11+	2.60	8	3.26
17+	2.16	11	3.49
19+	2.05	11	2.12
20+	2.01	12	1.50
25+	1.78	12	3.06
32+	2.20	15	2.30
32+	2.53	17	2.95
34+	1.47	22	2.73
35+	1.45	23	1.97

EXAMPLE: CONFOUNDING

Treatment group: $\overline{\log \text{WBC}} = 1.8$

Placebo group: $\overline{\log \text{WBC}} = 4.1$

Indicates **confounding** of treatment effect by log WBC

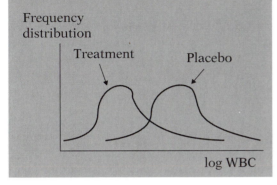

Need to adjust for imbalance in the distribution of log WBC

EXAMPLE: INTERACTION

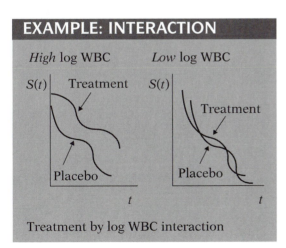

Treatment by log WBC interaction

Although a full exposition of the nature of confounding is not intended here, we provide a simple scenario to give you the basic idea. Suppose all of the subjects in the treatment group had very low log WBC, with an average, for example, of 1.8, whereas all of the subjects in the placebo group had very high log WBC, with an average of 4.1. We would have to conclude that the results we've seen so far that compare treatment with placebo groups may be misleading.

The additional information on log WBC would suggest that the treatment group is surviving longer simply because of their low WBC and not because of the efficacy of the treatment itself. In this case, we would say that **the treatment effect is confounded by the effect of log WBC.**

More typically, the distribution of log WBC may be quite different in the treatment group than in the control group. We have illustrated one extreme in the graph at the left. Even though such an extreme is not likely, and is not true for the data given here, the point is that some attempt needs to be made to adjust for whatever imbalance there is in the distribution of log WBC.

Another issue to consider regarding the effect of log WBC is **interaction.** What we mean by interaction is that the effect of the treatment may be different, depending on the level of log WBC. For example, suppose that for persons with high log WBC, survival probabilities for the treatment are consistently higher over time than for the placebo. This circumstance is illustrated by the first graph at the left. In contrast, the second graph, which considers only persons with low log WBC, shows no difference in treatment and placebo effect over time. In such a situation, we would say that **there is strong treatment by log WBC interaction,** and we would have to qualify the effect of the treatment as depending on the level of log WBC.

Need to consider:

- interaction;
- confounding.

The problem:

Compare two groups after adjusting for confounding and interaction.

The example of interaction we just gave is but one way interaction can occur; on the other hand, interaction may not occur at all. As with confounding, it is beyond our scope to provide a thorough discussion of interaction. In any case, the assessment of interaction is something to consider in one's analysis in addition to confounding that involves explanatory variables.

Thus, with our extended data example, the basic **problem** can be described as follows: to compare the survival experience of the two groups after adjusting for the possible confounding and/or interaction effects of log WBC.

The problem statement tells us that we are now considering two explanatory variables in our extended example, whereas we previously considered the single variable, group status. The data layout for the computer needs to reflect the addition of the second variable, log WBC. The extended table in computer layout form is given at the left. Notice that we have labeled the two explanatory variables X_1 (for group status) and X_2 (for log WBC). The variable X_1 is our primary study or exposure variable of interest here, and the variable X_2 is an extraneous variable that we are interested in adjusting for because of either confounding or interaction.

EXAMPLE

	Individual #	t (weeks)	δ	X_1 (Group)	X_2 (log WBC)
	1	6	1	1	2.31
	2	6	1	1	4.06
	3	6	1	1	3.28
	4	7	1	1	4.43
	5	10	1	1	2.96
	6	13	1	1	2.88
	7	16	1	1	3.60
	8	22	1	1	2.32
	9	23	1	1	2.57
	10	6	0	1	3.20
Group 1	11	9	0	1	2.80
	12	10	0	1	2.70
	13	11	0	1	2.60
	14	17	0	1	2.16
	15	19	0	1	2.05
	16	20	0	1	2.01
	17	25	0	1	1.78
	18	32	0	1	2.20
	19	32	0	1	2.53
	20	34	0	1	1.47
	21	35	0	1	1.45

EXAMPLE (continued)

Individual #	t (weeks)	δ	X_1 (Group)	X_2 (log WBC)
22	1	1	0	2.80
23	1	1	0	5.00
24	2	1	0	4.91
25	2	1	0	4.48
26	3	1	0	4.01
27	4	1	0	4.36
28	4	1	0	2.42
29	5	1	0	3.49
30	5	1	0	3.97
31	8	1	0	3.52
32	8	1	0	3.05
33	8	1	0	2.32
34	8	1	0	3.26
35	11	1	0	3.49
36	11	1	0	2.12
37	12	1	0	1.50
38	12	1	0	3.06
39	15	1	0	2.30
40	17	1	0	2.95
41	22	1	0	2.73
42	23	1	0	1.97

Group 2 (individuals 22–42)

Analysis alternatives:

- stratify on log WBC;
- use math modeling, e.g., proportional hazards model.

As implied by our extended example, which considers the possible confounding or interaction effect of log WBC, we need to consider methods for adjusting for log WBC and/or assessing its effect in addition to assessing the effect of treatment group. The two most popular alternatives for analysis are the following:

- to stratify on log WBC and compare survival curves for different strata; or
- to use mathematical modeling procedures such as the proportional hazards or other survival models; such methods will be described in subsequent chapters.

IX. Multivariable Example

- Describes general multivariable survival problem.
- Gives analogy to regression problems.

We now consider one other example. Our purpose here is to describe a more general type of multivariable survival analysis problem. The reader may see the analogy of this example to multiple regression or even logistic regression data problems.

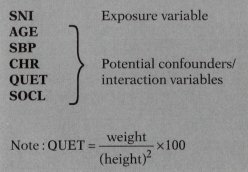

EXAMPLE

13-year follow-up of fixed cohort from Evans County, Georgia

$n = 170$ white males $(60+)$

T = years until death
Event = death

Explanatory variables:
- exposure variable
- confounders
- interaction variables

Exposure:
  Social Network Index (**SNI**)

```
|---+---+---+---+---|
0   1   2   3   4   5
```

Absence   Excellent
of social   social
network   network

Study goal: to determine whether **SNI** is protective against death,
i.e., **SNI** ↗ ⟹ $S(t)$ ↗

Explanatory variables:

SNI	Exposure variable
AGE	
SBP	
CHR	Potential confounders/
QUET	interaction variables
SOCL	

Note : $\text{QUET} = \dfrac{\text{weight}}{(\text{height})^2} \times 100$

We consider a data set developed from a 13-year follow-up study of a fixed cohort of persons in Evans County, Georgia, during the period 1967–1980 (Schoenbach et al., *Amer. J. Epid.*, 1986). From this data set, we focus on a portion containing $n = 170$ white males who are age 60 or older at the start of follow-up in 1967.

For this data set, the outcome variable is T, time in years until death from start of follow-up, so the event of interest is **death.** Several explanatory variables are measured, one of which is considered the primary exposure variable; the other variables are considered as potential confounders and/or interaction variables.

The primary exposure variable is a measure called Social Network Index (SNI). This is an ordinal variable derived from questionnaire measurement and is designed to assess the extent to which a study subject has social contacts of various types. With the questionnaire, a scale is used with values ranging from 0 (absence of any social network) to 5 (excellent social network).

The study's goal is to determine whether one's social network, as measured by SNI, is protective against death. If this study hypothesis is correct, then the higher the social network score, the longer will be one's survival time.

In evaluating this problem, several explanatory variables, in addition to SNI, are measured at the start of follow-up. These include AGE, systolic blood pressure (SBP), an indicator of the presence or absence of some chronic disease (CHR), body size as measured by Quetelet's index (QUET = weight over height squared times 100), and social class (SOCL).

These five additional variables are of interest because they are thought to have their own special or collective influence on how long a person will survive. Consequently, these variables are viewed as potential confounders and/or interaction variables in evaluating the effect of social network on time to death.

EXAMPLE (continued)

The problem:

To describe the relationship between **SNI** and time to death, after controlling for **AGE, SBP, CHR, QUET,** and **SOCL**.

Goals:

- Measure of effect (adjusted)
- Survivor curves for different SNI categories (adjusted)
- Decide on variables to be adjusted
- Determine method of adjustment

Computer layout: 13-year follow-up study (1967–1980) of a fixed cohort of $n = 170$ white males (60+) from Evans County, Georgia

#	t	δ	SNI	AGE	SBP	CHR	QUET	SOCL
1	t_1	δ_1	SNI_1	AGE_1	SBP_1	CHR_1	$QUET_1$	$SOCL_1$
2	t_2	δ_2	SNI_2	AGE_2	SBP_2	CHR_2	$QUET_2$	$SOCL_2$
.	.	.	.	.	.	.	.	.
.	.	.	.	.	.	.	.	.
.	.	.	.	.	.	.	.	.
170	t_{170}	δ_{170}	SNI_{170}	AGE_{170}	SBP_{170}	CHR_{170}	$QUET_{170}$	$SOCL_{170}$

We can now clearly state the problem being addressed by this study: To describe the relationship between SNI and time to death, controlling for AGE, SBP, CHR, QUET, and SOCL.

Our goals in using survival analysis to solve this problem are as follows:

- to obtain some measure of effect that will describe the relationship between SNI and time until death, after adjusting for the other variables we have identified;
- to develop survival curves that describe the probability of survival over time for different categories of social networks; in particular, we wish to compare the survival of persons with excellent networks to the survival of persons with poor networks. Such survival curves need to be adjusted for the effects of other variables.
- to achieve these goals, two intermediary goals are to decide which of the additional variables being considered need to be adjusted and to determine an appropriate method of adjustment.

The computer data layout for this problem is given at the left. The first column lists the 170 individuals in the data set. The second column lists the survival times, and the third column lists failure or censored status. The remainder of the columns list the 6 explanatory variables of interest, starting with the exposure variable SNI and continuing with the variables to be adjusted in the analysis.

X. Math Models in Survival Analysis

General framework

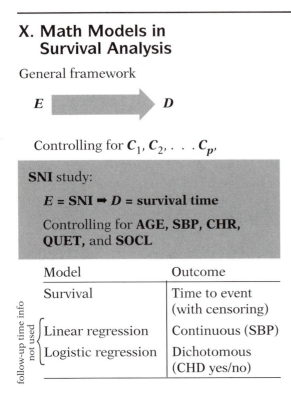

$$E \longrightarrow D$$

Controlling for $C_1, C_2, \ldots C_p$,

SNI study:

$E = \textbf{SNI} \Rightarrow D = \textbf{survival time}$

Controlling for **AGE, SBP, CHR, QUET,** and **SOCL**

	Model	Outcome
	Survival	Time to event (with censoring)
follow-up time info not used	Linear regression	Continuous (SBP)
	Logistic regression	Dichotomous (CHD yes/no)

Measure of effect:
Linear regression:
   regression coefficient β
Logistic regression:
   odds ratio e^{β}

Survival analysis:
   hazard ratio e^{β}

It is beyond the scope of this presentation to provide specific details of the survival analysis of these data. Nevertheless, the problem addressed by these data is closely analogous to the typical multivariable problem addressed by linear and logistic regression modeling. Regardless of which modeling approach is chosen, the typical problem concerns describing the relationship between an exposure variable (e.g., E) and an outcome variable (e.g., D) after controlling for the possible confounding and interaction effects of additional variables (e.g., C_1, C_2, and so on up to C_p). In our survival analysis example, E is the social network variable SNI, D is the survival time variable, and there are $p = 5$ C variables, namely, AGE, SBP, CHR, QUET, and SOCL.

Nevertheless, an important distinction among modeling methods is the type of outcome variable being used. In survival analysis, the outcome variable is "time to an event," the event being death, and there is censored data. In linear regression modeling, the outcome variable is generally a continuous variable, like blood pressure. In logistic modeling, the outcome variable is a dichotomous variable, like CHD status, yes or no. And with linear or logistic modeling, we usually do not have information on follow-up time available.

As with linear and logistic modeling, one statistical goal of a survival analysis is to obtain some measure of effect that describes the exposure–outcome relationship adjusted for relevant extraneous variables.

In linear regression modeling, the measure of effect is usually some regression coefficient β.

In logistic modeling, the measure of effect is an odds ratio expressed in terms of an exponential of one or more regression coefficients in the model, for example, e to the β.

In survival analysis, the measure of effect obtained is called a **hazard ratio;** as with the logistic model, this hazard ratio is expressed in terms of an exponential of a regression coefficient in the model.

EXAMPLE

SNI study: hazard ratio (HR) describes relationship between SNI and T, after controlling for covariates.

Thus, from the example of survival analysis modeling of the social network data, one can obtain a hazard ratio that describes the relationship between SNI and survival time (T), after controlling for the appropriate covariates.

Interpretation of HR (like OR):

HR $=1 \Rightarrow$ no relationship

HR $=10 \Rightarrow$ exposed hazard 10 times unexposed

HR $=1/10 \Rightarrow$ exposed hazard 1/10 times unexposed

The hazard ratio, although a different measure from an odds ratio, nevertheless has a similar interpretation of the strength of the effect. A hazard ratio of 1, like an odds ratio of 1, means that there is no effect; that is, 1 is the null value for the exposure–outcome relationship. A hazard ratio of 10, on the other hand, is interpreted like an odds ratio of 10; that is, the exposed group has ten times the hazard of the unexposed group. Similarly, a hazard ratio of 1/10 implies that the exposed group has one-tenth the hazard of the unexposed group.

Recall that the higher the survival probability at time t, the lower is the corresponding hazard rate, and vice versa.

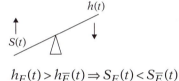

$$h_E(t) > h_{\overline{E}}(t) \Rightarrow S_E(t) < S_{\overline{E}}(t)$$

$$HR = \frac{h_E(t)}{h_{\overline{E}}(t)} > 1 \Rightarrow \frac{S_E(t)}{S_{\overline{E}}(t)} < 1$$

Similarly,

$$HR = \frac{h_E(t)}{h_{\overline{E}}(t)} < 1 \Rightarrow \frac{S_E(t)}{S_{\overline{E}}(t)} > 1$$

Therefore, if the hazard rate for an exposed group at time t is higher than that for the unexposed group at the same time, the corresponding survival probability for the exposed group is lower than the corresponding survival probability for the unexposed group. In other words, a hazard ratio greater than 1 corresponds to a ratio of survival probabilities that is less than 1. Similarly, a hazard ratio less than 1 corresponds to a ratio of survival probabilities greater than 1.

EXAMPLE

$$HR = \frac{h_E(t)}{h_{\overline{E}}(t)} = 10 \Rightarrow \frac{S_E(t)}{S_{\overline{E}}(t)} < 1;$$

i.e., $S_E(t) < S_{\overline{E}}(t)$

Thus, for example, if the hazard ratio comparing exposed to unexposed is 10, then the failure rate for the exposed is ten times higher than the failure rate for the unexposed. Consequently, the exposed group must have a lower (though not necessarily 1/10) survival probability than the unexposed. That is, if the hazard ratio is 10, then the exposed group has a poorer survival probability than the unexposed.

Chapters

This presentation is now complete. We suggest that you review the material covered here by reading the detailed outline that follows. Then do the practice exercises and test.

In Chapter 2 we describe how to estimate and graph survival curves using the Kaplan–Meier (KM) method. We also describe how to test whether two or more survival curves are estimating a common curve. The most popular such test is called the log–rank test.

Detailed Outline

 F. Examples of hazard curves:
  i. exponential
  ii. increasing Weibull
  iii. decreasing Weibull
  iv. log normal
 G. Uses of hazard function:
  • gives insight about conditional failure rates;
  • identifies specific model form;
  • math model for survival analysis is usually written in terms of hazard function;
 H. Relationship of $S(t)$ to $h(t)$: if you know one, you can determine the other.
  • example: $h(t) = \lambda$ if and only if $S(t) = e^{-\lambda t}$
  • general formulae:

$$S(t) = \exp\left[-\int_0^t h(u)\,du\right]$$

$$h(t) = -\left[\frac{dS(t)/dt}{S(t)}\right]$$

IV. Goals of survival analysis (page 15)
 A. Estimate and interpret survivor and/or hazard functions.
 B. Compare survivor and/or hazard functions.
 C. Assess the relationship of explanatory variables to survival time.

V. Basic data layout for computer (15–19)
 A. General layout:

#	t	δ	X_1	$X_2 \cdots X_p$
1	t_1	δ_1	X_{11}	$X_{12} \cdots X_{1p}$
2	t_2	δ_2	X_{21}	$X_{22} \cdots X_{2p}$
•	•	•		•
•	•	•		•
•	•	•		•
j	t_j	δ_j	X_{j1}	$X_{j2} \cdots X_{jp}$
•	•	•		•
•	•	•		•
•	•	•		•
n	t_n	δ_n	X_{n1}	$X_{n2} \cdots X_{np}$

 B. Example: Remission time data

VI. Basic data layout for understanding analysis (pages 19–24)

A. General layout:

Ordered failure times $(t_{(j)})$	# of failures (m_j)	# censored in $(t_{(j)}, t_{(j+1)})$ (q_j)	Risk set $R(t_{(j)})$
$t_{(0)} = 0$	$m_0 = 0$	q_0	$R(t_{(0)})$
$t_{(1)}$	m_1	q_1	$R(t_{(1)})$
$t_{(2)}$	m_2	q_2	$R(t_{(2)})$
•	•	•	•
•	•	•	•
•	•	•	•
$t_{(k)}$	m_k	q_k	$R(t_{(k)})$

Note: k = # of distinct times at which subjects failed; n = # of subjects ($k \leq n$); $R(t_{(j)})$, the risk set, is the set of individuals whose survival times are at least $t_{(j)}$ or larger.

B. Example: Remission time data

Group 1 ($n = 21$, 9 failures, $k = 7$); **Group 2** ($n = 21$, 21 failures, $k = 12$)

C. How to work with censored data:

Use all information up to the time of censorship; don't throw away information.

VII. Descriptive measures of survival experience (pages 24–26)

A. Average survival time (ignoring censorship status):

$$\overline{T} = \frac{\sum_{i=1}^{n} t_i}{n}$$

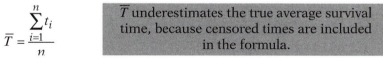

$\overline{T}$ underestimates the true average survival time, because censored times are included in the formula.

B. Average hazard rate:

$$\overline{h} = \frac{\text{\# failures}}{\sum_{i=1}^{n} t_i}$$

C. Descriptive measures $\overline{T}$ and $\overline{h}$ give overall comparison; estimated survivor curves give comparison over time.

D. Estimated survivor curves are step function graphs.

E. Median survival time: graphically, proceed horizontally from 0.5 on the *Y*-axis until reaching graph, then vertically downward until reaching the *X*-axis.

VIII. Example: Extended remission data (pages 26–29)

A. Extended data adds log WBC to previous remission data.

B. Need to consider **confounding** and **interaction.**

C. Extended data problem: compare survival experience of two groups, after adjusting for confounding and interaction effects of log WBC.

D. Analysis alternatives:

  i. stratify on log WBC and compare survival curves for different strata;

  ii. use math modeling, e.g., proportional hazards model.

IX. Multivariable example (pages 29–31)

A. The problem: to describe the relationship between social network index (**SNI**) and survival until death controlling for **AGE,** systolic blood pressure (**SBP**), presence or absence of chronic disease (**CHR**), Quetelet's index (**QUET**—a measure of body size), and social class (**SOCL**).

B. Goals:

• to obtain an adjusted measure of effect;

• to obtain adjusted survivor curves for different SNI categories;

• to decide on variables to be adjusted.

C. The data: 13-year follow-up study (1967–1980) of a fixed cohort of *n* = 170 white males (60+) from Evans County, Georgia.

#	t	δ	SNI	AGE	SBP	CHR	QUET	SOCL
1	t_1	δ_1	SNI_1	AGE_1	SBP_1	CHR_1	$QUET_1$	$SOCL_1$
2	t_2	δ_2	SNI_2	AGE_2	SBP_2	CHR_2	$QUET_2$	$SOCL_2$
·	·	·	·	·	·	·	·	·
·	·	·	·	·	·	·	·	·
·	·	·	·	·	·	·	·	·
170	t_{170}	δ_{170}	SNI_{170}	AGE_{170}	SBP_{170}	CHR_{170}	$QUET_{170}$	$SOCL_{170}$

X. Math models in survival analysis (pages 32–33)

A. Survival analysis problem is analogous to typical multivariable problem addressed by linear and/or logistic regression modeling: describe relationship of exposure to outcome, after controlling for possible confounding and interaction.

B. Outcome variable (time to event) for survival analysis is different from linear (continuous) or logistic (dichotomous) modeling.

C. Measure of effect in survival analysis: hazard ratio (**HR**).

D. Interpretation of HR: like OR. SNI study: HR describes relationship between SNI and T, after controlling for covariates.

Practice Exercises

True or False (Circle T or F):

T F 1. In a survival analysis, the outcome variable is dichotomous.

T F 2. In a survival analysis, the event is usually described by a (0,1) variable.

T F 3. If the study ends before an individual has gotten the event, then his or her survival time is censored.

T F 4. If, for a given individual, the event occurs **before** the person is lost to follow-up or withdraws from the study, then this person's survival time is censored.

T F 5. $S(t) = P(T > t)$ is called the hazard function.

T F 6. The hazard function is a probability.

T F 7. Theoretically, the graph of a survivor function is a smooth curve that decreases from $S(t) = 1$ at $t = 0$ to $S(t) = 0$ at $t = \infty$.

T F 8. The survivor function at time t gives the instantaneous potential per unit time for a failure to occur, given survival up to time t.

T F 9. The formula for a hazard function involves a conditional probability as one of its components.

T F 10. The hazard function theoretically has no upper bound.

T F 11. Mathematical models for survival analysis are frequently written in terms of a hazard function.

T F 12. One goal of a survival analysis is to compare survivor and/or hazard functions.

T F 13. Ordered failure times are censored data.

T F 14. Censored data are used in the analysis of survival data up to the time interval of censorship.

T F 15. A typical goal of a survival analysis involving several explanatory variables is to obtain an adjusted measure of effect.

16. Given the following survival time data (in weeks),

    1, 1, 1+, 1+, 1+, 2, 2, 2, 2+, 2+, 3, 3, 3+, 4+, 5+

    where + denotes censored data, complete the following table:

$t_{(j)}$	$m_{(j)}$	$q_{(j)}$	$R(t_{(j)})$
0	0	0	15 persons survive ≥ 0 weeks
1			
2			
3			

    Also, compute the average survival time ($\overline{T}$) and the average hazard rate ($\overline{h}$) using the raw data (ignoring + signs for $\overline{T}$).

17. Suppose that the estimated survivor curve for the above table is given by the following graph:

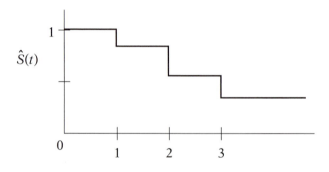

    What is the median survival time for this cohort?

Questions 18–20 consider the comparison of the following two survivor curves:

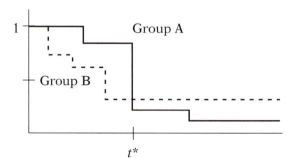

18. Which group has a better survival prognosis **before** time $t*$?

19. Which group has a better survival prognosis **after** time $t*$?

20. Which group has a longer median survival time?

Test

True or False (Circle T or F):

T F   1. Survival analysis is a collection of statistical procedures for data analysis for which the outcome variable is **time until an event occurs.**

T F   2. In survival analysis, the term "event" is synonymous with "failure."

T F   3. If a given individual is lost to follow-up or withdraws from the study before the end of the study without the event occurring, then the survival time for this individual is said to be "censored."

T F   4. In practice, the survivor function is usually graphed as a smooth curve.

T F   5. The survivor function ranges between 0 and ∞.

T F   6. The concept of instantaneous potential is illustrated by velocity.

T F   7. A hazard rate of one per day is equivalent to seven per week.

T F   8. If you know the form of a hazard function, then you can determine the corresponding survivor curve, and vice versa.

T F   9. One use of a hazard function is to gain insight about conditional failure rates.

T F   10. If the survival curve for group 1 lies completely above the survival curve for group 2, then the median survival time for group 2 is longer than that for group 1.

T F   11. The risk set at six weeks is the set of individuals whose survival times are less than or equal to six weeks.

T F   12. If the risk set at six weeks consists of 22 persons, and four persons fail and three persons are censored by the 7th week, then the risk set at seven weeks consists of 18 persons.

T F   13. The measure of effect used in survival analysis is an odds ratio.

T F   14. If a hazard ratio comparing group 1 relative to group 2 equals 10, then the potential for failure is ten times higher in group 1 than in group 2.

T F   15. The outcome variable used in a survival analysis is different from that used in linear or logistic modeling.

16. State two properties of a hazard function.

17. State three reasons why hazard functions are used.

18. State three goals of a survival analysis.

19. The following data are a sample from the 1967–1980 Evans County study. Survival times (in years) are given for two study groups, each with 25 participants. Group 1 has no history of chronic disease (CHR = 0), and group 2 has a positive history of chronic disease (CHR = 1):

Group 1 (CHR = 0):   12.3+, 5.4, 8.2, 12.2+, 11.7, 10.0, 5.7, 9.8, 2.6, 11.0, 9.2, 12.1+, 6.6, 2.2, 1.8, 10.2, 10.7, 11.1, 5.3, 3.5, 9.2, 2.5, 8.7, 3.8, 3.0

Group 2 (CHR = 1):   5.8, 2.9, 8.4, 8.3, 9.1, 4.2, 4.1, 1.8, 3.1, 11.4, 2.4, 1.4, 5.9, 1.6, 2.8, 4.9, 3.5, 6.5, 9.9, 3.6, 5.2, 8.8, 7.8, 4.7, 3.9

For group 1, complete the following table involving ordered failure times:

	$t_{(j)}$	$m_{(j)}$	$q_{(j)}$	$R(t_{(j)})$
Group 1:	0.0		0	0	25 persons survived $\geq$ 0 years
	1.8		1	0	25 persons survived $\geq$ 1.8 years
	2.2				
	2.5				
	2.6				
	3.0				
	3.5				
	3.8				
	5.3				
	5.4				
	5.7				
	6.6				
	8.2				
	8.7				
	9.2				
	9.8				
	10.0				
	10.2				
	10.7				
	11.0				
	11.1				
	11.7				

20. For the data of Problem 19, the average survival time ($\overline{T}$) and the average hazard rate ($\overline{h}$) for each group are given as follows:

	$\overline{T}$	$\overline{h}$
Group 1:	7.5	.1165
Group 2:	5.3	.1894

a. Based on the above information, which group has a better survival prognosis? Explain briefly.
b. How would a comparison of survivor curves provide additional information to what is provided in the above table?

Answers to Practice Exercises

1. F: the outcome is continuous; time until an event occurs.

2. T

3. T

4. F: the person fails, i.e., is not censored.

5. F: $S(t)$ is the survivor function.

6. F: the hazard is a rate, not a probability.

7. T

8. F: the hazard function gives instantaneous potential.

9. T

10. T

11. T

12. T

13. F: ordered failure times are data for persons who are failures.

14. T

15. T

16.

$t_{(j)}$	$m_{(j)}$	$q_{(j)}$	$R(t_{(j)})$
0	0	0	15 persons survive $\geq$ 0 weeks
1	2	3	15 persons survive $\geq$ 1 week
2	3	2	10 persons survive $\geq$ 2 weeks
3	2	3	5 persons survive $\geq$ 3 weeks

$$\bar{T} = \frac{33}{15} = 2.2; \quad \bar{h} = \frac{7}{33} = 0.2121$$

17.   Median = 3

18.   Group A

19.   Group B

20.   Group A

2

Kaplan–Meier
Survival Curves
and the
Log–Rank Test

Contents

Introduction

We begin with a brief review of the purposes of survival analysis, basic notation and terminology, and the basic data layout for the computer.

We then describe how to estimate and graph survival curves using the **Kaplan–Meier (KM)** method. The estimated survival probabilities are computed using a **product limit formula.**

Next, we describe how to compare two or more survival curves using the **log–rank test** of the null hypothesis of a common survival curve. For two groups, the log–rank statistic is based on the summed observed minus expected score for a given group and its variance estimate. For several groups, a computer should always be used because the log–rank formula is more complicated mathematically. The test statistic is approximately chi-square in large samples with G-1 degrees of freedom, where G denotes the number of groups being compared.

An alternative test is called the **Peto test,** which may be chosen if one wants to give more weight to the earlier part of the survival curves. This test is also a large sample chi-square test with G-1 degrees of freedom.

Abbreviated Outline

The outline below gives the user a preview of the material to be covered by the presentation. A detailed outline for review purposes follows the presentation.

Objectives

Upon completing the module, the learner should be able to:

1. Compute Kaplan–Meier (KM) probabilities of survival, given survival time and failure status information on a sample of subjects.
2. Interpret a graph of KM curves that compare two or more groups.
3. Draw conclusions as to whether or not two or more survival curves are the same based on computer results that provide a log–rank test.
4. Draw conclusions as to whether or not two or more survival curves are the same based on computer results that provide a Peto test.
5. Decide whether the log–rank test or the Peto test is more appropriate for a given set of survival data.

Presentation

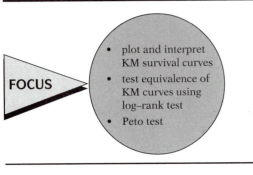

This presentation describes how to plot and interpret survival data using Kaplan–Meier (KM) survival curves and how to test whether or not two or more KM curves are equivalent using the log–rank test. We also describe an alternative test called the Peto test.

I. Review

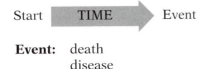

Event: death
             disease
             relapse

Time = survival time

Event = failure

Censoring: Don't know survival time exactly

We begin by reviewing the basics of survival analysis. Generally, survival analysis is a collection of statistical procedures for the analysis of data in which the outcome variable of interest is **time until an event occurs.** By **event,** we mean death, disease incidence, relapse from remission, or any designated experience of interest that may happen to an individual.

When doing a survival analysis, we usually refer to the time variable as **survival time.** We also typically refer to the event as a **failure.**

Most survival analyses consider a key data analytical problem called **censoring.** In essence, censoring occurs when we have some information about individual survival time, but **we don't know the survival time exactly.**

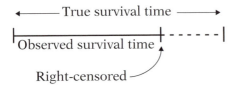

Most survival time data is right-censored, because the true survival time interval, which we don't really know, has been cut off (i.e., censored) at the right side of the time interval, giving us the survival time actually observed. We want to use the observed survival time to draw implications about the true survival time.

Notation

T = survival time

↖ random variable

t = specific value for T

As notation, we denote by a **capital T** the random variable for a person's survival time. Next, we denote by a **small letter t** any specific value of interest for the variable T.

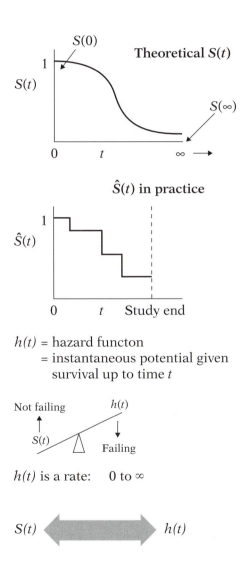

δ = (0,1) random variable

$$= \begin{cases} 1 \text{ if failure} \\ 0 \text{ if censored} \end{cases}$$

We let the Greek letter delta (δ) denote a (0,1) random variable indicating either censorship or failure. A person who does not fail, that is, does not get the event during the study period, must have been censored either before or at the end of the study.

$S(t)$ = survivor function
    = PR $(T > t)$

The survivor function, denoted by **S(t),** gives the probability that the random variable T exceeds the specified time t.

Theoretical S(t)

$S(0)$

$S(\infty)$

Theoretically, as t ranges from 0 up to infinity, the survivor function is graphed as a decreasing smooth curve, which begins at $S(t) = 1$ at $t = 0$ and heads downward toward zero as t increases toward infinity.

$\hat{S}(t)$ in practice

In practice, using data, we usually obtain survivor function graphs which are **step functions,** as illustrated here, rather than smooth curves.

$h(t)$ = hazard functon
    = instantaneous potential given survival up to time t

The hazard function, denoted by **h(t),** gives the **instantaneous potential** per unit time for the event to occur given that the individual has survived up to time t.

Not failing

$h(t)$

$S(t)$

Failing

$h(t)$ is a rate: 0 to ∞

In contrast to the survivor function, which focuses on **not** failing, the hazard function focuses on failing; in other words, as $S(t)$ goes up, $h(t)$ goes down, and vice versa. The hazard is a **rate,** rather than a probability. Thus, the values of the hazard function range between zero and infinity.

$S(t)$ ⟷ $h(t)$

Regardless of which function $S(t)$ or $h(t)$ one prefers, **there is a clearly defined relationship between the two.** In fact, if one knows the form of $S(t)$, one can derive the corresponding $h(t)$, and vice versa.

Data Layout:

Indiv. #	t	δ	X_1	$X_2 \cdots X_p$
1	t_1	δ_1	X_{11}	$X_{12} \cdots X_{1p}$
2	t_2	δ_2	X_{21}	$X_{22} \cdots X_{2p}$
.	.	.	.	.
.	.	.	.	.
.	.	.	.	.
n	t_n	δ_n	X_{n1}	$X_{n2} \cdots X_{np}$

The general data layout for a survival analysis is given by the table shown here. The first column of the table identifies the study subjects. The second column gives the observed survival time information. The third column gives the information for δ, the dichotomous variable that indicates censorship status. The remainder of the information in the table gives values for explanatory variables of interest.

Alternative (ordered) data layout:

Ordered failure times, $t_{(j)}$	# of failures m_j	# censored in $(t_{(j)}, t_{(j+1)})$, q_j	Risk set, $R(t_{(j)})$
$t_{(0)} = 0$	$m_0 = 0$	q_0	$R(t_{(0)})$
$t_{(1)}$	m_1	q_1	$R(t_{(1)})$
$t_{(2)}$	m_2	q_2	$R(t_{(2)})$
.	.	.	.
.	.	.	.
.	.	.	.
$t_{(k)}$	m_k	q_k	$R(t_{(k)})$

An alternative data layout is shown here. This layout is the basis upon which **Kaplan–Meier** survival curves are derived. The first column in the table gives ordered survival times from smallest to largest. The second column gives frequency counts of failures at each distinct failure time. The third column gives frequency counts, denoted by q_j, of those persons censored in the time interval starting with failure time $t_{(j)}$ up to but not including the next failure time denoted $t_{(j+1)}$. The last column gives the **risk set,** which denotes the collection of individuals who have survived at least to time $t_{(j)}$.

Table of ordered failures:
- Uses all information up to time of censorship;
- $S(t)$ is derived from $R(t)$.

To compute the survival probability at a given time, we make use of the risk set at that time to include the information we have on a censored person up to the time of censorship, rather than simply throw away all the information on a censored person.

Survival probability:
    Use **Kaplan–Meier (KM)** method.

The actual computation of such a survival probability can be carried out using the Kaplan–Meier (KM) method. We introduce the KM method in the next section by way of an example.

II. An Example of Kaplan–Meier Curves

EXAMPLE

The data: remission times (weeks) for two groups of leukemia patients

Group 1 ($n = 21$) treatment	Group 2 ($n = 21$) placebo
6, 6, 6, 7, 10,	1, 1, 2, 2, 3,
13, 16, 22, 23,	4, 4, 5, 5,
6+, 9+, 10+, 11+,	8, 8, 8, 8,
17+, 19+, 20+,	11, 11, 12, 12,
25+, 32+, 32+,	15, 17, 22, 23
34+, 35+	

Note: + denotes censored

	# failed	# censored	Total
Group 1	9	12	21
Group 2	21	0	21

Descriptive statistics:

$\overline{T}_1$ (ignoring + 's) = 17.1, $\overline{T}_2 = 8.6$

$\overline{h}_1 = .025$, $\overline{h}_2 = .115$, $\dfrac{\overline{h}_2}{\overline{h}_1} = 4.6$

The data for this example derive from a study of the remission times in weeks for two groups of leukemia patients, with 21 patients in each group. Group 1 is the treatment group and group 2 is the placebo group. The basic question of interest concerns comparing the survival experience of the two groups.

Of the 21 persons in group 1, 9 failed during the study period and 12 were censored. In contrast, none of the data in group 2 are censored; that is, all 21 persons in the placebo group went out of remission during the study period.

In Chapter 1, we observed for this data set that group 1 appears to have better survival prognosis than group 2, indicating that the treatment is effective. This conclusion was supported by descriptive statistics for the average survival time and average hazard rate shown here. Note, however, that descriptive statistics provide overall comparisons but do not compare the two groups at different times of follow-up.

| EXAMPLE (continued) | | | | A table of ordered failure times is shown here for each group. These tables provide the basic information for the computation of KM curves. |

EXAMPLE (continued)

Ordered failure times:

Group 1 (treatment)

$t_{(j)}$	n_j	m_j	q_j
0	21	0	0
6	21	3	1
7	17	1	1
10	15	1	2
13	12	1	0
16	11	1	3
22	7	1	0
23	6	1	5
>23	—	—	—

Group 2 (placebo)

$t_{(j)}$	n_j	m_j	q_j
0	21	0	0
1	21	2	0
2	19	2	0
3	17	1	0
4	16	2	0
5	14	2	0
8	12	4	0
11	8	2	0
12	6	2	0
15	4	1	③
17	3	1	0
22	2	1	0
23	1	1	0

Group 2: no censored subjects

A table of ordered failure times is shown here for each group. These tables provide the basic information for the computation of KM curves.

Each table begins with a survival time of zero, even though no subject actually failed at the start of follow-up. The reason for the zero is to allow for the possibility that some subjects might have been censored before the earliest failure time.

Also, each table contains a column denoted as n_j that gives the number of subjects in the risk set at the start of the interval. It is assumed that n_j includes those persons failing at time $t_{(j)}$; in other words, n_j counts those subjects at risk for failing instantaneously prior to time $t_{(j)}$.

We now describe how to compute the KM curve for the table for group 2. The computations for group 2 are quite straightforward because there are no censored subjects for this group.

EXAMPLE (continued)

Group 2 placebo

$t_{(j)}$	n_j	m_j	q_j	$\hat{S}(t_{(j)})$
0	21	0	0	1
1	21	2	0	19/21 = .90
2	19	2	0	17/21 = .81
3	17	1	0	16/21 = .76
4	16	2	0	14/21 = .67
5	14	2	0	12/21 = .57
8	12	4	0	8/21 = .38
11	8	2	0	6/21 = .29
12	6	2	0	4/21 = .19
15	4	1	3	3/21 = .14
17	3	1	0	2/21 = .10
22	2	1	0	1/21 = .05
23	1	1	0	0/21 = .00

The table of ordered failure times for group 2 is presented here again with the addition of another column that contains survival probability estimates. These estimates are the KM survival probabilities for this group. We will discuss the computations of these probabilities shortly.

KM Curve for Group 2 (Placebo)

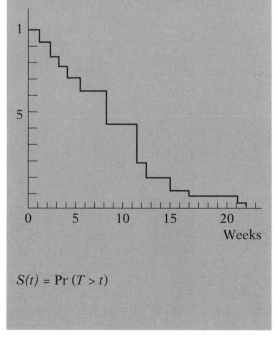

A plot of the KM survival probabilities corresponding to each ordered failure time is shown here for group 2. Empirical plots such as this one are typically plotted as a step function that starts with a horizontal line at a survival probability of 1 and then steps down to the other survival probabilities as we move from one ordered failure time to another.

$S(t) = \Pr(T > t)$

We now describe how the survival probabilities for the group 2 data are computed. Recall that a survival probability gives the probability that a study subject survives past a specified time.

EXAMPLE (continued)

Group 2 (placebo)

$t_{(j)}$	n_j	m_j	q_j	$\hat{S}(t_{(j)})$
0	21	0	0	1
1	21	2	0	19/21 = .90
2	19	2	0	17/21 = .81
3	17	1	0	16/21 = .76
4	16	2	0	14/21 = .67
5	14	2	0	12/21 = .57
8	12	4	0	8/21 = .38
11	8	2	0	6/21 = .29
12	6	2	0	4/21 = .19
15	4	1	0	3/21 = .14
17	3	1	0	2/21 = .10
22	2	1	0	1/21 = .05
23	1	1	0	0/21 = .00

$$\hat{S}(t_{(j)}) = \frac{\text{# surviving past } t_{(j)}}{21}$$

No censorship in group 2

Alternative formula: KM approach

EXAMPLE

$$\hat{S}(4) = 1 \times \frac{19}{21} \times \frac{17}{19} \times \frac{16}{17} \times \frac{14}{16} = \frac{14}{21} = .67$$

$$\Pr\left(T > t_{(j)} \mid T \ge t_{(j)}\right)$$

Thus, considering the group 2 data, the probability of surviving past zero is unity, as it will always be for any data set.

Next, the probability of surviving past the first ordered failure time of one week is given by 19/21 or (.91) because 2 people failed at one week, so that 19 people from the original 21 remain as survivors past one week.

Similarly, the next probability concerns subjects surviving past two weeks, which is 17/21 (or .81) because 2 subjects failed at one week and 2 subjects failed at two weeks leaving 17 out of the original 21 subjects surviving past two weeks.

The remaining survival probabilities in the table are computed in the same manner; that is, we count the number of subjects surviving past the specified time being considered and divide this number by 21, the number of subjects at the start of follow-up.

Recall that no subject in group 2 was censored, so the q column for group 2 consists entirely of zeros. If some of the q's had been nonzero, an alternative formula for computing survival probabilities would be needed. This alternative formula is called the Kaplan–Meier (KM) approach and can be illustrated using the group 2 data even though all values of q are zero.

For example, an alternative way to calculate the survival probability of exceeding four weeks for the group 2 data can be written using the KM formula shown here. This formula involves the product of terms each of which is a conditional probability of the type shown here. That is, each term in the product is the probability of exceeding a specific ordered failure time $t_{(j)}$ given that a subject survives up to that failure time.

$$\hat{S}(4) = 1 \times \boxed{\frac{19}{21}} \times \frac{17}{19} \times \boxed{\frac{16}{17}} \times \frac{14}{16} = \frac{14}{21} = .67$$

$$\frac{19}{21} = \Pr(T > 1 \mid T \geq 1)$$

$$\frac{16}{17} = \Pr(T > 3 \mid T \geq 3)$$

17 = # in risk set at week 3

$$\hat{S}(4) = 1 \times \frac{19}{21} \times \frac{17}{19} \times \frac{16}{17} \times \boxed{\frac{14}{16}}$$

$$\hat{S}(8) = 1 \times \frac{19}{21} \times \frac{17}{19} \times \frac{16}{17} \times \frac{14}{16} \times \frac{12}{14} \times \boxed{\frac{8}{12}}$$

KM formula = **product limit** formula

Next: Group 1

Group 1 (treatment)

$t_{(j)}$	n_j	m_j	q_j	$\hat{S}(t_{(j)})$
0	21	0	0	①
6	21	3	1	$1 \times \boxed{\frac{18}{21}} = .8571$
7	17	1	1	$.8571 \times \boxed{\frac{16}{17}} = .8067$
10	15	1	2	$.8067 \times \frac{14}{15} = .7529$
13	12	1	0	$.7529 \times \frac{11}{12} = .6902$
16	11	1	3	$.6902 \times \frac{10}{11} = .6275$
22	7	1	0	$.6275 \times \frac{6}{7} = .5378$
23	6	1	5	$.5378 \times \frac{5}{6} = .4482$

Thus, in the KM formula for survival past four weeks, the term 19/21 gives the probability of surviving past the first ordered failure time, one week, given survival up to the first week. Note that all 21 persons in group 2 survived up to one week, but that 2 failed at one week, leaving 19 persons surviving past one week.

Similarly, the term 16/17 gives the probability of surviving past the third ordered failure time at week 3, given survival up to week 3. There were 17 persons who survived up to week 3 and one of these then failed, leaving 16 survivors past week 3. Note that the 17 persons in the denominator represents the number in the risk set at week 3.

Notice that the product terms in the KM formula for surviving past four weeks stop at the fourth week with the component 14/16. Similarly, the KM formula for surviving past eight weeks stops at the eighth week.

More generally, any KM formula for a survival probability is limited to product terms up to the survival week being specified. That is why the KM formula is often referred to as a "product-limit" formula.

Next, we consider the KM formula for the data from group 1, where there are several censored observations.

The estimated survival probabilities obtained using the KM formula are shown here for group 1.

The first survival estimate on the list is $\hat{S}(0) = 1$, as it will always be, because this gives the probability of surviving past time zero.

The other survival estimates are calculated by multiplying the estimate for the immediately preceding failure time by a fraction. For example, the fraction is 18/21 for surviving past week 6, because 21 subjects remain up to week 6 and 3 of these subjects fail to survive past week 6. The fraction is 16/17 for surviving past week 7, because 17 people remain up to week 7 and one of these fails to survive past week 7. The other fractions are calculated similarly.

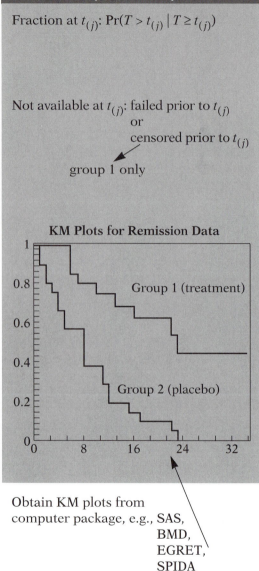

EXAMPLE (continued)

Fraction at $t_{(j)}$: $\Pr(T > t_{(j)} \mid T \geq t_{(j)})$

Not available at $t_{(j)}$: failed prior to $t_{(j)}$
or
censored prior to $t_{(j)}$

group 1 only

KM Plots for Remission Data

Group 1 (treatment)

Group 2 (placebo)

Obtain KM plots from
computer package, e.g., SAS,
BMD,
EGRET,
SPIDA

For a specified failure time $t_{(j)}$, the fraction may be generally expressed as the conditional probability of surviving past time $t_{(j)}$, given availability (i.e., in the risk set) at time $t_{(j)}$. This is exactly the same formula that we previously used to calculate each product term in the product limit formula used for the group 2 data.

Note that a subject might not be available at time $t_{(j)}$ for one of two reasons: (1) either the subject has failed prior to $t_{(j)}$, or (2) the subject has been censored prior to $t_{(j)}$. Group 1 has censored observations, whereas group 2 does not. Thus, for group 1, censored observations have to be taken into account when determining the number available at $t_{(j)}$.

Plots of the KM curves for groups 1 and 2 are shown here on the same graph. Notice that the KM curve for group 1 is consistently higher than the KM curve for group 2. These figures indicate that group 1, which is the treatment group, has better survival prognosis than group 2, the placebo group. Moreover, as the number of weeks increases, the two curves appear to get farther apart, suggesting that the beneficial effects of the treatment over the placebo are greater the longer one stays in remission.

The KM plots shown above can be easily obtained from most computer packages that perform survival analysis, including SAS, BMD, and EGRET. All the user needs to do is provide a KM computer program with the basic data layout and then provide appropriate commands to obtain plots. The above plots were obtained using the SPIDA package (from Macquarie University in Sydney, Australia). This package will also be used later to present results from log–rank tests.

III. General Features of KM Curves

General KM formula:

$$\hat{S}(t_{(j)}) = \hat{S}(t_{(j-1)}) \times \hat{\Pr}(T > t_{(j)} \mid T \geq t_{(j)})$$

The general formula for a KM survival probability at failure time $t_{(j)}$ is shown here. This formula gives the probability of surviving past the previous failure time $t_{(j-1)}$, multiplied by the conditional probability of surviving past time $t_{(j)}$, given survival to *at least* time $t_{(j)}$.

KM formula = product limit formula

$$\hat{S}(t_{(j-1)}) = \prod_{i=1}^{j-1} \hat{Pr}(T > t_{(i)} \mid T \ge t_{(i)})$$

The above KM formula can also be expressed as a product limit if we substitute for the survival probability $\hat{S}(t_{(j-1)})$, the product of all fractions that estimate the conditional probabilities for failure times $t_{(j-1)}$ and earlier.

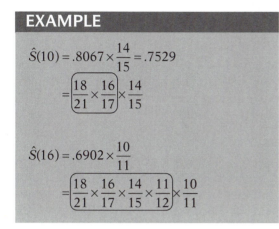

EXAMPLE

$$\hat{S}(10) = .8067 \times \frac{14}{15} = .7529$$

$$= \boxed{\frac{18}{21} \times \frac{16}{17}} \times \frac{14}{15}$$

$$\hat{S}(16) = .6902 \times \frac{10}{11}$$

$$= \boxed{\frac{18}{21} \times \frac{16}{17} \times \frac{14}{15} \times \frac{11}{12}} \times \frac{10}{11}$$

For example, the probability of surviving past ten weeks is given in the table for group 1 (page 55) by .8067 times 14/15, which equals .7529. But the .8067 can be alternatively written as the product of the fractions 18/21 and 16/17. Thus, the product limit formula for surviving past 10 weeks is given by the triple product shown here.

Similarly, the probability of surviving past sixteen weeks can be written either as .6902 × 10/11, or equivalently as the five-way product of fractions shown here.

$$\hat{S}(t_{(j)}) = \prod_{i=1}^{j} \hat{Pr}[T > t_{(i)} \mid T \ge t_{(i)}]$$

$$= \hat{S}(t_{(j-1)}) \times \hat{Pr}(T > t_{(j)} \mid T \ge t_{(j)})$$

The general expression for the product limit formula for the KM survival estimate is shown here together with the general KM formula given earlier. Both expressions are equivalent.

Math proof:

$$Pr(A \text{ and } B) = Pr(A) \times Pr(B \mid A) \text{ always}$$

A simple mathematical proof of the KM formula can be described in probability terms. One of the basic rules of probability is that the probability of a joint event, say A and B, is equal to the probability of one event, say A, times the conditional probability of the other event, B, given A.

$$A = "T \ge t_{(j)}"$$
$$B = "T > t_{(j)}" \quad \rightarrow A \text{ and } B = B$$

$$Pr(A \text{ and } B) = Pr(B) = \boxed{S(t_{(j)})}$$

If we let A be the event that a subject survives to at least time $t_{(j)}$ and we let B be the event that a subject survives past time $t_{(j)}$, then the joint event A and B simplifies to the event B, which is inclusive of A. It follows that the probability of A and B equals the probability of surviving past time $t_{(j)}$.

No failures during $t_{(j-1)} < T < t_{(j)}$

$$Pr(A) = Pr(T > t_{(j-1)}) = \boxed{S(t_{(j-1)})}$$

Also, because $t_{(j)}$ is the next failure time after $t_{(j-1)}$, there can be no failures after time $t_{(j-1)}$ and before time $t_{(j)}$. Therefore, the probability of A is equivalent to the probability of surviving past the $(j - 1)$th ordered failure time.

$$\Pr(B \mid A) = \boxed{\Pr(T > t_{(j)} \mid T \geq t_{(j)})}$$

Furthermore, the conditional probability of B given A is equivalent to the conditional probability in the KM formula.

Thus, from Pr(A and B) formula,

$$S(t_{(j)}) = S(t_{(j-1)}) \times \Pr(T > t_{(j)} \mid T \geq t_{(j)})$$

Thus, using the basic rules of probability, the KM formula can be derived.

IV. The Log–Rank Test for Two Groups

Are KM curves statistically equivalent?

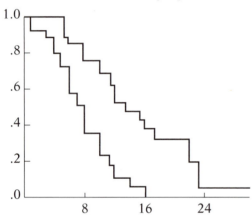

We now describe how to evaluate whether or not KM curves for two or more groups are statistically equivalent. In this section we consider two groups only. The most popular testing method is called the log–rank test.

When we state that two KM curves are "statistically equivalent," we mean that, based on a testing procedure that compares the two curves in some "overall sense," we do not have evidence to indicate that the true (population) survival curves are different.

- Chi-square test
- Overall comparison of KM curves
- Observed versus expected counts
- Categories defined by ordered failure times

The log–rank test is a large-sample chi-square test that uses as its test criterion a statistic that provides an overall comparison of the KM curves being compared. This (log–rank) statistic, like many other statistics used in other kinds of chi-square tests, makes use of observed versus expected cell counts over categories of outcomes. The categories for the log–rank statistic are defined by each of the ordered failure times for the entire set of data being analyzed.

EXAMPLE

Remission data: $n = 42$

$t_{(j)}$	# failures		# in risk set	
	m_{1j}	m_{2j}	n_{1j}	n_{2j}
1	0	2	21	21
2	0	2	21	19
3	0	1	21	17
④	0	2	21	16
5	0	2	21	14
6	3	0	21	12
7	1	0	17	12
8	0	4	16	12
⑩	1	0	15	8
11	0	2	13	8
12	0	2	12	6
13	1	0	12	4
15	0	1	11	4
16	1	0	11	3
17	0	1	10	3
22	1	1	7	2
23	1	1	6	1

As an example of the information required for the log–rank test, we again consider the comparison of the treatment (group 1) and placebo (group 2) subjects in the remission data on 42 leukemia patients.

Here, for each ordered failure time, $t_{(j)}$, in the entire set of data, we show the numbers of subjects (m_{ij}) failing at that time, separately by group (i), followed by the numbers of subjects (n_{ij}) in the risk set at that time, also separately by group.

Thus, for example, at week 4, no subjects failed in group 1, whereas two subjects failed in group 2. Also, at week 4, the risk set for group 1 contains 21 persons, whereas the risk set for group 2 contains 16 persons.

Similarly, at week 10, one subject failed in group 1, and no subjects failed at group 2; the risk sets for each group contain 15 and 8 subjects, respectively.

Expected cell counts:

$$e_{1j} = \left(\frac{n_{1j}}{n_{1j} + n_{2j}} \right) \times \left(m_{1j} + m_{2j} \right)$$

⬆ Proportion in risk set　　⬆ # of failures over both groups

$$e_{2j} = \left(\frac{n_{2j}}{n_{1j} + n_{2j}} \right) \times \left(m_{1j} + m_{2j} \right)$$

We now expand the previous table to include expected cell counts and observed minus expected values for each group at each ordered failure time. The formula for the expected cell counts is shown here for each group. For group 1, this formula computes the expected number at time j (i.e., e_{1j}) as the proportion of the total subjects in both groups who are at risk at time j, that is, $n_{1j}/(n_{1j} + n_{2j})$, multiplied by the total number of failures at that time over both groups (i.e., $m_{1j} + m_{2j}$). For group 2, e_{2j} is computed similarly.

EXAMPLE

Expanded Table (Remission Data)

		\# failures		\# in risk set		\# expected		Observed–expected	
j	$t_{(j)}$	m_{1j}	m_{2j}	n_{1j}	n_{2j}	e_{1j}	e_{2j}	$m_{1j}-e_{1j}$	$m_{2j}-e_{2j}$
1	1	0	2	21	21	$(21/42) \times 2$	$(21/42) \times 2$	−1.00	1.00
2	2	0	2	21	19	$(21/40) \times 2$	$(19/40) \times 2$	−1.05	1.05
3	3	0	1	21	17	$(21/38) \times 1$	$(17/38) \times 1$	−0.55	0.55
4	4	0	2	21	16	$(21/37) \times 2$	$(16/37) \times 2$	−1.14	1.14
5	5	0	2	21	14	$(21/35) \times 2$	$(14/35) \times 2$	−1.20	1.20
6	6	3	0	21	12	$(21/33) \times 3$	$(12/33) \times 3$	1.09	−1.09
7	7	1	0	17	12	$(17/29) \times 1$	$(12/29) \times 1$	0.41	−0.41
8	8	0	4	16	12	$(16/28) \times 4$	$(12/28) \times 4$	−2.29	2.29
9	10	1	0	15	8	$(15/23) \times 1$	$(8/23) \times 1$	0.35	−0.35
10	11	0	2	13	8	$(13/21) \times 2$	$(8/21) \times 2$	−1.24	1.24
11	12	0	2	12	6	$(12/18) \times 2$	$(6/18) \times 2$	−1.33	1.33
12	13	1	0	12	4	$(12/16) \times 1$	$(4/16) \times 1$	0.25	−0.25
13	15	0	1	11	4	$(11/15) \times 1$	$(4/15) \times 1$	−0.73	0.73
14	16	1	0	11	3	$(11/14) \times 1$	$(3/14) \times 1$	0.21	−0.21
15	17	0	1	10	3	$(10/13) \times 1$	$(3/13) \times 1$	−0.77	0.77
16	22	1	1	7	2	$(7/9) \times 2$	$(2/9) \times 2$	−0.56	0.56
17	23	1	1	6	1	$(6/7) \times 2$	$(1/7) \times 2$	−0.71	0.71
Totals		9	(21)			19.26	(10.74)	−10.26	(10.26)

\# of failure times

$$O_i - E_j = \sum_{j=1}^{17} \left(m_{ij} - e_{ij} \right), \qquad i = 1, 2$$

When two groups are being compared, the log–rank test statistic is formed using the sum of the observed minus expected counts over all failure times for one of the two groups. In this example, this sum is −10.26 for group 1 and 10.26 for group 2. We will use the group 2 value to carry out the test, but as we can see, except for the minus sign, the difference is the same for the two groups.

EXAMPLE

$$O_1 - E_1 = -10.26$$

$$O_2 - E_2 = 10.26$$

Two groups:

$O_2 - E_2$ = summed observed minus expected score for group 2

$$\text{Log} - \text{rank statistic} = \frac{(O_2 - E_2)^2}{\text{Var}(O_2 - E_2)}$$

$\text{Var}(O_i - E_i)$

$$= \sum_j \frac{n_{1j}n_{2j}(m_{1j} + m_{2j})(n_{1j} + n_{2j} - m_{1j} - m_{2j})}{(n_{1j} + n_{2j})^2(n_{1j} + n_{2j} - 1)}$$

$i = 1, 2$

H_0: no difference between survival curves

Log–rank statistic $\sim \chi^2$ with 1 df under H_0

For the two-group case, the log–rank statistic, shown here at the left, is computed by dividing the square of the summed observed minus expected score for one of the groups—say, group 2—by the estimated variance of the summed observed minus expected score.

The expression for the estimated variance is shown here. For two groups, the variance formula is the same for each group. This variance formula involves the number in the risk set in each group (n_{ij}) and the number of failures in each group (m_{ij}) at time j. The summation is over all distinct failure times.

The null hypothesis being tested is that there is no overall difference between the two survival curves. Under this null hypothesis, the log–rank statistic is approximately chi-square with one degree of freedom. Thus, a P-value for the log–rank test is determined from tables of the chi-square distribution.

Computer programs:
SPIDA's km:
- descriptive statistics for KM curves
- log–rank statistic
- Peto statistic

SAS's lifetest

Several computer programs are available for calculating the log–rank statistic. For example, the **SPIDA** package has a procedure called "**km**" that computes descriptive information about Kaplan–Meier curves, the log–rank statistic, and an alternative statistic called the Peto statistic, to be described later. Other packages, like **SAS** and **BMDP**, have procedures that provide results similar to those of SPIDA. A comparison of SPIDA, SAS, and BMDP procedures and output is provided in Appendix A at the back of this text.

EXAMPLE

Using SPIDA: Remission Data

Group	Size	% Cen.	LQ	Med.	UQ	0.95	Med CI
0	21	57.148	13	23		13.000	
1	21	0.000	4	8	12	4.000	8

df:1 (Log–rank: 16.793, P-value: 0.0), Peto: 9.954, P-value: 0.002

For the remission data, the printout from using the SPIDA "km" procedure is shown here. The log–rank statistic is 16.793 and the corresponding P-value is zero to three decimal places. This P-value indicates that the null hypothesis should be rejected. We can therefore conclude that the treatment and placebo groups have significantly different KM survival curves.

EXAMPLE

$$O_2 - E_2 = 10.26$$

$$\widehat{Var}(O_2 - E_2) = 6.2685$$

$$\text{Log-rank statistic} = \frac{(O_2 - E_2)^2}{\widehat{Var}(O_2 - E_2)}$$

$$= \frac{(10.26)^2}{6.2685} = 16.793$$

Although the use of a computer is the preferred way to calculate the log–rank statistic, we provide here some of the details of the calculation. We have already seen from earlier computations that the value of $O_2 - E_2$ is 10.26. The estimated variance of $O_2 - E_2$ is computed from the variance formula above to be 6.2685. The log–rank statistic then is obtained by squaring 10.26 and dividing by 6.285, which yields 16.793, as shown on the computer printout.

Approximate formula:

$$X^2 = \sum_{i}^{\text{\# of groups}} \frac{(O_i - E_i)^2}{E_i}$$

An approximation to the log–rank statistic, shown here, can be calculated using observed and expected values for each group without having to compute the variance formula. The approximate formula is of the classic chi-square form that sums over each group being compared the square of the observed minus expected value divided by the expected value.

EXAMPLE

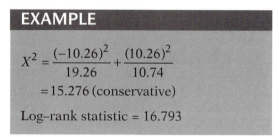

$$X^2 = \frac{(-10.26)^2}{19.26} + \frac{(10.26)^2}{10.74}$$

$$= 15.276 \text{ (conservative)}$$

Log–rank statistic = 16.793

The calculation of the approximate formula is shown here for the remission data. The expected values are 19.26 and 10.74 for groups 1 and 2, respectively. The chi-square value obtained is 15.276, which is slightly smaller than the log–rank statistic of 16.793. Thus, for these data, the approximate formula provides a more conservative test—i.e., it is less likely to reject the null hypothesis—than the (exact) log–rank statistic for these data.

V. The Log–Rank Test for Several Groups

H_0: All survival curves are the same.

The log–rank test can also be used to compare three or more survival curves. The null hypothesis for this more general situation is that all survival curves are the same.

Log–rank statistics for > 2 groups involves variances and covariances of $O_i - E_i$.

Matrix formula: See Appendix at end of this chapter.

Although the same tabular layout can be used to carry out the calculations when there are more than two groups, the test statistic is more complicated mathematically, involving both variances and covariances of summed observed minus expected scores for each group. A convenient mathematical formula can be given in matrix terms. We present the matrix formula for the interested reader in an Appendix at the end of this chapter.

Use computer program for calculations.

We will not describe further details about the calculation of the log–rank statistic, because a computer program can easily carry out the computations from the basic data file. Instead, we illustrate the use of this test with data involving more than two groups.

G (≥ 2) groups:
   log–rank statistic $\sim \chi^2$ with G –1 df

If the number of groups being compared is G (≥ 2), then the log–rank statistic has approximately a large sample distribution with $G - 1$ degrees of freedom. Therefore, the decision about significance is made using chi-square tables with the appropriate degrees of freedom.

Approximation formula:

$$X^2 = \sum_{i}^{\text{\# of groups}} \frac{(O_i - E_i)^2}{E_i}$$

Not required because computer program calculates the exact log–rank statistic

The approximate formula previously described involving only observed and expected values without variance or covariance calculations can also be used when there are more than two groups being compared. However, practically speaking, the use of this approximate formula is not required as long as a computer program is available to calculate the exact log–rank statistic.

We now provide an example to illustrate the use of the log–rank statistic to compare more than two groups.

EXAMPLE

vets.dat: survival time in days,

$$n = 137$$

Veteran's Administration Lung Cancer Trial

Column 1: Treatment standard = 1, test = 2)
Column 2: Cell type 1 (large = 1, other = 0)
Column 3: Cell type 2 (adeno = 1 other = 0)
Column 4: Cell type 3 (small = 1, other = 0)
Column 5: Cell type 4 (squamous = 1, other = 0)
Column 6: Survival time (days)
Column 7: Performance Status
           (0 = worst . . . 100 = best)
Column 8: Disease duration (months)
Column 9: Age
Column 10: Prior therapy (none = 0, some = 1)
Column 11: Status (0 = censored, 1 = died)

The data set "vets.dat" considers survival times in days for 137 patients from the Veteran's Administration Lung Cancer Trial cited by Kalbfleisch and Prentice in their text (*The Statistical Analysis of Survival Time Data*, John Wiley, pp. 223–224, 1980). Failure status is defined by the status variable (column 11). A complete list of the variables as stored in a SPIDA file is shown here; the actual data set is provided in an appendix.

Among the variables listed, we now focus on the performance status variable (column 7). This variable is an interval variable, so before we can obtain KM curves and the log–rank test, we need to categorize this variable.

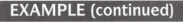

EXAMPLE (continued)

Performance Status Categories

Group #	Categories	Size
1	0–59	52
2	60–74	50
3	75–100	35

KM curves for performance status groups

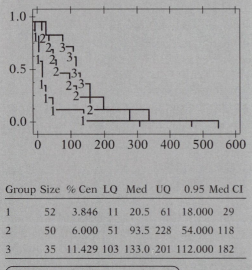

Group	Size	% Cen	LQ	Med	UQ	0.95 Med CI	
1	52	3.846	11	20.5	61	18.000	29
2	50	6.000	51	93.5	228	54.000	118
3	35	11.429	103	133.0	201	112.000	182

df:2 Log–rank: 29.181, P-value: 0.0 Peto: 32.558, P-value: 0.0

$G = 3$ groups; $df = G - 1 = 2$

Log–rank test is highly significant.

Conclude significant difference among three survival curves.

Peto test also significant.

If, for the performance status variable, we choose the categories 0–59, 60–74, and 75–100, we obtain three groups of sizes 52, 50, and 35, respectively.

The KM curves for each of three groups are shown here. Notice that these curves appear to be quite different. A test of significance of this difference is provided by the log–rank statistic.

A printout of descriptive information about the three KM curves together with the log–rank test and the Peto test results are shown here. These results were obtained using the **SPIDA** package.

Because three groups are being compared here, $G = 3$ and the degrees of freedom for the log–rank test is thus $G - 1$, or 2. The log–rank statistic is computed to be 29.181, which has a P-value of zero to three decimal places. Thus, the conclusion from the log–rank test is that there is a highly significant difference among the three survival curves for the performance status groups.

Note, also, that in this example, the Peto test is also highly significant.

VI. The Peto Test

An alternative to log–rank test

Log–rank uses:

$$O_i - E_i = \sum_j (m_{ij} - e_{ij}), \quad i = \text{group\#}$$
$$j = j\text{th failure time}$$

same weight = 1

Peto test: $\boxed{\text{weight} = n_j} = \sum_{i=1}^{G} n_{ij}$

Weighted average $= \dfrac{\sum_j n_j (m_{ij} - e_{ij})}{\sum_j n_j}$

Computer performs calculations.

Peto statistic $\sim \chi^2$ with $G - 1$ *df*

Peto test:
   Emphasizes beginning of survival curve;
   early failures receive larger weights.

Log–rank test:
   Emphasizes tail of the survival curve;
   equal weight given to each failure time.

The Peto test was suggested as an alternative to the log–rank test by Prentice and Marek ("A Qualitative Discrepancy Between Censored Rank Tests," *Biometrics* 35: 861–867, 1979).

In describing the difference between these two tests, recall that the log–rank test uses the summed observed minus expected score O–E in each group to form the test statistic. This simple sum gives the same weight—namely, unity—to each failure time when combining observed minus expected failures in each group.

In contrast, the Peto test weights the observed minus expected score at time t_j by the number at risk, n_j, over all groups at time t_j. Thus, instead of a simple sum, the Peto test uses a weighted average of observed minus expected score, as shown here.

The above formulae are not really important computationally, because a computer program can perform the calculations easily. The Peto test statistic, like the log–rank statistic, has approximately a large sample chi-square distribution with $G - 1$ degrees of freedom, where G is the number of survival curves being compared.

Nevertheless, the different formulae we have described indicate that the Peto test places more emphasis on the information at the beginning of the survival curve where the number at risk is large. Thus, early failures receive larger weights while failures in the tail of the survival curve receive smaller weights.

In contrast, the log–rank test emphasizes failures in the tail of the survival curve, where the number at risk decreases over time, yet equal weight is given to each failure time.

Peto test is not necessarily a conservative test (when compared to log–rank test).

Choose:
1. Peto test if we want more weight given to earlier part of survival curve;
2. log–rank test, if otherwise.

Despite the above differences between the log–rank and Peto tests, the Peto test is not necessarily a conservative test, because its numerical value may be either smaller or larger than the log–rank test, depending on the data being considered.

In choosing between the log–rank test and the Peto test, we suggest using the Peto test if we want to give more weight to the earlier part to the survival curve where there are larger numbers at risk. Otherwise, choose the log–rank test. This choice of emphasizing earlier failure times may rest on clinical features of one's study. A discussion of the relative merits of these tests as well as some other alternatives is described by Harris and Albert in *Survivorship Analysis for Clinical Studies,* Marcel Dekker, 1991.

EXAMPLE: Remission Data

Results for Treatment Status:

Group	Size	% Cen	LQ	Med	UQ	0.95 Med CI	
0	21	57.148	13	23		13.000	
1	21	0.000	4	8	12	4.000	8

*df:*2 log–rank: 16.793, P-value: 0.0, Peto: 9.954, P-value: 0.002

We illustrate the Peto test using examples shown earlier. For the remission data, a comparison of the treatment and placebo groups—with 21 subjects in each—yielded log–rank and Peto tests shown again here. Notice that both the log–rank and Peto tests are highly significant, although the Peto test yields a smaller chi-square value in this example.

EXAMPLE: vets.dat

Results for Performance Status (3 groups):

Group	Size	% Cen	LQ	Med	UQ	0.95 Med CI	
1	52	3.846	11	20.5	61	18.000	29
2	50	6.000	51	93.5	228	54.000	118
3	52	11.429	103	133.0	201	112.000	182

*df:*2 log–rank: 29.181, P-value: 0.0, Peto: 32.558, P-value: 0.0

As a second example, we consider the "vets.dat" data set previously described. The log–rank and Peto test results from comparing three groups of the variable performance status are again shown here. As in the above remission data example, both the log–rank and Peto tests are highly significant for the vets.dat data. Notice, however, that the Peto statistic of 32.558 is slightly higher than the log–rank statistic of 29.181.

VII. Summary

KM curves:

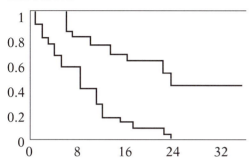

$t_{(j)}$: jth ordered failure time

$$\hat{S}\left(t_{(j)}\right) = \prod_{i=1}^{j} \hat{\Pr}\left[T > t_{(i)} \mid T \geq t_{(i)}\right]$$
$$= \hat{S}\left(t_{(j-1)}\right) \times \hat{\Pr}\left(T > t_{(j)} \mid T \geq t_{(j)}\right)$$

Log–rank test:
  H_0: common survival curve for all groups

$$\text{Log – rank statistic} = \frac{\left(O_2 - E_2\right)^2}{\widehat{\text{Var}}\left(O_2 - E_2\right)}$$

log–rank statistic $\sim \chi^2$ with $G - 1$ df under H_0

G = # of groups

Peto test: use if more weight to earlier part of survival curve.

We now briefly summarize this presentation. First, we described how to estimate and graph survival curves using the Kaplan–Meier (KM) method.

To compute KM curves, we must form a data layout that orders the failure times from smallest to largest. For each ordered failure time, the estimated survival probability is computed using the **product limit formula** shown here. Alternatively, this estimate can be computed as the product of the survival estimate for the previous failure time multiplied by the conditional probability of surviving past the current failure time.

When survival curves are being compared, the log–rank test gives a statistical test of the null hypothesis of a common survival curve. For two groups, the log–rank statistic is based on the summed observed minus expected scores for a given group and its variance estimate. For several groups, a computer should always be used since the log–rank formula is more complicated mathematically. The test statistic is approximately chi-square in large samples with $G - 1$ degrees of freedom, where G denotes the number of groups being compared.

An alternative test is called the Peto test, which may be chosen if one wants to give more weight to the earlier part of the survival curves. This test is also a large sample chi-square test with $G - 1$ degrees of freedom.

Chapters

This presentation is now complete. You can review this presentation using the detailed outline that follows and then try the practice exercises and test.

Chapter 3 introduces the Cox proportional hazards (PH) model, which is the most popular mathematical modeling approach for estimating survival curves when considering several explanatory variables simultaneously.

Detailed Outline

I. **Review** (pages 48–50)
   A. The outcome variable is (survival) time until an event (failure) occurs.
   B. Key problem: **censored data,** i.e., don't know survival time exactly.
   C. Notation: T = survival time random variable
      t = specific value of T
      δ = (0,1) variable for failure/censorship status
      $S(t)$ = survivor function
      $h(t)$ = hazard function
   D. Properties of survivor function:
      i. theoretically, graph is smooth curve, decreasing from $S(t) = 1$ at time $t = 0$ to $S(t) = 0$ at $t = \infty$;
      ii. in practice, graph is step function.
   E. Properties of $h(t)$:
      i. instantaneous potential for failing given survival up to time;
      ii. $h(t)$ is a rate; ranges from 0 to ∞.
   F. Relationship of $S(t)$ to $h(t)$: if you know one you can determine the other.
   G. Goals of survival analysis: estimation of survivor and hazard functions; comparisons and relationships of explanatory variables to survival.
   H. Data layouts
      i. for the computer;
      ii. for understanding the analysis: involves **risk sets.**

II. **An Example of Kaplan–Meier Curves** (pages 51–56)
   A. Data are from study of remission times in weeks for two groups of leukemia patients (21 in each group).
   B. Group 1 (treatment group) has several censored observations, whereas group 2 has no censored observations.
   C. Table of ordered failure times is provided for each group.
   D. For group 2 (all noncensored), survival probabilities are estimated directly and plotted. Formula used is

   $$\hat{S}\left(t_{(j)}\right) = \frac{\#\ \text{surviving past}\ t_{(j)}}{21}\ .$$

   E. Alternative formula for group 2 is given by a **product limit** formula.

F. For group 1, survival probabilities calculated by multiplying estimate for immediately preceding failure time by a conditional probability of surviving past current failure time, i.e.,

$$\hat{S}_{(j)} = \hat{S}_{(j-1)} \, \hat{\Pr}\left[T > t_{(j)} \,\middle|\, T \geq t_{(j)}\right].$$

III. General Features of KM Curves (pages 56–58)

A. Two alternative general formulae:

$$S_{(j)} = \prod_{i=1}^{j} \Pr\left[T > t_{(i)} \,\middle|\, T \geq t_{(i)}\right] \quad \text{(product limit formula)}$$

$$S_{(j)} = S_{(j-1)} \Pr\left[T > t_{(j)} \,\middle|\, T \geq t_{(j)}\right]$$

B. Second formula derived from probability rule:
$$\Pr(A \text{ and } B) = \Pr(A) \times \Pr(B \mid A)$$

IV. The Log–Rank Test for Two Groups (pages 58–62)

A. Large sample chi-square test; provides overall comparison of KM curves.

B. Uses observed versus expected counts over categories of outcomes, where categories are defined by ordered failure times for entire set of data.

C. Example provided using remission data involving two groups:

   i. expanded table described to show how expected and observed minus expected cell counts are computed.

   ii. for ith group at time j, where $i = 1$ or 2:
   observed counts = m_{ij},
   expected counts = e_{ij}, where
   expected counts = (proportion in risk set) $\times$ (# failures over both groups),

$$\text{i.e., } e_{ij} = \left(\frac{n_{ij}}{n_{1j} + n_{2j}}\right)\left(m_{1j} + m_{2j}\right).$$

D. Log–rank statistic for two groups:

$$\boxed{\frac{\left(O_i - E_i\right)^2}{\widehat{\mathrm{Var}}\left(O_i - E_i\right)},}$$

where $i = 1, 2,$

$$O_i - E_i = \sum_j \left(m_{ij} - e_{ij} \right), \text{and}$$

$$\widehat{\mathrm{Var}}\left(O_i - E_i \right) = \sum_j \frac{n_{1j} n_{2j} \left(m_{1j} + m_{2j} \right) \left(n_{1j} + n_{2j} - m_{1j} - m_{2j} \right)}{\left(n_{1j} + n_{2j} \right)^2 \left(n_{1j} + n_{2j} - 1 \right)}, i = 1, 2$$

E. H_0: no difference between survival curves.

F. Log–rank statistic $\sim \chi^2$ with 1 *df* under H_0.

G. Approximate formula:

$$X^2 = \sum_{i=1}^{G} \frac{\left(O_i - E_i \right)^2}{E_i}, \text{where } G = 2 = \text{\# of groups}$$

H. Remission data example: Log–rank statistic = 16.793, whereas X^2 = 15.276.

V. **The Log–Rank Test for Several Groups** (pages 62–64)

A. Involves variances and covariances; matrix formula in Appendix.

B. Use computer for calculations.

C. Under H_0, log–rank statistic $\sim \chi^2$ with $G - 1$ *df*, where G = # of groups.

D. Example provided using vets.dat with interval variable "performance status"; this variable is categorized into $G = 3$ groups, so *df* for log–rank test is $G - 1 = 2$, log–rank statistic is 29.181 ($P = 0.0$).

VI. **The Peto Test** (pages 65–66)

A. Peto test weights observed minus expected score at time j by number at risk, n_j, whereas log–rank test uses equal weights.

B. As with log–rank statistic, Peto statistic $\sim \chi^2$ with $G - 1$ *df*, where G = # of groups.

C. Use computer for calculations.

D. Peto test emphasizes beginning of survival curve; early failures receive larger weights; in contrast, log–rank test emphasizes tail of survival curve.

E. In practice, Peto and log–rank test give similar, but not necessarily equal, results.

VII. **Summary** (page 67)

Practice Exercises

1. The following data are a sample from the 1967–1980 Evans County study. Survival times (in years) are given for two study groups, each with 25 participants. Group 1 has no history of chronic disease (CHR = 0), and group 2 has a positive history of chronic disease (CHR = 1):

Group 1 (CHR = 0):   12.3+, 5.4, 8.2, 12.2+, 11.7, 10.0, 5.7, 9.8, 2.6, 11.0, 9.2, 12.1+, 6.6, 2.2, 1.8, 10.2, 10.7, 11.1, 5.3, 3.5, 9.2, 2.5, 8.7, 3.8, 3.0

Group 2 (CHR = 1):   5.8, 2.9, 8.4, 8.3, 9.1, 4.2, 4.1, 1.8, 3.1, 11.4, 2.4, 1.4, 5.9, 1.6, 2.8, 4.9, 3.5, 6.5, 9.9, 3.6, 5.2, 8.8, 7.8, 4.7, 3.9

a. Fill in the missing information in the following table of ordered failure times for groups 1 and 2:

	Group 1					Group 2			
$t_{(j)}$	n_j	m_j	q_j	$S(t_{(j)})$	$t_{(j)}$	n_j	m_j	q_j	$S(t_{(j)})$
0.0	25	0	0	1.00	0.0	25	1	0	1.00
1.8	25	1	0	.96	1.4	25	1	0	.96
2.2	24	1	0	.92	1.6	24	1	0	.92
2.5	23	1	0	.88	1.8	23	1	0	.88
2.6	22	1	0	.84	2.4	22	1	0	.84
3.0	21	1	0	.80	2.8	21	1	0	.80
3.5	20	⟨		⟩	2.9	20	1	0	.76
3.8	19	1	0	.72	3.1	19	1	0	.72
5.3	18	1	0	.68	3.5	18	1	0	.68
5.4	17	1	0	.64	3.6	17	1	0	.64
5.7	16	1	0	.60	3.9	⟨			⟩
6.6	15	1	0	.56	4.1				
8.2	14	1	0	.52	4.2				
8.7	13	1	0	.48	4.7	13	1	0	.48
9.2	⟨			⟩	4.9	12	1	0	.44
9.8	10	1	0	.36	5.2	11	1	0	.40
10.0	9	1	0	.32	5.8	10	1	0	.36
10.2	8	1	0	.28	5.9	9	1	0	.32
10.7	7	1	0	.24	6.5	8	1	0	.28
11.0	6	1	0	.20	7.8	7	1	0	.24
11.1	5	1	0	.16	8.3	6	1	0	.20
11.7	4	⟨		⟩	8.4	5	1	0	.16

(Continued on next page)

	Group 1				Group 2			
$t_{(j)}$	n_j	m_j	q_j	$S(t_{(j)})$	$t_{(j)}$	n_j	m_j	q_j	$S(t_{(j)})$
					8.8	4	1	0	.12
					9.1				
					9.9				
					11.4	1	1	0	.00

b. Based on your results in part a, plot the KM curves for groups 1 and 2 on the same graph. Comment on how these curves compare with each other.

c. Fill in the following expanded table of ordered failure times to allow for the computation of expected and observed minus expected values at each ordered failure time. Note that your new table here should combine both groups of ordered failure times into one listing and should have the following format:

$t_{(j)}$	m_{1j}	m_{2j}	n_{1j}	n_{2j}	e_{1j}	e_{2j}	$m_{1j}-e_{1j}$	$m_{2j}-e_{2j}$
1.4	0	1	25	25	.500	.500	−.500	.500
1.6	0	1	25	24	.510	.490	−.510	.510
1.8	1	1	25	23	1.042	.958	−.042	.042
2.2	1	0	24	22	.522	.478	.478	−.478
2.4.	0	1	23	22	.511	.489	−.511	.511
2.5.	1	0	23	21	.523	.477	.477	−.477
2.6	1	0	22	21	.516	.484	.484	−.484
2.8	0	1	21	21	.500	.500	−.500	.500
2.9	0	1	21	20	.512	.488	− .512	.512
3.0	1	0	21	19	.525	.475	.475	−.475
3.1								
3.5								
3.6								
3.8								
3.9	0	1	18	16	.529	.471	−.529	.529
4.1	0	1	18	15	.545	.455	−.545	.545
4.2	0	1	18	14	.563	.437	−.563	.563

(Continued on next page)

$t_{(j)}$	m_{1j}	m_{2j}	n_{1j}	n_{2j}	e_{1j}	e_{2j}	$m_{1j}-e_{1j}$	$m_{2j}-e_{2j}$
4.7	0	1	18	13	.581	.419	−.581	.581
4.9	0	1	18	12	.600	.400	−.600	.600
5.2	0	1	18	11	.621	.379	−.621	.621
5.3	1	0	18	10	.643	.357	.357	−.357
5.4	1	0	17	10	.630	.370	.370	−.370
5.7	1	0	16	10	.615	.385	.385	−.385
5.8	0	1	15	10	.600	.400	−.600	.600
5.9	0	1	15	9	.625	.375	−.625	.625
6.5	0	1	15	8	.652	.348	−.652	.652
6.6	1	0	15	7	.682	.318	.318	−.318
7.8	0	1	14	7	.667	.333	−.667	.667
8.2	1	0	14	6	.700	.300	.300	−.300
8.3	0	1	13	6	.684	.316	−.684	.684
8.4	0	1	13	5	.722	.278	−.722	.722
8.7	1	0	13	4	.765	.235	.335	−.335
8.8	0	1	12	4	.750	.250	−.750	.750
9.1	0	1	12	3	.800	.200	−.800	.800
9.2								
9.8								
9.9								
10.0	1	0	9	1	.900	.100	.100	−.100
10.2	1	0	8	1	.888	.112	.112	−.112
10.7	1	0	7	1	.875	.125	.125	−.125
11.0	1	0	6	1	.857	.143	.143	−.143
11.1	1	0	5	1	.833	.167	.167	−.167
11.4	0	1	4	1	.800	.200	−.800	.800
11.7	1	0	4	0	1.000	.000	.000	.000
Totals	22	25			30.79	16.21		

d. Use the results in part c to compute the log–rank statistic. Use this statistic to carry out the log–rank test for these data. What is your null hypothesis and how is the test statistic distributed under this null hypothesis? What are your conclusions from the test?

2. The following data set called "anderson.dat" consists of remission survival times on 42 leukemia patients, half of whom get a certain new treatment therapy and the other half of whom get a standard treatment therapy. The exposure variable of interest is treatment status ($Rx = 0$ if new treatment, $Rx = 1$ if standard treatment). Two other variables for control as potential confounders are log white blood cell count (i.e., logwbc) and sex. Failure status is defined by the relapse variable (0 if censored, 1 if failure). The data set is listed as follows:

Subj	Survt	Relapse	Sex	log WBC	Rx
1	35	0	1	1.45	0
2	34	0	1	1.47	0
3	32	0	1	2.20	0
4	32	0	1	2.53	0
5	25	0	1	1.78	0
6	23	1	1	2.57	0
7	22	1	1	2.32	0
8	20	0	1	2.01	0
9	19	0	0	2.05	0
10	17	0	0	2.16	0
11	16	1	1	3.60	0
12	13	1	0	2.88	0
13	11	0	0	2.60	0
14	10	0	0	2.70	0
15	10	1	0	2.96	0
16	9	0	0	2.80	0
17	7	1	0	4.43	0
18	6	0	0	3.20	0
19	6	1	0	2.31	0
20	6	1	1	4.06	0
21	6	1	0	3.28	0
22	23	1	1	1.97	1
23	22	1	0	2.73	1
24	17	1	0	2.95	1
25	15	1	0	2.30	1
26	12	1	0	1.50	1

(Continued on next page)

Subj	Survt	Relapse	Sex	log WBC	Rx
27	12	1	0	3.06	1
28	11	1	0	3.49	1
29	11	1	0	2.12	1
30	8	1	0	3.52	1
31	8	1	0	3.05	1
32	8	1	0	2.32	1
33	8	1	1	3.26	1
34	5	1	1	3.49	1
35	5	1	0	3.97	1
36	4	1	1	4.36	1
37	4	1	1	2.42	1
38	3	1	1	4.01	1
39	2	1	1	4.91	1
40	2	1	1	4.48	1
41	1	1	1	2.80	1
42	1	1	1	5.00	1

a. Suppose we wish to describe KM curves for the variable logwbc. Because logwbc is continuous, we need to categorize this variable before we compute KM curves. Suppose we categorize logwbc into three categories—low, medium, and high—as follows:

low (0 – 2.30), $n = 11$;
medium (2.31–3.00), $n = 14$;
high (> 3.00), $n = 17$.

Based on this categorization, compute and graph KM curves for each of the three categories of logwbc. (You may use a computer program to assist you or you can form three tables of ordered failure times and compute KM probabilities directly.)

b. Compare the three KM plots you obtained in part a. How are they different?

c. Below is a printout of the log–rank test and the Peto test for comparing the three groups.

Group	Size	% Cen	LQ	Median	UQ	0.95	Med CI
1	11	63.636	15			15.000	
2	14	28.571	8	17	22	8.000	17
3	17	5.882	4	6	8	4.000	7

df: 2, log–rank: 26.391, P-value: 0, Peto: 16.067, P-value: 0.

What do you conclude about whether or not the three KM curves are the same?

Test

To answer the questions below, you will need to use a computer program (from **SAS**, **BMD**, **SPIDA**, **EGRET**, **S+** or any other package you are familiar with) that computes and plots KM curves and computes the log–rank test.

1. For the vets.dat data set described in the presentation (and listed in Appendix B at the end of this book):
   a. Obtain KM plots for the two categories of the variable cell type 1 (1 = large, 0 = other). Comment on how the two curves compare with each other. Carry out the log–rank and/or Peto tests, and draw conclusions from the test(s).
   b. Obtain KM plots for the four categories of cell type—large, adeno, small, and squamous. Note that you will need to recode the data to define a single variable which numerically distinguishes the four categories (e.g., 1 = large, 2 = adeno, etc.). As in part a, compare the four KM curves. Also, carry out the log–rank and/or Peto tests for the equality of the four curves and draw conclusions.

2. The following questions consider a data set from a study by Caplehorn et al. ("Methadone Dosage and Retention of Patients in Maintenance Treatment," *Med. J. Aust.,* 1991). These data comprise the times in days spent by heroin addicts from entry to departure from one of two methadone clinics. There are two further covariates, namely, prison record and methadone dose, believed to affect the survival times. The data set name is addicts.dat. A listing of the data as stored in a **SPIDA** file is given in Appendix B. A listing of the variables is given below:

   Column 1: Subject ID
   Column 2: Clinic (1 or 2)
   Column 3: Survival status (0 = censored, 1 = departed from clinic)
   Column 4: Survival time in days
   Column 5: Prison record (0 = none, 1 = any)
   Column 6: Methadone dose (mg/day)

a. Compute and plot the KM plots for the two categories of the "clinic" variable and comment on the extent to which they differ.

b. A printout of the log–rank and Peto tests (using **SPIDA**) is provided below. What are your conclusions from this printout?

Group	Size	% Cen	LQ	Median	UQ	0.95	Med CI
1	163	25.153	192	428	652	341.000	504
2	75	62.667	280			661.000	

df: 1, log–rank: 27.893, P-value: 0, Peto: 11.078, P-value: 0.001.

c. Compute and evaluate KM curves and the log–rank and/or Peto test for comparing suitably chosen categories of the variable "Methadone dose." Explain how you determined the categories for this variable.

Answers to Practice Exercises

1. a.

	Group 1				Group 2			
$t_{(j)}$	n_j	m_j	q_j	$S(t_{(j)})$	$t_{(j)}$	n_j	m_j	q_j	$S(t_{(j)})$
0.0	25	0	0	1.00	0.0	25	1	0	1.00
1.8	25	1	0	.96	1.4	25	1	0	.96
2.2	24	1	0	.92	1.6	24	1	0	.92
2.5	23	1	0	.88	1.8	23	1	0	.88
2.6	22	1	0	.84	2.4	22	1	0	.84
3.0	21	1	0	.80	2.8	21	1	0	.80
3.5	20	1	0	.76	2.9	20	1	0	.76
3.8	19	1	0	.72	3.1	19	1	0	.72
5.3	18	1	0	.68	3.5	18	1	0	.68
5.4	17	1	0	.64	3.6	17	1	0	.64
5.7	16	1	0	.60	3.9	16	1	0	.60
6.6	15	1	0	.56	4.1	15	1	0	.56
8.2	14	1	0	.52	4.2	14	1	0	.52
8.7	13	1	0	.48	4.7	13	1	0	.48
9.2	12	2	0	.40	4.9	12	1	0	.44
9.8	10	1	0	.36	5.2	11	1	0	.40
10.0	9	1	0	.32	5.8	10	1	0	.36
10.2	8	1	0	.28	5.9	9	1	0	.32

(Continued on next page)

	Group 1					Group 2			
$t_{(j)}$	n_j	m_j	q_j	$S(t_{(j)})$	$t_{(j)}$	n_j	m_j	q_j	$S(t_{(j)})$
10.7	7	1	0	.24	6.5	8	1	0	.28
11.0	6	1	0	.20	7.8	7	1	0	.24
11.1	5	1	0	.16	8.3	6	1	0	.20
11.7	4	1	3	.12	8.4	5	1	0	.16
					8.8	4	1	0	.12
					9.1	3	1	0	.08
					9.9	2	1	0	.04
					11.4	1	1	0	.00

b. KM curves for CHR data:

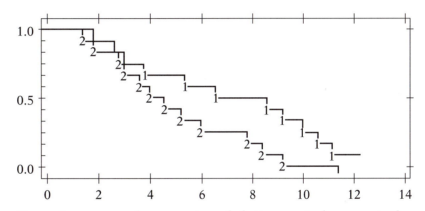

Group 1 appears to have consistently better survival prognosis than group 2. However, the KM curves are very close during the first four years, but are quite separate after four years, although they appear to come close again around twelve years.

c. Using the expanded table format, the following information is obtained:

$t_{(j)}$	m_{1j}	m_{2j}	n_{1j}	n_{2j}	e_{1j}	e_{2j}	$m_{1j}-e_{1j}$	$m_{2j}-e_{2j}$
1.4	0	1	25	25	.500	.500	−.500	.500
1.6	0	1	25	24	.510	.490	−.510	.510
1.8	1	1	25	23	1.042	.958	−.042	.042
2.2	1	0	24	22	.522	.478	.478	−.478
2.4.	0	1	23	22	.511	.489	−.511	.511
2.5.	1	0	23	21	.523	.477	.477	−.477
2.6	1	0	22	21	.516	.484	.484	−.484

(Continued on next page)

$t_{(j)}$	m_{1j}	m_{2j}	n_{1j}	n_{2j}	e_{1j}	e_{2j}	$m_{1j}-e_{1j}$	$m_{2j}-e_{2j}$
2.8	0	1	21	21	.500	.500	−.500	.500
2.9	0	1	21	20	.512	.488	−.512	.512
3.0	1	0	21	19	.525	.475	.475	−.475
3.1	0	1	20	19	.513	.487	−.513	.513
3.5	1	1	20	18	1.053	.947	−.053	.053
3.6	0	1	19	17	.528	.472	−.528	.528
3.8	1	0	19	16	.543	.457	.457	−.457
3.9	0	1	18	16	.529	.471	−.529	.529
4.1	0	1	18	15	.545	.455	−.545	.545
4.2	0	1	18	14	.563	.437	−.563	.563
4.7	0	1	18	13	.581	.419	−.581	.581
4.9	0	1	18	12	.600	.400	−.600	.600
5.2	0	1	18	11	.621	.379	−.621	.621
5.3	1	0	18	10	.643	.357	.357	−.357
5.4	1	0	17	10	.630	.370	.370	−.370
5.7	1	0	16	10	.615	.385	.385	−.385
5.8	0	1	15	10	.600	.400	−.600	.600
5.9	0	1	15	9	.625	.375	−.625	.625
6.5	0	1	15	8	.652	.348	−.652	.652
6.6	1	0	15	7	.682	.318	.318	−.318
7.8	0	1	14	7	.667	.333	−.667	.667
8.2	1	0	14	6	.700	.300	.300	−.300
8.3	0	1	13	6	.684	.316	−.684	.684
8.4	0	1	13	5	.722	.278	−.722	.722
8.7	1	0	13	4	.765	.235	.335	−.335
8.8	0	1	12	4	.750	.250	−.750	.750
9.1	0	1	12	3	.800	.200	−.800	.800
9.2	2	0	12	2	1.714	.286	.286	−.286
9.8	1	0	10	2	.833	.167	.167	−.167
9.9	0	1	9	2	.818	.182	−.818	.818
10.0	1	0	9	1	.900	.100	.100	−.100
10.2	1	0	8	1	.888	.112	.112	−.112
10.7	1	0	7	1	.875	.125	.125	−.125
11.0	1	0	6	1	.857	.143	.143	−.143
11.1	1	0	5	1	.833	.167	.167	−.167
11.4	0	1	4	1	.800	.200	−.800	.800
11.7	1	0	4	0	1.000	.000	.000	.000
Totals	22	25			30.79	16.21	−8.690	8.690

d. The log–rank statistic can be computed from the totals of the expanded table using the formulae:

$$\text{log-rank statistic} = \frac{(O_i - E_i)^2}{\widehat{\text{Var}}(O_i - E_i)}$$

$$\text{Var}(O_i - E_i) = \sum_j \frac{n_{1j} n_{2j}(m_{1j} + m_{2j})(n_{1j} + n_{2j} - m_{1j} - m_{2j})}{(n_{1j} + n_{2j})^2(n_{1j} + n_{2j} - 1)}$$

The variance turns out to be 9.448, so that the log–rank statistic is $(8.69)^2/9.448 = 7.993$.

Using SPIDA, the results for the log–rnak and Peto tests are given as follows:

Group	Size	%Cen	LQ	Median	UQ	0.95	Med CI
1	25	12.000	3.8	8.700	10.7	5.300	10.0
2	25	0.000	3.1	4.700	7.8	3.500	5.9

df: 1, log–rank: 7.993, P-value: 0.005, Peto: 3.516, P-value: 0.061.

The log–rank test gives highly significant results, whereas the Peto test is almost significant at the .05 level. These results indicate that there is a significant difference in survival between the two groups.

2. a. For the Anderson dataset, the KM plots for the three categories of log WBC are shown below:

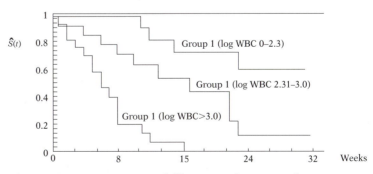

  b. The KM curves are quite different with group 1 having consistently better survival prognosis than group 2, and group 2 having consistently better survival prognosis than group 3. Note also that the difference between group 1 and 2 is about the same over time, whereas group 2 appears to diverge from group 3 as time increases.

  c. Both the log–rank statistic (26.391) and the Peto statistic (16.067) are highly significant with P-values equal to zero to three decimal places. Because there are three groups being compared, each statistic is approximately chi-square with two degrees of freedom under the null hypothesis that all three groups have a common survival curve.

Appendix: Matrix Formula for the Log–Rank Statistic for Several Groups

For $i=1, 2, \ldots, G$ and $j=1, 2, \ldots, k$, where $G=$ # of groups and $k=$ # of distinct failure times,

$n_{ij} =$ # at risk in ith group at jth ordered failure time

$m_{ij} =$ observed # of failures in ith group at jth ordered failure time

$e_{ij} =$ expected # of failures in ith group at jth ordered failure time

$$= \left(\frac{n_{ij}}{n_{1j} + n_{2j}} \right) (m_{1j} + m_{2j})$$

$$n_j = \sum_{i=1}^{G} n_{ij}$$

$$m_j = \sum_{i=1}^{G} m_{ij}$$

$$O_i - E_i = \sum_{j=1}^{k} (m_{ij} - e_{ij})$$

$$\widehat{\text{Var}}(O_i - E_i) = \sum_{j=1}^{k} \frac{n_{ij}(n_j - n_{ij}) m_j (n_j - m_j)}{n_j^2 (n_j - 1)}$$

$$\widehat{\text{Cov}}(O_i - E_i, O_l - E_l) = \sum_{j=1}^{k} \frac{-n_{ij} n_{lj} m_j (n_j - m_j)}{n_j^2 (n_j - 1)}$$

$$\mathbf{d} = (O_1 - E_1, O_2 - E_2, \ldots, O_{G-1} - E_{G-1})'$$

$$\mathbf{V} = ((v_{il}))'$$

where $v_{ii} = \widehat{\text{Var}}(O_i - E_i)$ and $v_{il} = \widehat{\text{Cov}}(O_i - E_i, O_l - E_l)$ for $i = 1, 2, \ldots, G-1$; $l = 1, 2, \ldots, G-1$.

Then, the log–rank statistic is given by the matrix product formula:

$$\boxed{\text{Log–rank statistic} = \mathbf{d}' \mathbf{V}^{-1} \mathbf{d}}$$

which has approximately a chi-square distribution with $G-1$ degrees of freedom under the null hypothesis that all G groups have a common survival curve.

3

The Cox Proportional Hazards Model and Its Characteristics

Introduction

We begin by discussing some computer results using the Cox PH model, without actually specifying the model; the purpose here is to show the similarity between the Cox model and standard linear regression or logistic regression.

We then introduce the Cox model and describe why it is so popular. In addition, we describe its basic properties, including the meaning of the proportional hazards assumption.

Abbreviated Outline

The outline below gives the user a preview of the material to be covered by the presentation. A detailed outline for review purposes follows the presentation.

Objectives   Upon completing the module, the learner should be able to:

1. State or recognize the general form of the Cox PH model.
2. State the specific form of a Cox PH model appropriate for the analysis, given a survival analysis scenario involving one or more explanatory variables.
3. State or recognize the form and properties of the baseline hazard function in the Cox PH model.
4. Give three reasons for the popularity of the Cox PH model.
5. State the formula for a designated hazard ratio of interest given a scenario describing a survival analysis using a Cox PH model, when
   a. there are confounders but no interaction terms in the model;
   b. there are both confounders and interaction terms in the model.
6. State or recognize the meaning of the PH assumption.
7. Determine and explain whether the PH assumption is satisfied when the graphs of the hazard functions for two groups cross each other over time.
8. State or recognize what is an adjusted survival curve.
9. Compare and/or interpret two or more adjusted survival curves.
10. Given a computer printout involving one or more fitted Cox PH models,
    a. compute or identify any hazard ratio(s) of interest;
    b. carry out and interpret a designated test of hypothesis;
    c. carry out, identify or interpret a confidence interval for a designated hazard ratio;
    d. evaluate interaction and confounding involving one or more covariates.

Presentation

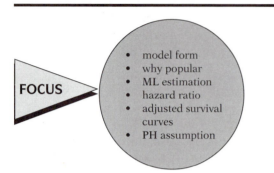

- model form
- why popular
- ML estimation
- hazard ratio
- adjusted survival curves
- PH assumption

FOCUS

This presentation describes the **Cox proportional hazards (PH) model,** a popular mathematical model used for analyzing survival data. Here, we focus on the model form, why the model is popular, maximum likelihood (ML) estimation of the model parameters, the formula for the hazard ratio, how to obtain adjusted survival curves, and the meaning of the PH assumption.

I. A Computer Example Using the Cox PH Model

We introduce the Cox PH model using computer output from the analysis of remission time data (Freireich et al., *Blood*, 1963), which we previously discussed in Chapters 1 and 2. The data set is listed here at the left.

EXAMPLE

Leukemia Remission Data

Group 1($n = 21$)		Group 2($n = 21$)	
t(weeks)	log WBC	t(weeks)	log WBC
6	2.31	1	2.80
6	4.06	1	5.00
6	3.28	2	4.91
7	4.43	2	4.48
10	2.96	3	4.01
13	2.88	4	4.36
16	3.60	4	2.42
22	2.32	5	3.49
23	2.57	5	3.97
6+	3.20	8	3.52
9+	2.80	8	3.05
10+	2.70	8	2.32
11+	2.60	8	3.26
17+	2.16	11	3.49
19+	2.05	11	2.12
20+	2.01	12	1.50
25+	1.78	12	3.06
32+	2.20	15	2.30
32+	2.53	17	2.95
34+	1.47	22	2.73
35+	1.45	23	1.97

+ denotes censored observation

These data involve two groups of leukemia patients, with 21 patients in each group. Group 1 is the treatment group, and group 2 is the placebo group. The data set also contains the variable log WBC, which is a well-known prognostic indicator of survival for leukemia patients.

For this example, the basic question of interest concerns comparing the survival experience of the two groups adjusting for the possible confounding and/or interaction effects of log WBC.

EXAMPLE (continued)

T = weeks until going out of remission
X_1 = group status = E
X_2 = log WBC (confounding?)

Interaction?
$X_3 = X_1 \times X_2$ = group status × log WBC

Computer results for three Cox PH models using the SPIDA package

Other computer packages provide similar information.

Appendix A: uses SPIDA, SAS, and BMDP on the same dataset.

We are thus considering a problem involving two explanatory variables as predictors of survival time T, where T denotes "weeks until going out of remission." We label the explanatory variables X_1 (for group status) and X_2 (for log WBC). The variable X_1 is the primary study or exposure variable of interest. The variable X_2 is an extraneous variable that we are including as a possible confounder or effect modifier.

Note that if we want to evaluate the possible interaction effect of log WBC on group status, we would also need to consider a third variable, that is, the product of X_1 and X_2.

For this dataset, the computer results from fitting three different Cox proportional hazards models are presented below. The computer package used is **SPIDA.** This is one of several packages that have procedures for carrying out a survival analysis using the Cox model. The information printed out by different packages will not have exactly the same format, but they will provide similar information. A comparison of output using SPIDA, SAS, and BMDP procedures on the same dataset is provided in Appendix A at the back of this text.

Output from Spida

Model 1:

Column name	Coeff	StErr	p-value	HR	0.95	CI	P(PH)
Rx	1.509	0.410	0	4.523	2.027	10.094	0.794
n:42	%Cen: 28.571		−2 log L: 172.759				

Model 2:

Column name	Coeff	StErr	p-value	HR	0.95	CI	P(PH)
Rx	1.294	0.422	0.002	3.648	1.505	8.343	0.944
log WBC	1.604	0.329	0.000	4.975	2.609	9.486	0.917
n:42	%Cen: 28.571		−2 log L: 144.559				

Model 3:

Column name	Coeff	StErr	p-value	HR	0.95	CI	P(PH)
Rx	2.355	1.681	0.161	10.537	0.391	284.200	0.628
log WBC	1.803	0.447	0.000	6.067	2.528	14.561	0.996
Rx × log WBC	−0.342	0.520	0.510	0.710	0.256	1.967	0.410
n:42	%Cen: 28.571		−2 log L: 144.131				

OUTPUT FROM SPIDA

Model 1:

Column name	Coeff	StErr	p-value	HR
Rx	1.509	0.410	0	4.523
n:42	%Cen: 28.571	−2 log L: 172.759		

Model 2:   **Hazard ratios**

Column name	Coeff	StErr	p-value	HR
Rx	1.294	0.422	0.002	3.648
log WBC	1.604	0.329	0.000	4.975
n:42	%Cen: 28.571	−2 log L: 144.559		

Model 3:

Column name	Coeff	StErr	p-value	HR
Rx	2.355	1.681	0.161	10.537
log WBC	1.803	0.447	0.000	6.067
Rx × log WBC	−0.342	0.520	0.510	0.710
n:42	%Cen: 28.571	−2 log L: 144.131		

EXAMPLE (continued)

Same dataset for each model
$n = 42$ subjects
T = time (weeks) until out of remission

Model 1: Rx only

Model 2: Rx and log WBC

Model 3: Rx, log WBC, and
         Rx × log WBC

We now describe how to use the computer printout to evaluate the possible effect of treatment status on remission time adjusted for the potential confounding and interaction effects of the covariate log WBC. For now, we focus only on the first five columns of information provided in the printout, as presented at the left for all three models.

For each model, the first column identifies the **variables** that have been included in the model. The second column gives **regression coefficients** corresponding to each variable in the model. The third column gives **standard errors** of the regression coefficients. The fourth column gives **p-values** for testing the significance of each coefficient. The fifth column, labeled as *HR*, gives **hazard ratios** for the effect of each variable adjusted for the other variables in the model.

Except for the *HR* column, these computer results are typical of output found in standard linear regression printouts. As the printout suggests, we can analyze the results from a Cox model in a manner similar to the way we would analyze a linear regression model.

We now distinguish among the output for the three models shown here. All three models are using the same set of remission time data on 42 subjects. The outcome variable for each model is the same—time in weeks until a subject goes out of remission. However, the independent variables are different for each model. Model 1 contains only the treatment status variable, indicating whether a subject is in the treatment or placebo group. Model 2 contains two variables—treatment status and log WBC. And model 3 contains an interaction term defined as the product of group status and log WBC.

OUTPUT: ML ESTIMATION

Model 3:

Column name	Coeff	StErr	p-value	HR
Rx	2.355	1.681	0.161	10.537
log WBC	1.803	0.447	0.000	6.067
Rx× log WBC	−0.342	0.520	(0.510)	0.710

n:42	%Cen: 28.571	−2 log L: 144.131

EXAMPLE (continued)

$$P = 0.510: \frac{-0.342}{0.520} = -0.66 = Z \qquad \text{Wald statistic}$$

LR statistic: uses $-2 \log L = 144.131$

(i.e., log likelihood value)

OUTPUT

Model 2:

Column name	Coeff	StErr	p-value	HR
Rx	1.294	0.422	0.002	3.648
log WBC	1.604	0.329	0.000	4.975

n:42	%Cen: 28.571	−2 log L: 144.559

EXAMPLE (continued)

LR (interaction in model 3)

$= -2 \log L_{\text{model 2}} - (-2 \log L_{\text{model 3}})$

$= 144.559 - 144.131 = 0.428$

(LR is χ^2 with 1 d.f. under H_0:
 no interaction.)

$0.40 < P < 0.50$, **not significant**

Wald test $P = 0.510$

We now focus on the output for model 3. The method of estimation used to obtain the coefficients for this model, as well as the other two models, is maximum likelihood (ML) estimation. Note that a p-value of 0.510 is obtained for the coefficient of the product term for the interaction of treatment with log WBC. This p-value indicates that there is no significant interaction effect, so that we can drop the product term from the model and consider the other two models instead.

two-tailed test

The p-value of 0.510 that we have just described is obtained by dividing the coefficient –0.342 of the product term by its standard error of 0.520, which gives –0.66, and then assuming that this quantity is approximately a standard normal or Z variable. This Z statistic is known as a **Wald statistic,** which is one of two test statistics typically used with ML estimates. The other test statistic, called the **likelihood ratio,** or LR statistic, makes use of the log likelihood value. This is given by $-2 \log L$ in the output, which has the value 144.131 for model 3.

We now look at the printout for model 2, which contains two variables. The treatment status variable *(Rx)* represents the exposure variable of primary interest. The log WBC variable is being considered as a confounder. Our goal is to describe the effect of treatment status adjusted for log WBC.

Notice first that the log likelihood value for model 2 is given by $-2 \log L = 144.559$. We can use this value together with the $-2 \log L$ value from model 3 to obtain the LR statistic for testing the significance of the interaction term in model 3.

We compute 144.559 minus 144.131 to obtain 0.428. This test statistic has a chi-square distribution under the null hypothesis of no interaction effect. The p-value for this test is between 0.40 and 0.50, which indicates no significant interaction. Although the p-values for the Wald test (0.510) and the LR test are not exactly the same, both p-values lead to the same conclusion.

−2 log L must measure change

LR ≠ Wald

When in doubt, use the LR test.

In general, the LR and Wald statistics may not give exactly the same answer. Statisticians have shown that of the two test procedures, the LR statistic has better statistical properties, so when in doubt, you should use the LR test.

We now focus on how to assess the effect of treatment status adjusting for log WBC using the model 2 output, again shown here.

OUTPUT

Model 2:

Column name	Coeff	StErr	p-value	HR
Rx	1.294	0.422	0.002	3.648
log WBC	1.604	0.329	0.000	4.975

n:42   %Cen: 28.571 $-2 \log L$: 144.559

Three statistical objectives:
1. **test for significance of effect**
2. **point estimate of effect**
3. **confidence interval for effect**

There are three statistical objectives typically considered. One is to **test for the significance** of the treatment status variable, adjusted for log WBC. Another is to obtain a **point estimate of the effect** of treatment status, adjusted for log WBC. And a third is to obtain a **confidence interval for this effect.** We can accomplish these three objectives using the output provided, without having to explicitly describe the formula for the Cox model being used.

EXAMPLE (continued)

Test for treatment effect:
Wald statistic: $P = 0.002$ (highly significant)
LR statistic: compare
    $-2 \log L$ from model 2 with
    $-2 \log L$ from model without Rx
        variable
            Printout not provided here

Conclusion: treatment effect is significant, after adjusting for log WBC

Point estimate:
$$\widehat{HR} = 3.648$$
$$= e^{1.294}$$

Coefficient of treatment variable

To test for the significance of the treatment effect, the p-value provided in the table for the Wald statistic is 0.002, which is highly significant. Alternatively, a likelihood ratio (LR) test could be performed comparing the log likelihood statistic (144.559) for model 2, with the log likelihood for a model which does not contain the treatment variable. This latter model, which should contain only the log WBC variable, is not provided here, so we will not report on it other than to note that the LR test is also very significant. Thus, these test results show that using model 2, the treatment effect is significant, after adjusting for log WBC.

A point estimate of the effect of the treatment is provided in the *HR* column by the value 3.648. This value gives the estimated hazard ratio (HR) for the effect of the treatment; in particular, we see that the hazard for the placebo group is 3.6 times the hazard for the treatment group. Note that the value 3.648 is calculated as e to the coefficient of the treatment variable; that is, e to the 1.294 equals 3.648.

To describe the confidence interval for the effect of treatment status, we consider the output for the extended table for model 2 given earlier.

OUTPUT

Model 2:

Column name	Coeff	StErr	p-value	HR	0.95	CI	P(PH)
Rx	1.294	0.422	0.002	3.648	1.505	8.343	0.944
log WBC	1.604	0.329	0.000	4.975	2.609	9.486	0.917
n:42		%Cen: 28.571		−2 log L: 144.559			

EXAMPLE (continued)

95% confidence interval for the *HR*: (1.505, 8.343)

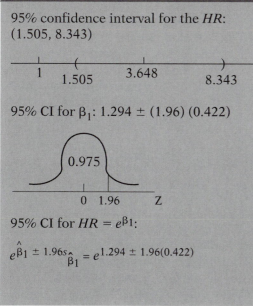

95% CI for β_1: $1.294 \pm (1.96)(0.422)$

95% CI for $HR = e^{\beta_1}$:

$$e^{\hat{\beta}_1 \pm 1.96 s_{\hat{\beta}_1}} = e^{1.294 \pm 1.96(0.422)}$$

SPIDA: provides CI directly

Other packages: provide $\hat{\beta}$'s and $s_{\hat{\beta}}$'s

From the table, we see that a 95% confidence interval for the treatment effect is given by the range of values 1.505–8.343. This is a confidence interval for the hazard ratio (HR), which surrounds the point estimate of 3.648 previously described. Notice that this confidence interval is fairly wide, indicating that the point estimate is somewhat unreliable. As expected from the low p-value of 0.002, the confidence interval for HR does not contain the null value of 1.

The calculation of the confidence interval for HR is carried out as follows:

1. Compute a 95% confidence interval for the regression coefficient of the *Rx* variable ($\hat{\beta}_1$). The large sample formula is 1.294 plus or minus 1.96 times the standard error 0.422, where 1.96 is the 97.5 percentile of the standard normal or *Z* distribution.

2. Exponentiate the two limits obtained for the confidence interval for the regression coefficient of *Rx*.

The SPIDA program output provides the required confidence interval directly, so that the user does not have to carry out the computations required by the large sample formula. Other computer packages may not provide the confidence interval directly, but, rather, may provide only the regression coefficients and their standard errors.

OUTPUT

Model 1:

Column name	Coeff	StErr	p-value	HR
Rx (crude model)	1.509	0.410	0	4.523

n:42   %Cen: 28.571 $-2 \log L$: 172.759

Model 2:

Column name	Coeff	StErr	p-value	HR
Rx	1.294	0.422	0.002	3.648
log WBC	1.604	0.329	0.000	4.975

n:42   %Cen: 28.571 $-2 \log L$: 144.559

EXAMPLE (continued)

HR for model 1 (4.523) is higher than HR for model 2 (3.648).

Confounding: crude versus adjusted $\widehat{HR}$'s are meaningfully different.

Confounding due to log WBC
$\Rightarrow$ must control for log WBC, i.e., prefer model 2 to model 1.

If no confounding, then consider precision: e.g., if 95% CI is narrower for model 2 than model 1, we prefer model 2.

OUTPUT: Confidence Intervals

Column name ...	0.95	CI
Rx model 1	2.027	10.094
	width = **8.067**	
	width = **6.838**	
Rx model 2	1.505	8.343
log WBC	2.609	9.486

To this point, we have made use of information from outputs for models 2 and 3, but have not yet considered the model 1 output, which is shown again here. Note that model 1 contains only the treatment status variable, whereas model 2, shown below, contains log WBC in addition to treatment status. Model 1 is sometimes called the "crude" model because it ignores the effect of potential covariates of interest, like log WBC.

Model 1 can be used in comparison with model 2 to evaluate the potential confounding effect of the variable log WBC. In particular, notice that the value in the HR column for the treatment status variable is 4.523 for model 1, but only 3.648 for model 2. Thus, the crude model yields an estimated hazard ratio that is somewhat higher than the corresponding estimate obtained when we adjust for log WBC. If we decide that the crude and adjusted estimates are meaningfully different, we then say that there is confounding due to log WBC.

Once we decide that confounding is present, we then **must** control for the confounder—in this case, log WBC—in order to obtain a valid estimate of the effect. Thus, we prefer model 2, which controls for log WBC, to model 1, which does not.

Note that if we had decided that there is no "meaningful" confounding, then we would not need to control for log WBC to get a valid answer. Nevertheless, we might wish to control for log WBC anyhow, to obtain a more precise estimate of the hazard ratio. That is, if the confidence interval for the HR is narrower when using model 2 than when using model 1, we would prefer model 2 to model 1 for **precision** gain.

The confidence intervals for Rx in each model are shown here at the left. The interval for Rx in model 1 has width equal to 10.094 minus 2.027, or **8.067**; for model 2, the width is 8.343 minus 1.505, or **6.838**. Therefore, model 2 gives a more precise estimate of the hazard ratio than does model 1.

EXAMPLE (continued)

Model 2 is best model.

$\widehat{HR} = 3.648$ statistically significant

95% CI for HR: (1.5, 8.3)

Our analysis of the output for the three models has led us to conclude that model 2 is the best of the three models and that, using model 2, we get a statistically significant hazard ratio of 3.648 for the effect of the treatment, with a 95% confidence interval ranging between 1.5 and 8.3.

Cox model formulae not specified

Analysis strategy and methods for Cox model analogous to those for logistic and classical linear models.

Note that we were able to carry out this analysis without actually specifying the formulae for the Cox PH models being fit. Also, the strategy and methods used with the output provided have been completely analogous to the strategy and methods one uses when fitting logistic regression models (see Kleinbaum, *Logistic Regression*, Chapters 6 and 7, 1994), and very similar to carrying out a classical linear regression analysis (see Kleinbaum et al., *Applied Regression Analysis*, 2d ed., Chapter 16, 1987).

EXAMPLE (continued)

Survival Curves Adjusted for log WBC (Model 2)

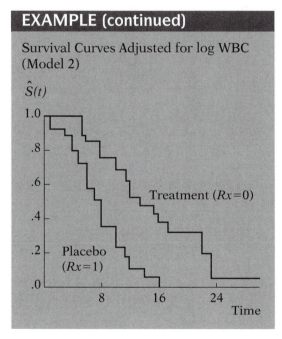

In addition to the above analysis of this data, we can also obtain survival curves for each treatment group, **adjusted** for the effects of log WBC and based on the model 2 output. Such curves, sketched here at the left, give additional information to that provided by estimates and tests about the hazard ratio. In particular, these curves describe how the treatment groups compare over the time period of the study.

For these data, the survival curves show that the treatment group consistently has higher survival probabilities than the placebo group after adjusting for log WBC. Moreover, the difference between the two groups appears to widen over time.

Adjusted survival curves	KM curves
Adjusted for covariates Use fitted Cox model	No covariates No Cox model fitted

Note that adjusted survival curves are mathematically different from Kaplan–Meier (KM) curves. KM curves do not adjust for covariates and, therefore, are not computed using results from a fitted Cox PH model.

EXAMPLE (continued)

For these data, KM and adjusted survival plots have similar appearance.

Nevertheless, for these data, the plotted KM curves (which were described in Chapter 2) are similar in appearance to the adjusted survival curves.

P(PH) OUTPUT

Model 2:

Column name ...	P(PH)
Rx	0.944
log WBC	0.917

Before concluding this section, we point out one other piece of information provided in the output that we have not mentioned until now. We refer to the *P(PH)* values provided in the last column of the printout, as shown here for model 2.

P(PH): gives p-value for evaluating PH assumption for each variable in model; derived from $N(0,1)$ statistic

The *P(PH)* information allows one to evaluate the proportional hazards (PH) assumption. The value given is a p-value derived from a standard normal statistic computed from the model output. A nonsignificant (i.e., large) p-value, say greater than 0.10, indicates that the PH assumption is satisfied, whereas a small p-value, say less than 0.05, indicates that the variable being tested does not satisfy this assumption. We discuss the PH assumption in more detail later in this presentation.

$$\begin{array}{l} P(PH) \text{ large} \\ \text{(e.g., } P > 0.10) \end{array} \Rightarrow PH \text{ satisfied}$$

$$\begin{array}{l} P(PH) \text{ small} \\ \text{(e.g., } P < 0.05) \end{array} \Rightarrow PH \text{ not satisfied}$$

EXAMPLE (continued)

Model 2:
P(PH) nonsignificant for both variables, i.e., PH is satisfied

The *P(PH)* output for model 2 yields nonsignificant p-values for both variables, thus indicating that the PH assumption is satisfied for both variables.

Three approaches for evaluating PH (Chapter 4)

Procedures when PH not satisfied (Chapters 5 and 6)

The *P(PH)* information provides one of three approaches for evaluating the PH assumption. All three approaches will be discussed and compared in Chapter 4. In addition, Chapters 5 and 6 describe procedures to use when the PH assumption is not satisfied.

Remainder:
• Cox model formula
• basic characteristics of Cox model
• meaning of PH assumption

In the remainder of this presentation, we describe the Cox PH formula and its basic characteristics, including what is the meaning of the PH assumption.

II. The Formula for the Cox PH Model

$$h(t, \mathbf{X}) = h_0(t) \, e^{\sum_{i=1}^{p} \beta_i X_i}$$

$$\mathbf{X} = (X_1, X_2, \ldots, X_p)$$
explanatory/predictor variables

The Cox PH model is usually written in terms of the hazard model formula shown here at the left. This model gives an expression for the hazard at time t for an individual with a given specification of a set of explanatory variables denoted by the bold **X**. That is, the bold **X** represents a collection (sometimes called a "vector") of predictor variables that is being modeled to predict an individual's hazard.

$$\underbrace{h_0(t)}_{\substack{\text{Baseline hazard} \\ \text{Involves } t \text{ but} \\ \text{not } X\text{'s}}} \times \underbrace{e^{\sum\limits_{i=1}^{p} \beta_i X_i}}_{\substack{\text{Exponential} \\ \text{Involves } X\text{'s but} \\ \text{not } t \ (X\text{'s are time-} \\ \text{independent)}}}$$

The Cox model formula says that the hazard at time t is the product of two quantities. The first of these, $h_0(t)$, is called the **baseline hazard** function. The second quantity is the exponential expression e to the linear sum of $\beta_i X_i$, where the sum is over the p explanatory X variables.

An important feature of this formula, which concerns the proportional hazards *(PH)* assumption, is that the baseline hazard is a function of t, but does not involve the X's. In contrast, the exponential expression shown here, involves the X's, but does not involve t. The X's here are called **time-independent** X's.

X's involving t: time-dependent

Requires extended Cox model (no PH)

It is possible, nevertheless, to consider X's which do involve t. Such X's are called **time-dependent** variables. If time-dependent variables are considered, the Cox model form may still be used, but such a model no longer satisfies the PH assumption, and is called the **extended Cox model.**

Time-dependent variables: Chapter 6

The use of time-dependent variables is discussed in Chapter 6. For the remainder of this presentation, we will consider time-independent X's only.

Time-independent variable:
Values for a given individual do not change over time; e.g., SEX and SMK

Assumed not to change
once measured

A time-independent variable is defined to be any variable whose values for a given individual do not change over time. Examples are SEX and smoking status (SMK). Note, however, that a person's smoking status may actually change over time, but for purposes of the analysis, the SMK variable is assumed not to change once it is measured, so that only one value per individual is used.

AGE and WGT values do not change much, or effect on survival depends on one measurement.

Also note that although variables like AGE and weight (WGT) change over time, it may be appropriate to treat such variables as time-independent in the analysis if their values do not change much over time or if the effect of such variables on survival risk depends essentially on the value at only one measurement.

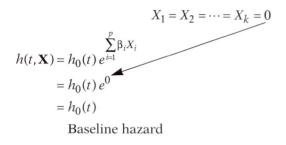

$$X_1 = X_2 = \cdots = X_k = 0$$

$$h(t, \mathbf{X}) = h_0(t)\, e^{\sum_{i=1}^{p} \beta_i X_i}$$

$$= h_0(t)\, e^0$$

$$= h_0(t)$$

Baseline hazard

No X's in model: $h(t, \mathbf{X}) = h_0(t)$.

$h_0(t)$ is unspecified.

Cox model: **nonparametric**

The Cox model formula has the property that if all the X's are equal to zero, the formula reduces to the baseline hazard function. That is, the exponential part of the formula becomes e to the zero, which is 1. This property of the Cox model is the reason why $h_0(t)$ is called the baseline function.

Or, from a slightly different perspective, the Cox model reduces to the baseline hazard when no X's are in the model. Thus, $h_0(t)$ may be considered as a starting or "baseline" version of the hazard function, prior to considering any of the X's.

Another important property of the Cox model is that the baseline hazard, $h_0(t)$, is an unspecified function. It is this property that makes the Cox model a **nonparametric** model.

EXAMPLE: Parametric Model

Weibull:

$$h(t, \mathbf{X}) = \lambda t^{\alpha-1}\, e^{\sum_{i=1}^{p} \beta_i X_i}$$

where $h_0(t) = \lambda t^{\alpha-1}$.

Nonparametric property
⇓
Popularity of the Cox model

In contrast, a **parametric** model is one whose functional form is completely specified, except for the values of the unknown parameters. For example, the Weibull hazard model is a parametric model and has the form shown here, where the unknown parameters are λ, α, and the β_i's. Note that for the Weibull model, $h_0(t)$ is given by $\lambda t^{\alpha-1}$.

One of the reasons why the Cox model is so popular is that it is nonparametric. We discuss this and other reasons in the next section (III) concerning why the Cox model is so widely used.

III. Why the Cox PH Model Is Popular

Cox PH model is "robust":
Will closely approximate correct parametric model

A key reason for the popularity of the Cox model is that, even though the baseline hazard is not specified, reasonably good estimates of regression coefficients, hazard ratios of interest, and adjusted survival curves can be obtained for a wide variety of data situations. Another way of saying this is that the Cox PH model is a "robust" model, so that the results from using the Cox model will closely approximate the results for the correct parametric model.

If correct model is:

$$\text{Weibull} \Rightarrow \begin{array}{l} \text{Cox model will} \\ \text{approximate Weibull} \end{array}$$

$$\text{Exponential} \Rightarrow \begin{array}{l} \text{Cox model will} \\ \text{approximate exponential} \end{array}$$

Prefer parametric model if sure of correct model, e.g., use goodness-of-fit test (Lee, 1982).

When in doubt, the Cox model is a "safe" choice.

$$h(t,\mathbf{X}) = \underbrace{h_0(t)}_{\begin{array}{c}\text{Baseline} \\ \text{hazard}\end{array}} \times \underbrace{e^{\sum\limits_{i=1}^{p} \beta_i X_i}}_{\begin{array}{c}\text{Exponential} \\ \Downarrow\end{array}}$$

$0 \le h(t,\mathbf{X}) < \infty$ always

$$h_0(t) \times \underbrace{\sum_{i=1}^{k} \beta_i X_i}_{\begin{array}{c}\text{Linear} \\ \Downarrow \\ \text{Might be} < 0\end{array}}$$

For example, if the correct parametric model is Weibull, then use of the Cox model typically will give results comparable to those obtained using a Weibull model. Or, if the correct model is exponential, then the Cox model results will closely approximate the results from fitting an exponential model.

We would prefer to use a parametric model if we were sure of the correct model. Although there are various methods for assessing goodness of fit of a parametric model (for example, see Lee, *Statistical Methods for Survival Data Analysis*, 1982), we may not be completely certain that a given parametric model is appropriate.

Thus, when in doubt, as is typically the case, the Cox model will give reliable enough results so that it is a "safe" choice of model, and the user does not need to worry about whether the wrong parametric model is chosen.

In addition to the general "robustness" of the Cox model, the specific form of the model is attractive for several reasons.

As described previously, the specific form of the Cox model gives the hazard function as a product of a baseline hazard involving t and an exponential expression involving the X's without t. The exponential part of this product is appealing because it ensures that the fitted model will always give estimated hazards that are nonnegative.

We want such nonnegative estimates because, by definition, the values of any hazard function must range between zero and plus infinity, that is, a hazard is always nonnegative. If, instead of an exponential expression, the X part of the model were, for example, linear in the X's, we might obtain negative hazard estimates, which are not allowed.

Even though $h_0(t)$ is unspecified, we can estimate the β's.

Measure of effect: hazard ratio (HR) involves only β's, without estimating $h_0(t)$.

Another appealing property of the Cox model is that, even though the baseline hazard part of the model is unspecified, it is still possible to estimate the β's in the exponential part of the model. As we will show later, all we need are estimates of the β's to assess the effect of explanatory variables of interest. The measure of effect, which is called a hazard ratio, is calculated without having to estimate the baseline hazard function.

Can estimate $h(t,\mathbf{X})$ and $S(t,\mathbf{X})$ for Cox model using a minimum of assumptions.

Note that the hazard function $h(t,\mathbf{X})$ and its corresponding survival curves $S(t,X)$ can be estimated for the Cox model even though the baseline hazard function is not specified. Thus, with the Cox model, using a minimum of assumptions, we can obtain the primary information desired from a survival analysis, namely, a hazard ratio and a survival curve.

Cox model preferred to **logistic** model.
⇓   ⇓

| Uses survival times and censoring | Uses (0,1) outcome; ignores survival times and censoring |

One last point about the popularity of the Cox model is that it is preferred over the logistic model when survival time information is available and there is censoring. That is, the Cox model uses more information—the survival times—than the logistic model, which considers a (0,1) outcome and ignores survival times and censoring.

IV. ML Estimation of the Cox PH Model

$$h(t,\mathbf{X}) = h_0(t)\, e^{\sum_{i=1}^{p} \beta_i X_i}$$

ML estimates: $\hat{\beta}_i$

Column name	Coeff	StErr	p-value	HR
Rx	1.294	0.422	0.002	3.648
log WBC	1.604	0.329	0.000	4.975
n:42		%Cen: 28.571		$-2 \log L$: 144.559

Model 2:
$$h(t,\mathbf{X}) = h_0(t)e^{\beta_1 Rx + \beta_2 \log WBC}$$

Estimated model:
$$\hat{h}(t,\mathbf{X}) = \hat{h}_0(t)e^{1.294Rx + 1.604 \log WBC}$$

We now describe how estimates are obtained for the parameters of the Cox model. The parameters are the β's in the general Cox model formula shown here. The corresponding estimates of these parameters are called maximum likelihood (ML) estimates and are denoted as β_i "hat."

As an example of ML estimates, we consider once again the computer output for one of the models (model 2) fitted previously from remission data on 42 leukemia patients.

The Cox model for this example involves two parameters, one being the coefficient of the treatment variable (denoted here as Rx) and the other being the coefficient of the log WBC variable. The expression for this model is shown at the left, and below this formula we show the estimated model, which contains the estimated coefficients 1.294 for Rx and 1.604 for log white blood cell count.

ML estimates: maximize likelihood function L

L = joint probability of observed data
  = $L(\beta)$

As with logistic regression, the ML estimates of the Cox model parameters are derived by maximizing a likelihood function, usually denoted as L. The likelihood function is a mathematical expression which describes the joint probability of obtaining the data actually observed on the subjects in the study as a function of the unknown parameters (the β's) in the model being considered. L is sometimes written notationally as $L(\beta)$ where β denotes the collection of unknown parameters.

L is
- complicated mathematically
- formula built into computer program
- capable of obtaining estimates without seeing formula

We will **not** show you here the explicit mathematical expression for L for the Cox model. This expression is quite complicated mathematically; moreover, in practice, the formula for L is built into the computer program you will be using, so you never have to see it in order to obtain the ML estimates.

L is a partial likelihood:
- considers probabilities only for subjects who fail
- does not consider probabilities for subjects who are censored

The formula for the Cox model likelihood function is actually called a "partial" likelihood function rather than a (complete) likelihood function. The term "partial" likelihood is used because the likelihood formula considers probabilities only for those subjects who fail, and does not explicitly consider probabilities for those subjects who are censored. Thus the likelihood for the Cox model does not consider probabilities for all subjects, and so it is called a "partial" likelihood.

Number of failure times

$$L = L_1 \times L_2 \times L_3 \times \cdots \times L_k = \prod_{j=1}^{k} L_j$$

where

L_j = portion of L for the jth failure time given the risk set $R(t_{(j)})$

In particular, the partial likelihood can be written as the product of several likelihoods, one for each of, say, k failure times. Thus, at the jth failure time, L_j denotes the likelihood of failing at this time, given survival up to this time. Note that the set of individuals at risk at the jth failure time is called the "risk set," $R(t_{(j)})$, and this set will change—actually get smaller in size—as the failure time increases.

Information on censored subjects used prior to censorship.

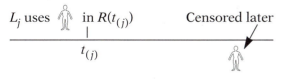

L_j uses ⚊ in $R(t_{(j)})$ Censored later

$t_{(j)}$

Thus, although the partial likelihood focuses on subjects who fail, survival time information prior to censorship is used for those subjects who are censored. That is, a person who is censored *after* the jth failure time is part of the risk set used to compute L_j, even though this person is censored later.

Steps for obtaining ML estimates:
- form L from model
- maximize $\ln L$ by solving

$$\frac{\partial L}{\partial \beta_i} = 0, \ i = 1, \ldots, p(\# \text{of parameters})$$

Once the likelihood function is formed for a given model, the next step for the computer is to maximize this function. This is generally done by maximizing the natural log of L, which is computationally easier.

Solution by iteration:
- guess at solution
- modify guess in successive steps
- stop when solution is obtained

The maximization process is carried out by taking partial derivatives of L with respect to each parameter in the model, and then solving a system of equations as shown here. This solution is carried out using **iteration.** That is, the solution is obtained in a stepwise manner, which starts with a guessed value for the solution, and then successively modifies the guessed value until a solution is finally obtained.

Statistical inferences for hazard ratios:
(See Section I, pages 84–92)

Test hypotheses	Confidence intervals
Wald test	Large sample 95% CI
LR test	

$\widehat{HR} = e^{\hat{\beta}}$ for a (0,1) exposure variable (no interaction)

Once the ML estimates are obtained, we are usually interested in carrying out statistical inferences about hazard ratios defined in terms of these estimates. We illustrated previously how to test hypotheses and form confidence intervals for the hazard ratio in Section I above. There, we described how to compute a Wald test and a likelihood ratio (LR) test. We also illustrated how to calculate a large sample 95% confidence interval for a hazard ratio. The estimated hazard ratio (HR) was computed by exponentiating the coefficient of a (0,1) exposure variable of interest. Note that the model contained no interaction terms involving exposure.

V. Computing the Hazard Ratio

$$\widehat{HR} = \frac{\hat{h}(t, \mathbf{X^*})}{\hat{h}(t, \mathbf{X})}$$

where

and $\begin{aligned} \mathbf{X^*} &= \left(X_1^*, X_2^*, \cdots, X_p^*\right) \\ \mathbf{X} &= \left(X_1, X_2, \cdots, X_p\right) \end{aligned}$

denote the set of X's for two individuals

In general, a hazard ratio (HR) is defined as the hazard for one individual divided by the hazard for a different individual. The two individuals being compared can be distinguished by their values for the set of predictors, that is, the X's.

We can write the hazard ratio as the estimate of $h(t, \mathbf{X^*})$ divided by the estimate of $h(t, \mathbf{X})$, where $\mathbf{X^*}$ denotes the set of predictors for one individual, and $\mathbf{X}$ denotes the set of predictors for the other individual.

To interpret $\widehat{HR}$, want $\widehat{HR} \geq 1$, i.e.,
$\hat{h}(t,\mathbf{X}^*) \geq \hat{h}(t,\mathbf{X})$.

Typical coding: $\mathbf{X}^*$: unexposed group
$\mathbf{X}$: exposed group

EXAMPLE: Remission Data

$\mathbf{X}^* = (X_1^* = 1, X_2^*,...,X_p^*)$, where $X_1^* = 1$
denotes **placebo** group.

$\mathbf{X} = (X_1 = 0, X_2,...,X_p)$, where $X_1 = 0$
denotes **treatment** group.

Note that, as with an odds ratio, it is easier to interpret an HR that exceeds the null value of 1 than an HR that is less than 1. Thus, the X's are typically coded so that the group with the larger hazard—typically an unexposed or placebo group—corresponds to $\mathbf{X}^*$, and the group with the smaller hazard corresponds to $\mathbf{X}$. As an example, for the remission data described previously, the placebo group is coded as $X_1^* = 1$, and the treatment group is coded as $X_1 = 0$.

$$\widehat{HR} = \frac{\hat{h}(t,\mathbf{X}^*)}{\hat{h}(t,\mathbf{X})} = \frac{\widehat{h_0(t)}\, e^{\sum_{i=1}^{p} \hat{\beta}_i X_i^*}}{\widehat{h_0(t)}\, e^{\sum_{i=1}^{p} \hat{\beta}_i X_i}}$$

We now obtain an expression for the HR formula in terms of the regression coefficients by substituting the Cox model formula into the numerator and denominator of the hazard ratio expression. This substitution is shown here. Notice that the only difference in the numerator and denominator are the X^*'s versus the X's. Notice also that the baseline hazards will cancel out.

$$\widehat{HR} = \frac{\hat{h}_0(t)\, e^{\sum_{i=1}^{p} \hat{\beta}_i X_i^*}}{\hat{h}_0(t)\, e^{\sum_{i=1}^{p} \hat{\beta}_i X_i}} = e^{\sum_{i=1}^{p} \hat{\beta}_i \left(X_i^* - X_i \right)}$$

Using algebra involving exponentials, the hazard ratio formula simplifies to the exponential expression shown here. Thus, the hazard ratio is computed by exponentiating the sum of each β_i "hat" times the difference between X_i^* and X_i.

$$\boxed{\widehat{HR} = \exp\left[\sum_{i=1}^{p} \hat{\beta}_i \left(X_i^* - X_i \right) \right]}$$

An alternative way to write this formula, using exponential notation, is shown here. We will now illustrate the use of this general formula through a few examples.

EXAMPLE

$\mathbf{X} = (X_1, X_2,...,X_p) = (X_1)$, where X_1
denotes $(0,1)$ exposure status $(p = 1)$

$X_1^* = 1, X_1 = 0$
$\widehat{HR} = \exp[\hat{\beta}_1(X_1^* - X_1)]$
$\quad = \exp[\hat{\beta}_1(1-0)] = e^{\hat{\beta}_1}$

Suppose, for example, there is only one X variable of interest, X_1, which denotes $(0,1)$ exposure status, so that $p = 1$. Then, the hazard ratio comparing exposed to unexposed persons is obtained by letting $X_1^* = 1$ and $X_1 = 0$ in the hazard ratio formula. The estimated hazard ratio then becomes e to the quantity β_1 "hat" times 1 minus 0, which simplifies to e to the β_1 "hat."

EXAMPLE (continued)

Model 1:

Column name	Coeff	StErr	p-value	HR
Rx	1.509	0.410	0	4.523

Recall the remission data printout for model 1, which contains only the *Rx* variable, again shown here. Then the estimated hazard ratio is obtained by exponentiating the coefficient 1.509, which gives the value 4.523 shown in the *HR* column of the output.

EXAMPLE 2

Model 2:

Column name	Coeff	StErr	p-value	RRisk
Rx	1.294	0.422	0.002	3.648
log WBC	1.604	0.329	0.000	4.975

$\mathbf{X}^* = (1, \log \text{WBC})$, $\mathbf{X} = (0, \log \text{WBC})$

HR for effect of *Rx* adjusted for log WBC:

$$\widehat{HR} = \exp[\hat{\beta}_1(X_1^* - X_1) + \hat{\beta}_2(X_2^* - X_2)]$$
$$= \exp[1.294(1-0)$$
$$+ 1.604 (\log \text{WBC} - \log \text{WBC})]$$
$$= \exp[1.294(1) + 1.604(0)] = e^{1.294}$$

As a second example, consider the output for model 2, which contains two variables, the *Rx* variable and log WBC. Then to obtain the hazard ratio for the effect of the *Rx* variable adjusted for the log WBC variable, we let the vectors $\mathbf{X}^*$ and $\mathbf{X}$ be defined as $\mathbf{X}^* = (1, \log \text{WBC})$ and $\mathbf{X} = (0, \log \text{WBC})$. Here we assume that log WBC is fixed, though unspecified.

The estimated hazard ratio is then obtained by exponentiating the sum of two quantities, one involving the coefficient 1.294 of the *Rx* variable, and the other involving the coefficient 1.604 of the log WBC variable. Since the log WBC value is fixed, however, this portion of the exponential is zero, so that the resulting estimate is simply *e* to the 1.294.

General rule: If X_1 is a (0,1) exposure variable, then

$$\widehat{HR} = e^{\hat{\beta}_1} \quad (= \text{effect of exposure adjusted for other } X\text{'s})$$

provided no other *X*'s are product terms involving exposure.

This second example illustrates the general rule that the hazard ratio for the effect of a (0,1) exposure variable which adjusts for other variables is obtained by exponentiating the estimated coefficient of the exposure variable. This rule has the proviso that the model does not contain any product terms involving exposure.

EXAMPLE 3

Model 3:

Column name	Coeff	StErr	p-value	RRisk
Rx	2.355	1.681	0.161	10.537
log WBC	1.803	0.447	0.000	6.067
Rx × log WBC	−0.342	0.520	0.510	0.710

We now give a third example which illustrates how to compute a hazard ratio when the model does contain product terms. We consider the printout for model 3 of the remission data shown here.

EXAMPLE 3 (continued)

Want *HR* for effect of *Rx* adjusted for log WBC.

Placebo subject:
$X^* = (X_1^* = 1, X_2^* = \log \text{WBC}, X_3^* = 1 \times \log \text{WBC})$

Treated subject:
$X = (X_1 = 0, X_2 = \log \text{WBC}, X_3 = 0 \times \log \text{WBC})$

$$\widehat{HR} = \exp\left[\sum_{i=1}^{3} \hat{\beta}_i \left(X_i^* - X_i \right) \right]$$

$\widehat{HR} = \exp[2.355(1 - 0)$
$\qquad + 1.803 \, (\log \text{WBC} - \log \text{WBC})$
$\qquad + (-0.342)(1 \times \log \text{WBC} -$
$\qquad 0 \times \log \text{WBC})]$

$\boxed{= \exp[2.355 - 0.342 \log \text{WBC}]}$

log WBC = 2:
$\quad \widehat{HR} = \exp[2.355 - 0.342 \, (2)]$
$\qquad = e^{1.671} = 5.32$

log WBC = 4:
$\quad \widehat{HR} = \exp[2.355 - 0.342 \, (4)]$
$\qquad = e^{0.987} = 2.68$

To obtain the hazard ratio for the effect of *Rx* adjusted for log WBC using model 3, we consider *X** and *X* vectors which have three components, one for each variable in the model. The *X** vector, which denotes a treated subject, has components $X_1^* = 1$, $X_2^* = \log \text{WBC}$ and $X_3^* = 1$ times log WBC. The *X* vector, which denotes a placebo subject, has components $X_1 = 0$, $X_2 = \log$ WBC and $X_3 = 0$ times log WBC. Note again that, as with the previous example, the value for log WBC is treated as fixed, though unspecified.

Using the general formula for the hazard ratio, we must now compute the exponential of the sum of three quantities, corresponding to the three variables in the model. Substituting the values from the printout and the values of the vectors *X** and *X* into this formula, we obtain the exponential expression shown here. Using algebra, this expression simplifies to the exponential of 2.355 minus 0.342 times log WBC.

In order to get a numerical value for the hazard ratio, we must specify a value for log WBC. For instance, if log WBC = 2, the estimated hazard ratio becomes 5.32, whereas if log WBC = 4, the estimated hazard ratio becomes 2.68. Thus, we get different hazard ratio values for different values of log WBC, which should make sense since log WBC is an effect modifier in model 3.

General rule for (0,1) exposure variables when there are product terms:

$$\boxed{\widehat{HR} = \exp\left[\hat{\beta} + \sum \hat{\delta}_j W_j \right]}$$

where
$\quad \hat{\beta} = \text{coefficient of } E$
$\quad \hat{\delta}_j = \text{coefficient of } E \times W_j$

($\widehat{HR}$ does not contain coefficients of non-product terms)

The example we have just described using model 3 illustrates a general rule which states that the hazard ratio for the effect of a (0,1) exposure variable in a model which contains product terms involving this exposure with other *X*'s can be written as shown here. Note that β "hat" denotes the coefficient of the exposure variable and the δ "hats" are coefficients of product terms in the model of the form ExW_j. Also note that this formula does not contain coefficients of nonproduct terms other than *E*.

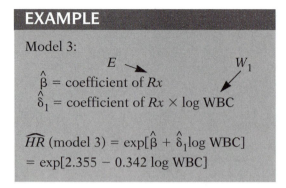

EXAMPLE

Model 3:

$$E \searrow \qquad W_1$$
$$\hat{\beta} = \text{coefficient of } Rx$$
$$\hat{\delta}_1 = \text{coefficient of } Rx \times \log \text{WBC}$$

$$\widehat{HR} \text{ (model 3)} = \exp[\hat{\beta} + \hat{\delta}_1 \log \text{WBC}]$$
$$= \exp[2.355 - 0.342 \log \text{WBC}]$$

For model 3, β "hat" is the coefficient of the *Rx* variable, and there is only one δ "hat" in the sum, which is the coefficient of the product term *Rx* × log WBC. Thus, there is only one *W*, namely W_1 = log WBC. The hazard ratio formula for the effect of exposure is then given by exponentiating β "hat" plus δ_1 "hat" times log WBC. Substituting the estimates from the printout into this formula yields the expression obtained previously, namely the exponential of 2.355 minus 0.342 times log WBC.

VI. Adjusted Survival Curves Using the Cox PH Model

Two primary quantities:
1. estimated hazard ratios
2. estimated survival curves

The two primary quantities desired from a survival analysis point of view are estimated hazard ratios and estimated survival curves. Having just described how to compute hazard ratios, we now turn to estimation of survival curves using the Cox model.

No model: use KM curves

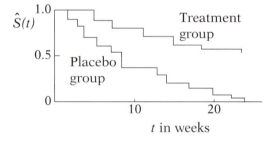

t in weeks

Recall that if no model is used to fit survival data, a survival curve can be estimated using a Kaplan–Meier method. Such KM curves are plotted as step functions as shown here for the remission data example.

Cox model: adjusted survival curves (also step functions).

When a Cox model is used to fit survival data, survival curves can be obtained that adjust for the explanatory variables used as predictors. These are called **adjusted survival curves,** and, like KM curves, these are also plotted as step functions.

Cox model hazard function:

$$h(t, \mathbf{X}) = \hat{h}_0(t)\, e^{\sum_{i=1}^{p} \beta_i X_i}$$

Cox model survival function:

$$S(t, \mathbf{X}) = [S_0(t)]^{e^{\sum \beta_i X_i}}$$

Estimated survival function:

$$\hat{S}(t, \mathbf{X}) = [\hat{S}_0(t)]^{e^{\sum \hat{\beta}_i X_i}}$$

$\hat{S}_0(t)$ and $\hat{\beta}_i$ are provided by the computer program. The X_i must be specified by the investigator.

The hazard function formula for the Cox PH model, shown here again, can be converted to a corresponding survival function formula as shown below. This survival function formula is the basis for determining adjusted survival curves. Note that this formula says that the survival function at time t for a subject with vector $\mathbf{X}$ as predictors is given by a baseline survival function $S_0(t)$ raised to a power equal to the exponential of the sum of β_i times X_i.

The expression for the estimated survival function can then be written with the usual "hat" notation as shown here.

The estimates of $\hat{S}_0(t)$ and $\hat{\beta}_i$ are provided by the computer program that fits the Cox model. The X's, however, must first be specified by the investigator before the computer program can compute the estimated survival curve.

EXAMPLE: Model 2 Remission Data

$$\hat{h}(t, \mathbf{X}) = \hat{h}_0(t)e^{1.294\,Rx\,+\,1.604\,\log WBC}$$
$$\hat{S}(t, \mathbf{X}) = [\hat{S}_0(t)]e^{1.294\,Rx\,+\,1.604\,\log WBC}$$

Specify values for $\mathbf{X} = (Rx, \log WBC)$:

$Rx = 1$, $\log WBC = 2.93$:
$$\hat{S}(t, \mathbf{X}) = [\hat{S}_0(t)]e^{1.294\,(1)\,+\,1.604\,(2.93)}$$
$$= [\hat{S}_0(t)]e^{5.99} = \left([\hat{S}_0(t)]^{400.9}\right)$$

$Rx = 0$, $\log WBC = 2.93$:
$$\hat{S}(t, \mathbf{X}) = [\hat{S}_0(t)]e^{1.294\,(0)\,+\,1.604\,(2.93)}$$
$$= [\hat{S}_0(t)]e^{4.70} = \left([\hat{S}_0(t)]^{109.9}\right)$$

For example, if we consider model 2 for the remission data, the fitted model written in terms of both the hazard function and corresponding survival function is given here.

We can obtain a specific survival curve by specifying values for the vector $\mathbf{X}$, whose component variables are Rx and $\log WBC$.

For instance, if $Rx = 1$ and $\log WBC = 2.93$, the estimated survival curve is obtained by substituting these values in the formula as shown here, and carrying out the algebra to obtain the expression circled. Note that the value 2.93 is the overall mean log WBC for the entire dataset of 42 subjects.

Also, if $Rx = 0$ and $\log WBC = 2.93$, the estimated survival curve is obtained as shown here.

EXAMPLE (continued)

Adjusted Survival Curves

$Rx = 1$, log WBC $= 2.93$:
$$\hat{S}(t,\mathbf{X}) = [\hat{S}_0(t)]^{400.9}$$
$Rx = 0$, log WBC $= 2.93$:
$$\hat{S}(t,\mathbf{X}) = [\hat{S}_0(t)]^{109.9}$$

Typically, use $X = \overline{X}$ or X_{median}.

Computer uses $\overline{X}$.

Each of the circled expressions gives **adjusted** survival curves, where the adjustment is for the values specified for the X's. Note that for each expression, a survival probability can be obtained for any value of t.

The two formulae just obtained, again shown here, allow us to compare survival curves for different treatment groups adjusted for the covariate log WBC. Both curves describe estimated survival probabilities over time assuming the same value of log WBC, in this case, the value 2.93.

Typically, when computing adjusted survival curves, the value chosen for a covariate being adjusted is an average value like an arithmetic mean or a median. In fact, most computer programs for the Cox model automatically use the mean value over all subjects for each covariate being adjusted.

EXAMPLE (continued)

Remission data ($n = 42$):

$\overline{\text{log WBC}} = 2.93$

In our example, the mean log WBC for all 42 subjects in the remission data set is 2.93. That is why we chose this value for log WBC in the formulae for the adjusted survival curve.

General formulae for adjusted survival curves comparing two groups:

Exposed subjects:

$$\hat{S}(t,\mathbf{X}_1) = \left[\hat{S}_0(t)\right]^{e^{\hat{\beta}_1(1)+\sum_{i\neq1}\hat{\beta}_i\overline{X}_i}}$$

Unexposed subjects:

$$\hat{S}(t,\mathbf{X}_0) = \left[\hat{S}_0(t)\right]^{e^{\hat{\beta}_1(0)+\sum_{i\neq1}\hat{\beta}_i\overline{X}_i}}$$

More generally, if we want to compare survival curves for two levels of an exposure variable, and we want to adjust for several covariates, we can write the formula for each curve as shown here. Note that we are assuming that the exposure variable is variable X_1, whose estimated coefficient is β_1 "hat," and the value of X_1 is 1 for exposed and 0 for unexposed subjects.

General formula for adjusted survival curve for all covariates in the model:

$$\hat{S}(t,\overline{\mathbf{X}}) = \left[\hat{S}_0(t)\right]^{e^{\sum\hat{\beta}_i\overline{X}_i}}$$

Also, if we want to obtain an adjusted survival curve which adjusts for all covariates in the model, the general formula which uses the mean value for each covariate is given as shown here. This formula will give a single adjusted survival curve rather than different curves for each exposure group.

EXAMPLE (continued)

Single survival curve for Cox model containing Rx and log WBC:

$\overline{Rx} = 0.50$

$\overline{\log \text{WBC}} = 2.93$

$$\hat{S}(t, \mathbf{X}) = [\hat{S}_0(t)]^{e^{\hat{\beta}_1 \overline{Rx} + \hat{\beta}_2 \overline{\log \text{WBC}}}}$$

$$= [\hat{S}_0(t)]^{e^{1.294(0.5) + 1.604(2.93)}}$$

$$= [\hat{S}_0(t)]^{e^{5.35}} = \left([\hat{S}_0(t)]^{210.6}\right)$$

Compute survival probability by specifying value for t in $\hat{S}(t, \mathbf{X}) = [\hat{S}_0(t)]^{210.6}$

Computer uses t's which are failure times.

To illustrate this formula, suppose we again consider the remission data, and we wish to obtain a single survival curve that adjusts for both Rx and log WBC in the fitted Cox model containing these two variables. Using the mean value of each covariate, we find that the mean value for Rx is 0.5 and the mean value for log WBC is 2.93, as before.

To obtain the single survival curve that adjusts for Rx and log WBC, we then substitute the mean values in the formula for the adjusted survival curve for the model fitted. The formula and the resulting expression for the adjusted survival curve are shown here. (Note that for the remission data, where it is of interest to compare two exposure groups, the use of a single survival curve is not appropriate.)

From this expression for the survival curve, a survival probability can be computed for any value of t that is specified. When graphing this survival curve using a computer package, the values of t that are chosen are the failure times of all persons in the study who got the event. This process is automatically carried out by the computer without having the user specify each failure time.

The graph of adjusted survival curves obtained from fitting a Cox model is usually plotted as a step function. For example, we show here the step functions for the two adjusted survival curves obtained by specifying either 1 or 0 for treatment status and letting log WBC be the mean value 2.93.

EXAMPLE

Adjusted Survival Curves for Treatment and Placebo Groups

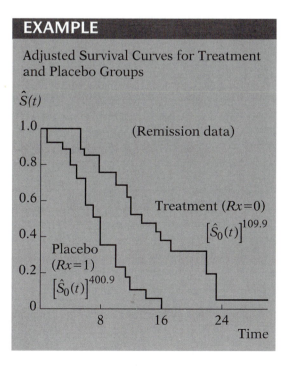

$\hat{S}(t)$

(Remission data)

Treatment $(Rx=0)$

$\left[\hat{S}_0(t)\right]^{109.9}$

Placebo $(Rx=1)$

$\left[\hat{S}_0(t)\right]^{400.9}$

Time

Next section: PH assumption
- explain meaning
- when PH **not** satisfied

We now turn to the concept of the proportional hazard (PH) assumption. In the next section, we explain the meaning of this assumption and we give an example of when this assumption is not satisfied.

Later presentations:
- how to evaluate PH
- analysis when PH not met

In later presentations, we expand on this subject, describing how to evaluate statistically whether the assumption is met and how to carry out the analysis when the assumption is not met.

VII. The Meaning of the PH Assumption

The PH assumption requires that the HR is constant over time, or equivalently, that the hazard for one individual is proportional to the hazard for any other individual, where the proportionality constant is independent of time.

PH: HR is constant over time, i.e.,
$$\hat{h}(t, \mathbf{X^*}) = \text{constant} \times \hat{h}(t, \mathbf{X})$$

$$\widehat{HR} = \frac{\hat{h}(t, \mathbf{X^*})}{\hat{h}(t, \mathbf{X})} = \frac{\hat{h}_0(t)\, e^{\sum\limits_{i=1}^{p} \hat{\beta}_i X_i^*}}{\hat{h}_0(t)\, e^{\sum\limits_{i=1}^{p} \hat{\beta}_i X_i}}$$

$$= \exp\left[\sum_{i=1}^{p} \hat{\beta}_i \left(X_i^* - X_i\right)\right]$$

where $\mathbf{X^*} = (X_1^*, X_2^*, \ldots, X_p^*)$
and $\mathbf{X} = (X_1, X_2, \ldots, X_p)$
denote the set of X's for two individuals.

To understand the PH assumption, we need to reconsider the formula for the HR that compares two different specifications $\mathbf{X^*}$ and $\mathbf{X}$ for the explanatory variables used in the Cox model. We derived this formula previously in Section V, page 99, and we show this derivation again here. Notice that the baseline hazard function $\hat{h}_0(t)$ appears in both the numerator and denominator of the hazard ratio and cancels out of the formula.

$$\frac{\hat{h}(t, \mathbf{X^*})}{\hat{h}(t, \mathbf{X})} = \exp\left[\sum_{i=1}^{p} \hat{\beta}_i \left(X_i^* - X_i\right)\right]$$

does not involve t.

The final expression for the hazard ratio therefore involves the estimated coefficients β_1 "hat" and the values of $\mathbf{X^*}$ and $\mathbf{X}$ for each variable. However, because the baseline hazard has canceled out, the final expression does not involve time t.

Let
$$\hat{\theta} = \exp\left[\sum_{i=1}^{p} \hat{\beta}_i \left(X_i^* - X_i\right)\right]$$
Constant

then
$$\frac{\hat{h}(t, \mathbf{X^*})}{\hat{h}(t, \mathbf{X})} = \hat{\theta}$$

Thus, once the model is fitted and the values for $\mathbf{X^*}$ and $\mathbf{X}$ are specified, the value of the exponential expression for the estimated hazard ratio is a constant, which does not depend on time. If we denote this constant by θ "hat," then we can write the hazard ratio as shown here. This is a mathematical expression which states the proportional hazards assumption.

$\widehat{HR}$ (**X*** versus **X**)

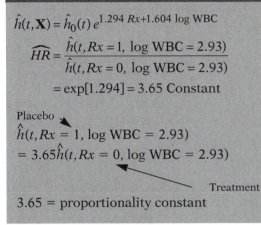

$$\hat{h}(t, X^*) = \hat{\theta}\hat{h}(t, X)$$

Proportionality constant (not dependent on time)

Graphically, this expression says that the estimated hazard ratio comparing any two individuals, plots as a constant over time.

Another way to write the proportional hazards assumption mathematically expresses the hazard function for individual **X*** as θ "hat" times the hazard function for individual **X,** as shown here. This expression says that the hazard function for one individual is proportional to the hazard function for another individual, where the proportionality constant is θ "hat," which does not depend on time.

EXAMPLE: Remission Data

$$\hat{h}(t, \mathbf{X}) = \hat{h}_0(t)\, e^{1.294\, Rx + 1.604\, \log WBC}$$

$$\widehat{HR} = \frac{\hat{h}(t, Rx = 1,\ \log WBC = 2.93)}{\hat{h}(t, Rx = 0,\ \log WBC = 2.93)}$$

$$= \exp[1.294] = 3.65 \text{ Constant}$$

Placebo

$$\hat{h}(t, Rx = 1,\ \log WBC = 2.93)$$
$$= 3.65\,\hat{h}(t, Rx = 0,\ \log WBC = 2.93)$$

Treatment

3.65 = proportionality constant

To illustrate the proportional hazard assumption, we again consider the Cox model for the remission data involving the two variables Rx and log WBC. For this model, the estimated hazard ratio that compares placebo ($Rx = 1$) with treated ($Rx = 0$) subjects controlling for log WBC is given by e to the 1.294, which is 3.65, a constant.

Thus, the hazard for placebo group ($Rx = 1$) is 3.65 times the hazard for the treatment group ($Rx = 0$), and the value, 3.65, is the same regardless of time. In other words, using the above model, the hazard for the placebo group is proportional to the hazard for the treatment group, and the proportionality constant is 3.65.

EXAMPLE: PH Not Satisfied

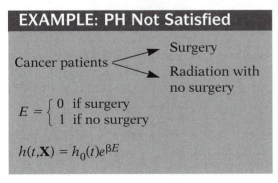

Cancer patients → Surgery
→ Radiation with no surgery

$$E = \begin{cases} 0 & \text{if surgery} \\ 1 & \text{if no surgery} \end{cases}$$

$$h(t, \mathbf{X}) = h_0(t)e^{\beta E}$$

To further illustrate the concept of proportional hazards, we now provide an example of a situation for which the proportional hazards assumption is *not* satisfied.

For our example, we consider a study in which cancer patients are randomized to either surgery or radiation therapy without surgery. Thus, we have a (0,1) exposure variable denoting surgery status, with 0 if a patient receives surgery and 1 if not. Suppose further that this exposure variable is the only variable of interest, so that a Cox PH model for the analysis of this data, as shown here, will contain only the one variable E, denoting exposure.

EXAMPLE (continued)

Is the above Cox PH model appropriate?

Note:

$$\frac{\text{Serious}}{\text{surgery}} \Rightarrow \text{High risk for death early}$$

$h(t,X)$

Hazards cross

$E=0$ (surgery)

$E=1$

$E=1$ (no surgery)

$E=0$

3   t(days)

2 days: $\dfrac{\hat{h}(t=2,E=1)}{\hat{h}(t=2,E=0)}<1$

but

5 days: $\dfrac{\hat{h}(t=5,E=1)}{\hat{h}(t=5,E=0)}>1$

Given the above description, **HR is not constant over time.**

Cox PH model inappropriate because PH model assumes constant HR:

$$h(t,\mathbf{X})=h_0(t)\,e^{\beta E}$$

$$\widehat{HR}=\frac{\hat{h}(t,E=1)}{\hat{h}(t,E=0)}=e^{\hat{\beta}}$$

Now the question we consider here is whether the above Cox model containing the variable E is an appropriate model to use for this situation. To answer this question we note that when a patient undergoes serious surgery, as when removing a cancerous tumor, there is usually a high risk for complications from surgery or perhaps even death early in the recovery process, and once the patient gets past this early critical period, the benefits of surgery, if any, can then be observed.

Thus, in a study that compares surgery to no surgery, we might expect to see hazard functions for each group that appear as shown here. Notice that these two functions cross at about three days, and that prior to three days the hazard for the surgery group is higher than the hazard for the no surgery group, whereas after three days, the hazard for the surgery group is lower than the hazard for the no surgery group.

Looking at the above graph more closely, we can see that at 2 days, when $t = 2$, the hazard ratio of nonsurgery ($E = 1$) to surgery ($E = 0$) patients yields a value less than 1. In contrast, at $t = 5$ days, the hazard ratio of nonsurgery to surgery yields a value greater than 1.

Thus, if the above description of the hazard functions for each group is accurate, the hazard ratios are not constant over time. That is, the hazard ratio is some number less than 1 before three days and greater than 1 after three days.

It is therefore inappropriate to use a Cox PH model for this situation, because the PH model assumes a constant hazard ratio across time, whereas our situation yields a hazard ratio that varies with time.

In fact, if we use a Cox PH model, shown here again, the estimated hazard ratio comparing exposed to unexposed patients at any time is given by the constant value e to the β "hat," which does not vary over time.

General rule:
  If the hazards cross, then a Cox PH model
  is not appropriate.

Analysis when Cox PH model not appropriate? See Chapters 5 and 6.

EXAMPLE (continued)

Surgery study analysis options:
• stratify by exposure (use KM curves)
• start analysis at three days; use Cox PH model
• fit PH model for < 3 days and for > 3 days; get $\widehat{HR}$ (< 3 days) and $\widehat{HR}$ (> 3 days)
• include time-dependent variable (e.g., $E \times t$); use extended Cox model

Different options may lead to different conclusions.

Hazards
  cross $\Rightarrow$ PH not met
but

  ? $\Rightarrow$ PH met

See Chapter 4: Evaluating PH Assumption

This example illustrates the general rule that if the hazards cross, then the PH assumption cannot be met, so that a Cox PH model is inappropriate.

It is natural to ask at this point, if the Cox PH model is inappropriate, how should we carry out the analysis? The answer to this question is discussed in Chapters 5 and 6. However, we will give a brief reply with regard to the surgery study example just described.

Actually, for the surgery study there are several options available for the analysis. These include:

• analyze by stratifying on the exposure variable; that is, do not fit any model, and, instead obtain Kaplan–Meier curves for each exposure group separately;
• start the analysis at three days, and use a Cox PH model on three-day survivors;
• fit Cox model for less than three days and a different Cox model for greater than three days to get two different hazard ratio estimates, one for each of these two time periods;
• fit a modified Cox model that includes a time-dependent variable which measures the interaction of exposure with time. This model is called an **extended Cox model.**

Further discussion of these options is beyond the scope of this presentation. We point out, however, that different options may lead to different conclusions, so that the investigator may have to weigh the relative merits of each option in light of the data actually obtained before deciding on any particular option as best.

One final comment before concluding this section: although we have shown that when the hazards cross, the PH assumption is not met, we have not shown how to decide when the PH assumption is met. This is the subject of Chapter 4 entitled, "Evaluating the PH Assumption."

VIII. Summary

In this section we briefly summarize the content covered in this presentation.

1. Review: $S(t)$, $h(t)$, data layout, etc.
2. Computer example of Cox model:
   - estimate HR
   - test hypothesis about HR
   - obtain confidence intervals

- We began with a computer example that uses the Cox PH model. We showed how to use the output to estimate the HR, and how to test hypotheses and obtain confidence intervals about the hazard ratio.

3. Cox model formula:

$$h(t, \mathbf{X}) = h_0(t)\, e^{\sum_{i=1}^{p} \beta_i X_i}$$

- We then provided the formula for the hazard function for the Cox PH model and described basic features of this model. The most important feature is that the model contains two components, namely, a baseline hazard function of time and an exponential function involving X's but not time.

4. Why popular: Cox PH model is "robust"

- We discussed reasons why the Cox model is popular, the primary reason being that the model is "robust" for many different survival analysis situations.

5. ML estimation: maximize a partial likelihood
   L = joint probability of observed data = $L(\beta)$

- We then discussed ML estimation of the parameters in the Cox model, and pointed out that the ML procedure maximizes a "partial" likelihood that focuses on probabilities at failure times only.

6. Hazard ratio formula:

$$\widehat{HR} = \exp\left[\sum_{i=1}^{p} \hat{\beta}_i \left(X_i^* - X_i \right) \right]$$

- Next, we gave a general formula for estimating a hazard ratio that compared two specifications of the X's, defined as $\mathbf{X^*}$ and $\mathbf{X}$. We illustrated the use of this formula when comparing two exposure groups adjusted for other variables.

7. Adjusted survival curves:
   Comparing E groups:

$$\hat{S}(t, \mathbf{X}) = \left[\hat{S}_0(t) \right]^{e^{\hat{\beta}_1 (E) + \sum_{i \neq 1} \hat{\beta}_1 \bar{X}_i}}$$

     0 or 1

Single curve:

$$\hat{S}(t, \overline{\mathbf{X}}) = \left[\hat{S}_0(t) \right]^{e^{\sum \hat{\beta}_i \bar{X}_i}}$$

- We then defined an adjusted survival curve and presented formulas for adjusted curves comparing two groups adjusted for other variables in the model and a formula for a single adjusted curve that adjusts for all X's in the model. Computer packages for these formulae use the mean value of each X being adjusted in the computation of the adjusted curve.

8. PH assumption:

$$\frac{\hat{h}(t, \mathbf{X^*})}{\hat{h}(t, \mathbf{X})} = \hat{\theta} \quad \text{(a constant over } t\text{)}$$

i.e., $\hat{h}(t, \mathbf{X^*}) = \hat{\theta}\hat{h}(t, \mathbf{X})$

Hazards cross $\Rightarrow$ PH not met

- Finally, we described the PH assumption as meaning that the hazard ratio is constant over time, or equivalently that the hazard for one individual is proportional to the hazard for any other individual, where the proportionality constant is independent of time. We also showed that for study situations in which the hazards cross, the PH assumption is not met.

Chapters

This presentation is now complete. We recommend that the reader review the detailed outline that follows and then do the practice exercises and test.

The next Chapter (4) describes how to evaluate the PH assumption. Chapters 5 and 6 describe methods for carrying out the analysis when the PH assumption is not met.

<table>
<tr><td>**Detailed Outline**</td><td>

I. A computer example using the Cox PH model (pages 86–94)

A. Printout shown for three models involving leukemia remission data.

B. Three explanatory variables of interest: treatment status, log WBC, and product term; outcome is time until subject goes out of remission.

C. Discussion of how to evaluate which model is best.

D. Similarity to classical regression and logistic regression.

II. The formula for the Cox PH model (pages 94–96)

A.
$$h(t,\mathbf{X}) = h_0(t)\exp\left[\sum_{i=1}^{p}\beta_i X_i\right]$$

B. $h_0(t)$ is called the **baseline hazard function.**

C. $\mathbf{X}$ denotes a collection of p explanatory variables $X_1, X_2, \ldots, X_p$.

D. The model is **nonparametric** because $h_0(t)$ is unspecified.

E. Examples of the Cox model using the leukemia remission data.

F. Survival curves can be derived from the Cox PH model.

III. Why the Cox PH model is popular (pages 96–98)

A. Can get an estimate of effect (the hazard ratio) without needing to know $h_0(t)$.

B. Can estimate $h_0(t)$, $h(t,\mathbf{X})$, and survivor functions, even though $h_0(t)$ is not specified.

C. The e part of the formula is used to ensure that the fitted hazard is nonnegative.

D. The Cox model is "robust": it usually fits the data well no matter which parametric model is appropriate.

IV. ML estimation of the Cox PH model (pages 98–100)

A. Likelihood function is maximized.

B. L is called a partial likelihood, because it uses survival time information only on failures, and does not use censored information explicitly.

C. L makes use of the risk set at each time that a subject fails.

D. Inferences are made using standard large sample ML techniques, e.g., Wald or likelihood ratio tests and large sample confidence intervals based on asymptotic normality assumptions

V. Computing the hazard ratio (pages 100–104)

A. Formula for hazard ratio comparing two individuals, $\mathbf{X}^* = (X_1^*, X_2^*, \ldots, X_p^*)$ and $\mathbf{X} = (X_1, X_2, \ldots, X_p)$:
</td></tr>
</table>

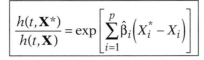

$$\frac{h(t,\mathbf{X}^*)}{h(t,\mathbf{X})} = \exp\left[\sum_{i=1}^{p}\hat{\beta}_i\left(X_i^* - X_i\right)\right]$$

  B. Examples are given using a (0,1) exposure variable, potential confounders, and potential effect modifiers.
  C. Typical coding identifies $\mathbf{X}^*$ as unexposed group and $\mathbf{X}$ as exposed group, i.e., $X_1^* = 1$ for unexposed group and $X_1 = 0$ for exposed group; such coding allows $\mathbf{X}^*$ to indicate the group with the larger hazard.

 VI. **Adjusted survival curves using the Cox PH model** (pages 104–108)
  A. Survival curve formula can be obtained from hazard ratio formula:

$$S(t,\mathbf{X}) = \left[S_0(t)\right]^{e^{\sum \beta_i X_i}}$$

   where $S_0(t)$ is the baseline survival function that corresponds to the baseline hazard function $h_0(t)$.
  B. To graph $S(t,\mathbf{X})$, must specify values for $\mathbf{X} = (X_1, X_2, \ldots, X_p)$.
  C. To obtain "adjusted" survival curves, usually use overall mean values for the X's being adjusted.
  D. Examples of "adjusted" $S(t,\mathbf{X})$ using leukemia remission data.

VII. **The meaning of the PH assumption** (pages 108–111)
  A. Hazard ratio formula shows that hazard ratio is independent of time:

$$\frac{h(t,\mathbf{X}^*)}{h(t,\mathbf{X})} = \theta$$

  B. Baseline hazard function not involved in the HR formula.
  C. Hazard ratio for two $\mathbf{X}$'s are proportional: $h(t, \mathbf{X}^*) = \theta \, h(t, \mathbf{X})$
  D. An example when the PH assumption is not satisfied: hazards cross

VIII. **Summary** (page 112)

Practice Exercises

 1. In a 10-year follow-up study conducted in Evans County, Georgia, involving persons 60 years or older, one research question concerned evaluating the relationship of social support to mortality status. A Cox proportional hazards model was fit to describe the relationship of a measure of social network to time until death. The social network index was denoted as SNI, and took on integer values between 0 (poor social network) to 5 (excellent social network). Variables to be considered for control in the analysis as either potential confounders or potential effect modifiers were AGE (treated continuously), RACE (0,1), and SEX (0,1).

a. State an initial PH model that can be used to assess the relationship of interest, which considers the potential confounding and interaction effects of the AGE, RACE, and SEX (assume no higher than two-factor products involving SNI with AGE, RACE, and SEX).

b. For your model in part 1a, give an expression for the hazard ratio that compares a person with SNI = 4 to a person with SNI = 2 and the same values of the covariates being controlled.

c. Describe how you would test for interaction using your model in part 1a. In particular, state the null hypothesis, the general form of your test statistic, with its distribution and degrees of freedom under the null hypothesis.

d. Assuming a revised model containing no interaction terms, give an expression for a 95% interval estimate for the adjusted hazard ratio comparing a person with SNI = 4 to a person with SNI = 2 and the same values of the covariates in your model.

e. For the no-interaction model described in part 1d, give an expression (i.e., formula) for the estimated survival curve for a person with SNI = 4, adjusted for AGE, RACE, and SEX, where the adjustment uses the overall mean value for each of the three covariates.

f. Using the no-interaction model described in part 1d, if the estimated survival curves for persons with SNI = 4 and SNI = 2 adjusted for (mean) AGE, RACE, and SEX are plotted over time, will these two estimated survival curves cross? Explain briefly.

2. For this question, we consider the survival data for 137 patients from the Veteran's Administration Lung Cancer Trial cited by Kalbfleisch and Prentice in their book (*The Statistical Analysis of Survival Time Data*, Wiley, 1980). The variables in this dataset are listed as follows:

Variable #	Variable name	Coding
1	Treatment	Standard = 1, test = 2
2	Cell type 1	Large = 1, other = 0
3	Cell type 2	Adeno = 1, other = 0
4	Cell type 3	Small = 1, other = 0
5	Cell type 4	Squamous = 1, other = 0
6	Survival time	(Days) integer counts
7	Performance status	0 = worst, . . . , 100 = best
8	Disease duration	(Months) integer counts
9	Age	(Years) integer counts
10	Prior therapy	None = 0, some = 10
11	Status	0 = censored, 1 = died

Four indicator variables for cell type { 2, 3, 4, 5 }

For these data, a Cox PH model was fitted yielding the following computer results:

Response: survival time

Variable name	Coeff	S.E.	p-value	*HR*	95%	CI	*P(PH)*
1 Treatment	0.290	0.207	0.162	1.336	0.890	2.006	0.628
3 Adeno cell	0.789	0.303	0.009	2.200	1.216	3.982	0.083
4 Small cell	0.457	0.266	0.086	1.579	0.937	2.661	0.080
5 Squamous cell	−0.400	0.283	0.157	0.671	0.385	1.167	0.089
7 Perf. status	−0.033	0.006	0.000	0.968	0.958	0.978	0.000
8 Disease dur.	0.000	0.009	0.992	1.000	0.982	1.018	0.919
9 Age	−0.009	0.009	0.358	0.991	0.974	1.010	0.199
10 Prior therapy	0.007	0.023	0.755	1.007	0.962	1.054	0.147

$-2 \ln L$: 950.359

a. State the Cox PH model used to obtain the above computer results.

b. Using the printout above, what is the hazard ratio that compares persons with adeno cell type with persons with large cell type? Explain your answer using the general hazard ratio formula for the Cox PH model.

c. Using the printout above, what is the hazard ratio that compares persons with adeno cell type with persons with squamous cell type? Explain your answer using the general hazard ratio formula for the Cox PH model.

d. Based on the computer results, is there an effect of treatment on survival time? Explain briefly.

e. Give an expression for the estimated survival curve for a person who was given the test treatment and who had a squamous cell type, where the variables to be adjusted are performance status, disease duration, age, and prior therapy.

f. Is there any suggestion from the printout that the PH assumption may not be appropriate for some of the variables in the model? Explain.

g. Suppose a revised Cox model is used which contains, in addition to the variables already included, the product terms: treatment × performance status; treatment × disease duration; treatment × age; and treatment × prior therapy. For this revised model, give an expression for the hazard ratio for the effect of treatment, adjusted for the other variables in the model.

3. The data for this question contain survival times of 65 multiple myeloma patients (references: *SPIDA manual*, Sydney, Australia, 1991; and Krall et al., "A Step-up Procedure for Selecting Variables Associated with Survival Data," *Biometrics*, vol. 31, pp. 49–57, 1975). A partial list of the variables in the dataset is given below:

Variable 1: observation number
Variable 2: survival time (in months) from time of diagnosis
Variable 3: survival status (0 = alive, 1 = dead)
Variable 4: platelets at diagnosis (0 = abnormal, 1 = normal)
Variable 5: age at diagnosis (years)
Variable 6: sex (1 = male, 2 = female)

Below, we provide computer results for several different Cox models that were fit to this dataset. A number of questions will be asked about these results starting on the next page.

Model 1:

Variable	Coeff	S.E.	p-value	*HR*	0.95	CI	*P(PH)*
Platelets	0.470	2.854	.869	1.600	0.006	429.689	0.729
Age	0.000	0.037	.998	1.000	0.930	1.075	0.417
Sex	0.183	0.725	.801	1.200	0.290	4.969	0.405
Platelets × age	−0.008	0.041	.850	0.992	0.915	1.075	0.561
Platelets × sex	−0.503	0.804	.532	0.605	0.125	2.924	0.952

−2 ln *L*: 306.080

Model 2:

Variable	Coeff	S.E.	p-value	*HR*	0.95	CI	*P(PH)*
Platelets	−0.725	0.401	.071	0.484	0.221	1.063	0.863
Age	−0.005	0.016	.740	0.995	0.965	1.026	0.405
Sex	−0.221	0.311	.478	0.802	0.436	1.476	0.487

−2 ln *L*: 306.505

Model 3:

Variable	Coeff	S.E.	p-value	*HR*	0.95	CI	*P(PH)*
Platelets	−0.706	0.401	.078	0.493	0.225	1.083	0.792
Age	−0.003	0.015	.828	0.997	0.967	1.027	0.450

−2 ln *L*: 307.018

Model 4:

Variable	Coeff	S.E.	p-value	*HR*	0.95	CI	*P(PH)*
Platelets	−0.705	0.397	.076	0.494	0.227	1.075	0.860
Sex	−0.204	0.307	.506	0.815	0.447	1.489	0.473

−2 ln *L*: 306.616

Model 5:

Variable	Coeff	S.E.	p-value	*HR*	0.95	CI	*P(PH)*
Platelets	−0.694	0.397	.080	0.500	0.230	1.088	0.793

−2 ln *L*: 307.065

a. Considering any of the above computer results, do you find any evidence that the proportional hazards assumption is not satisfied for any variable being considered?

b. For model 1, give an expression for the hazard ratio for the effect of the platelet variable adjusted for age and sex.

c. Using your answer to part 3b, compute the estimated hazard ratio for a 40-year-old male. Also compute the estimated hazard ratio for a 50-year-old female.

d. Carry out an appropriate test of hypothesis to evaluate whether there is any significant interaction in model 1. What is your conclusion?

e. Considering models 2–5, evaluate whether age and sex need to be controlled as confounders?

f. Which of the five models do you think is the best model and why?

g. Based on your answer to part 3f, summarize the results that describe the effect of the platelet variable on survival adjusted for age and sex.

Test

1. Consider a hypothetical two-year study to investigate the effect of a passive smoking intervention program on the incidence of upper respiratory infection (URI) in newborn infants. The study design involves the random allocation of one of three intervention packages (A, B, C) to all healthy newborn infants in Orange County, North Carolina, during 1985. These infants are followed for two years to determine whether or not URI develops. The variables of interest for using a survival analysis on these data are:

T = time (in weeks) until URI is detected or time until censored

s = censorship status (= 1 if URI is detected, = 0 if censored)

PS = passive smoking index of family during the week of birth of the infant

DC = daycare status (= 1 if outside daycare, = 0 if only daycare is in home)

BF = breastfeeding status (= 1 if infant is breastfed, = 0 if infant is not breastfed)

T_1 = first dummy variable for intervention status (= 1 if A, = 0 if B, = –1 if C)

T_2 = second dummy variable for intervention status (= 1 if B, = 0 if A, = –1 if C).

a. State the Cox PH model that would describe the relationship between intervention package and survival time, controlling for PS, DC, and BF as confounders and effect modifiers. In defining your model, use only two factor product terms involving exposure (i.e., intervention) variables multiplied by control variables in your model.

b. Assuming that the Cox PH model is appropriate, give a formula for the hazard ratio that compares a person in intervention group A with a person in intervention group C, adjusting for PS, DC, and BF, and assuming interaction effects.

c. Assuming that the PH model in part 1a is appropriate, describe how you would carry out a chunk test for interaction; i.e., state the null hypothesis, describe the test statistic and give the distribution of the test statistic and its degrees of freedom under the null hypothesis.

d. Assuming no interaction effects, how would you test whether packages A, B, and C are equally effective, after controlling for *PS, DC,* and *BF* in a Cox PH model without interaction terms (i.e., state the two models being compared, the null hypothesis, the test statistic, and the distribution of the test statistic under the null hypothesis).

e. For the no-interaction model considered in parts 1c and 1d, give an expression for the estimated survival curves for the effect of intervention A adjusted for *PS, DC,* and *BF.* Also, give similar (but different) expressions for the adjusted survival curves for interventions B and C.

2. The data for this question consists of a sample of 50 persons from the 1967–1980 Evans County Study. There are two basic independent variables of interest: AGE and chronic disease status (CHR), where CHR is coded as 0 = none, 1 = chronic disease. A product term of the form AGE × CHR is also considered. The dependent variable is time until death, and the event is death. The primary question of interest concerns whether CHR, considered as the exposure variable, is related to survival time, controlling for AGE. The output of computer results for this question is given as follows:

Model 1:

Variable	Coeff	S.E.	Chi-sq	p-value
CHR	0.8595	0.3116	7.61	.0058

$-2 \ln L = 285.74$

Model 2:

CHR	0.8051	0.3252	6.13	.0133
AGE	0.0856	0.0193	19.63	.0000

$-2 \ln L = 264.90$

Model 3:

CHR	1.0009	2.2556	0.20	.6572
AGE	0.0874	0.0276	10.01	.0016
CHR × AGE	−0.0030	0.0345	0.01	.9301

$-2 \ln L = 264.89$

a. State the Cox PH model that allows for main effects of CHR and AGE as well as the interaction effect of CHR with AGE.

b. Carry out the test for significant interaction; i.e., state the null hypothesis, the test statistic, and its distribution under the null hypothesis. What are your conclusions about interaction?

c. Assuming no interaction, should AGE be controlled? Explain your answer on the basis of confounding and/or precision considerations.

d. If, when considering plots of various hazard functions over time, the hazard function for persons with CHR = 1 crosses the hazard function for persons with CHR = 0, what does this indicate about the use of any of the three models provided in the printout?

e. Using model 2, give an expression for the estimated survival curve for persons with CHR = 1, adjusted for AGE. Also, give an expression for the estimated survival curve for persons with CHR = 0, adjusted for AGE.

f. What is your overall conclusion about the effect of CHR on survival time based on the computer results provided from this study?

3. The data for this question contain remission times of 42 multiple leukemia patients in a clinical trial of a new treatment. The variables in the dataset are given below:

Variable 1: survival time (in weeks)
Variable 2: status (1 = in remission, 0 = relapse)
Variable 3: sex (1 = female, 0 = male)
Variable 4: log WBC
Variable 5: Rx status (1 = placebo, 0 = treatment)

Below, we provide computer results for several different Cox models that were fit to this dataset. A number of questions will be asked about these results starting below.

Model 1:

Variable	Coeff	S.E.	p-value	HR	0.95	CI	P(PH)
Rx	0.894	1.815	.622	2.446	0.070	85.812	0.391
Sex	−1.012	0.752	.178	0.363	0.083	1.585	0.058
log WBC	1.693	0.441	.000	5.437	2.292	12.897	0.482
Rx × Sex	1.952	0.907	.031	7.046	1.191	41.702	0.011
Rx × log WBC	−0.151	0.531	.776	0.860	0.304	2.433	0.443

−2 ln L: 139.029

Model 2:

	Coeff	S.E.	p-value	HR	0.95	CI	P(PH)
Rx	0.405	0.561	.470	1.500	0.499	4.507	0.483
Sex	−1.070	0.725	.140	0.343	0.083	1.422	0.068
log WBC	1.610	0.332	.000	5.004	2.610	9.592	0.461
Rx × Sex	2.013	0.883	.023	7.483	1.325	42.261	0.016

−2 in L: 139.110

Model 3:

	Coeff	S.E.	p-value	HR	0.95	CI	P(PH)
Rx	0.587	0.542	.279	1.798	0.621	5.202	0.340
Sex	−1.073	0.701	.126	0.342	0.087	1.353	0.003
Rx × Sex	1.906	0.815	.019	6.726	1.362	33.213	0.000

−2 ln L: 166.949

Model 4:

	Coeff	S.E.	p-value	HR	0.95	CI	P(PH)
Rx	1.391	0.457	.002	4.018	1.642	9.834	0.935
Sex	0.263	0.449	.558	1.301	0.539	3.139	0.038
log WBC	1.594	0.330	.000	4.922	2.578	9.397	0.828

−2 ln L: 144.218

a. Use the above computer results to carry out a chunk test to evaluate whether the two interaction terms in model 1 are significant. What are your conclusions?

b. Evaluate whether you would prefer model 1 or model 2. Explain your answer.

c. Using model 2, give an expression for the hazard ratio for the effect of the *Rx* variable adjusted for SEX and log WBC.

d. Using your answer in part 3c, compute the hazard ratio for the effect of *Rx* for males and for females separately.

e. [obscured] confounding of log WBC, determine [obscured]

[obscured] you consider to be best?

[obscured] the *P(PH)* column suggest [obscured] ut? Explain.

Answers to Practice Exercises

[handwritten note on sticky:]
DR. JARVINEN —
I STOPPED BY, BUT MUST
HAVE MISSED YOU.
HERE'S YOUR BOOK -- SORRY
I DIDN'T RETURN IT
THURSDAY.
— ANDREA

[partially obscured equation:] $+ \beta_3 \text{RACE} + \beta_4 \text{SEX} + \beta_7 \text{SNI} \times \text{SEX}]$

[partially obscured:] $\text{ACE})\beta_6 + 2(\text{SEX})\beta_7]$

c. $H_0: \beta_5$ [obscured]

Likelihood ratio test statistic $-2 \ln \hat{L}_R - (-2 \ln \hat{L}_F)$, which is approximately χ^2_3 under H_0, where R denotes the reduced model (containing no product terms) under H_0, and F denotes the full model (given in part 1a above).

d. 95% CI for adjusted HR: $\exp\left[2\hat{\beta}_1 \pm 1.96 \times 2\sqrt{\text{var}(\hat{\beta}_1)}\right]$

e. $\hat{S}(t,\mathbf{X}) = \left[\hat{S}_0(t)\right]^{\exp[4\hat{\beta}_1+(\overline{\text{AGE}})\hat{\beta}_2+(\overline{\text{RACE}})\hat{\beta}_3+(\overline{\text{SEX}})\hat{\beta}_4]}$

f. The two survival curves will **not** cross, because both are computed using the same proportional hazards model, which has the property that the hazard functions, as well as their corresponding estimated survivor functions, will not cross.

2.   a. $h(t,\mathbf{X}) = h_0(t)\,\exp\,[\beta_1X_1 + \beta_3X_3 + \beta_4X_4 + \beta_5X_5 + \beta_7X_7 + \ldots + \beta_{10}X_{10}]$

b. Adeno cell type: $\mathbf{X}^* = $ (treatment, 1, 0, 0, perfstat, disdur, age, prther)

Large cell type: $\mathbf{X} = $ (treatment, 0, 0, 0, perfstat, disdur, age, prther)

$$HR = \frac{h(t,\mathbf{X}^*)}{h(t,\mathbf{X})} = \exp\left[\sum_{i=1}^{k}\beta_i(\mathbf{X}^*-X_i)\right] = \exp\left[0+\hat{\beta}_3(1-0)+\hat{\beta}_4(0-0)+\hat{\beta}_5(0-0)+0+\cdots+0\right]$$
$$= \exp\left[\hat{\beta}_3\right] = \exp[0.789] = 2.20$$

c. Adeno cell type: $\mathbf{X}^* = $ (treatment, 1, 0, 0, perfstat, disdur, age, prther)

Squamous cell type: $\mathbf{X} = $ (treatment, 0, 0, 1, perfstat, disdur, age, prther)

$$HR = \frac{h(t,\mathbf{X}^*)}{h(t,\mathbf{X})} = \exp\left[\sum_{i=1}^{k}\beta_i(\mathbf{X}^*-X_i)\right] = \exp\left[0+\hat{\beta}_3(1-0)+\hat{\beta}_4(0-0)+\hat{\beta}_5(0-1)+0+\cdots+0\right]$$
$$= \exp\left[\hat{\beta}_3 - \hat{\beta}_5\right] = \exp[0.789-(-0.400)] = \exp[1.189] = 3.28$$

d. There does not appear to be an effect of treatment on survival time, adjusted for the other variables in the model. The hazard ratio is 1.3, which is close to the null value of one, the p-value of 0.162 for the Wald test for treatment is not significant, and the 95% confidence interval for the treatment effect correspondingly includes the null value.

e. $\hat{S}(t,\mathbf{X}) = \left[\hat{S}_0(t)\right]^{\exp[\hat{\beta}_1+\hat{\beta}_5+(\overline{\text{perfstat}})\hat{\beta}_7+(\overline{\text{disdur}})\hat{\beta}_8+(\overline{\text{age}})\hat{\beta}_9+(\overline{\text{prther}})\hat{\beta}_9]}$

f. The $P(PH)$ values for the variables "adeno cell," "small cell," "squamous cell," and "perf. status" are all below 0.05, suggesting that the PH assumption may not be satisfied for some or all of these variables. Moreover, "perf. status" has $P(PH) = 0.000$.

g. $HR = \dfrac{h(t, \mathbf{X}^*)}{h(t, \mathbf{X})} = \exp\left[\beta_1 + (\text{perfstat})\beta_{11} + (\text{disdur})\beta_{12} + (\text{age})\beta_{13} + (\text{prther})\beta_{14}\right]$

where β_1 is the coefficient of the treatment variable and β_{11}, β_{12}, β_{13}, and β_{14} are the coefficients of product terms involving treatment with the four variables indicated.

3.   a. None of the $P(PH)$ values for any variable in any of the models fitted is approaching statistical significance. Thus, there is no evidence from the results provided that the PH assumption is not satisfied.

   b. $\widehat{HR} = \exp[0.470 + (-0.008)\text{age} + (-0.503)\text{sex}]$

   c. 40-year-old male: $\widehat{HR} = \exp[0.470 + (-0.008)40 + (-0.503)1] = 0.70$

   50-year-old female: $\widehat{HR} = \exp[0.470 + (-0.008)50 + (-0.503)2] = 0.39$

   d. The LR (chunk) test for the significance of both interaction terms simultaneously yields the following likelihood ratio statistic which compares models 1 and 2:

   $LR = 306.505 - 306.080 = 0.425$

   This statistic is approximately chi-square with 2 degrees of freedom under the null hypothesis of no interaction. This LR statistic is highly nonsignificant. Thus, we conclude that there is no significant interaction in the model (1).

   e. The gold-standard hazard ratio is 0.484, which is obtained for model 2. Note that model 2 contains no interaction terms and controls for both covariates of interest. When either age or sex or both are dropped from the model, the hazard ratio (for platelets) does not change appreciably. Therefore, it appears that neither age nor sex need to be controlled for confounding.

   f. Models 2–5 are all more or less equivalent, since they all give essentially the same hazards ratio and confidence interval for the effect of the platelet variable. A political choice for best model would be the gold-standard model (2), because the critical reviewer can see both age and sex being controlled in model 2.

g.
- The point estimate of the hazard ratio for normal versus abnormal platelet count is .484 = 1/2.07, so that the hazard for an abnormal count is twice that for a normal count.
- There is no significant effect of platelet count on survival adjusted for age and sex ($P = .863$).
- The 95% CI for the hazard ratio is given by $0.221 < HR < 1.063$, which is quite wide and therefore shows a very imprecise estimate.

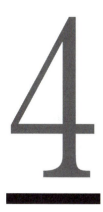

4

Evaluating the Proportional Hazards Assumption

Introduction

We begin with a brief review of the characteristics of the Cox proportional hazards (PH) model. We then give an overview of three methods for checking the PH assumption: graphical, goodness-of-fit (GOF), and time-dependent variable approaches.

We then focus on each of the above approaches, starting with graphical methods. The most popular graphical approach involves the use of "log–log" survival curves. A second graphical approach involves the comparison of "observed" with "expected" survival curves.

The GOF approach uses a test statistic or equivalent p-value to assess the significance of the PH assumption. We illustrate this test and describe some of its advantages and drawbacks.

Finally, we discuss the use of time-dependent variables in an extended Cox model as a third method for checking the PH assumption. A more detailed description of the use of time-dependent variables is provided in Chapter 6.

Abbreviated Outline

The outline below gives the user a preview of the material to be covered by the presentation. A detailed outline for review purposes follows the presentation.

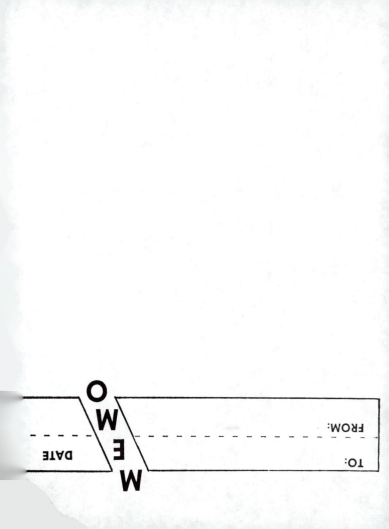

Objectives

Upon completing this chapter, the learner should be able to:

1. State or recognize three general approaches for evaluating the PH assumption.
2. Summarize how log–log survival curves may be used to assess the PH assumption.
3. Summarize how observed versus expected plots may be used to assess the PH assumption.
4. Summarize how GOF tests may be used to assess the PH assumption.
5. Summarize how time-dependent variables may be used to assess the PH assumption.
6. Describe—given survival data or computer output from a survival analysis that uses a Cox PH model—how to assess the PH assumption for one or more variables in the model using
   a. a graphical approach
   b. the GOF approach
   c. an extended Cox model with time-dependent covariates
7. State the formula for an extended Cox model that provides a method for checking the PH assumption for one more of the time-independent variables in the model, given survival analysis data or computer output that uses a Cox PH model.

Presentation

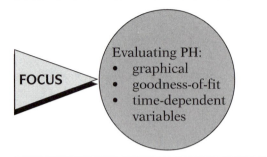

FOCUS

Evaluating PH:
- graphical
- goodness-of-fit
- time-dependent variables

This presentation describes three approaches for evaluating the proportional hazards (PH) assumption of the Cox model—a graphical procedure, a goodness-of-fit testing procedure, and a procedure that involves the use of time-dependent variables.

I. Background

Cox PH model:

$$h(t, \mathbf{X}) = h_0(t)\, e^{\sum_{i=1}^{p} \beta_i X_i}$$

$X = (X_1, X_2, \ldots, X_p)$ explanatory/predictor variables

$h_0(t)$	$\times$	$e^{\sum_{i=1}^{p} \beta_i X_i}$
Baseline hazard		Exponential
Involves t but not X's		Involves X's but not t (X's are time-independent)

X's involving t: **time-dependent**

Requires **extended Cox model** (no PH)
↑
Chapter 6

Recall from the previous chapter that the general form of the Cox PH model gives an expression for the hazard at time t for an individual with a given specification of a set of explanatory variables denoted by the bold **X**.

The Cox model formula says that the hazard at time t is the product of two quantities. The first of these, $h_0(t)$, is called the **baseline hazard** function. The second quantity is the exponential expression e to the linear sum of $\beta_i X_i$, where the sum is over the p explanatory X variables.

An important feature of this formula, which concerns the proportional hazards (PH) assumption, is that the baseline hazard is a function of t, but does not involve the X's, whereas the exponential expression involves the X's, but does not involve t. The X's here are called **time-independent** X's.

It is possible, nevertheless, to consider X's that do involve t. Such X's are called **time-dependent** variables. If time-dependent variables are considered, the Cox model form may still be used, but such a model no longer satisfies the PH assumption, and is called the **extended Cox model.** We will discuss this extended Cox model in Chapter 6 of this series.

Hazard ratio formula:

$$\widehat{HR} = \exp\left[\sum_{i=1}^{p} \hat{\beta}_i \left(X_i^* - X_i\right)\right]$$

where $\mathbf{X}^* = (X_1^*, X_2^*, \ldots, X_p^*)$
and $\mathbf{X} = (X_1, X_2, \ldots, X_p)$
denote the two sets of X's.

From the Cox PH model, we can obtain a general formula, shown here, for estimating a hazard ratio that compares two specifications of the X's, defined as **X*** and **X.**

Adjusted survival curves: 0 or 1
Comparing E groups:

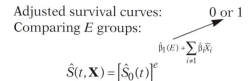

$$\hat{S}(t,\mathbf{X}) = \left[\hat{S}_0(t)\right]^{e^{\hat{\beta}_1(E) + \sum_{i \neq 1} \hat{\beta}_i \bar{X}_i}}$$

Single curve:

$$\hat{S}(t,\overline{\mathbf{X}}) = \left[\hat{S}_0(t)\right]^{e^{\sum \hat{\beta}_i \bar{X}_i}}$$

PH assumption:

$$\frac{\hat{h}(t,\mathbf{X}^*)}{\hat{h}(t,\mathbf{X})} = \hat{\theta}, \text{ constant over } t$$

i.e., $\hat{h}(t,\mathbf{X}^*) = \hat{\theta}\,\hat{h}(t,\mathbf{X})$

Hazards cross $\Rightarrow$ PH not met

Hazards don't cross $\not\Rightarrow$ PH met

We can also obtain from the Cox model an expression for an adjusted survival curve. Here we show a general formula for obtaining adjusted survival curves comparing two groups adjusted for other variables in the model. Below this, we give a formula for a single adjusted survival curve that adjusts for all X's in the model. Computer packages for these formulae use the mean value of each X being adjusted in the computation of the adjusted curve.

The Cox PH model assumes that the hazard ratio comparing any two specifications of predictors is constant over time. Equivalently, this means that the hazard for one individual is proportional to the hazard for any other individual, where the proportionality constant is independent of time.

The PH assumption is not met if the graph of the hazards cross for two or more categories of a predictor of interest. However, even if the hazard functions do not cross, it is possible that the PH assumption is not met. Thus, rather than checking for crossing hazards, we must use other approaches to evaluate the reasonableness of the PH assumption.

II. Checking the Proportional Hazards Assumption: Overview

Three approaches:
- (• graphical)
- • goodness-of-fit test
- • time-dependent variables

Graphical techniques:
$-\ln(-\ln)\ S$ curves parallel?
$-\ln(-\ln)\ \hat{S}$

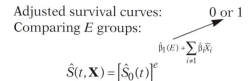

                     Males

                 Females

                     Time

There are three general approaches for assessing the PH assumption, again listed here. We now briefly overview each approach, starting with graphical techniques.

There are two types of graphical techniques available. The most popular of these involves comparing **estimated –ln(–ln) survivor curves** over different (combinations of) categories of variables being investigated. We will describe such curves in detail in the next section. Parallel curves, say comparing males with females, indicate that the PH assumption is satisfied, as shown in this illustration for the variable GENDER.

Observed vs. predicted: Close?

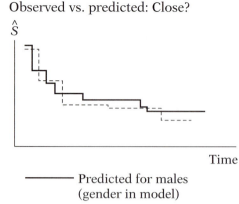

——— Predicted for males
       (gender in model)

------- Observed for males

Goodness-of-fit (GOF) tests:
Large sample Z or chi-square statistics

An alternative graphical approach is to compare **observed with predicted** survivor curves. The observed curves are derived for categories of the variable being assessed, say, GENDER, without putting this variable in a PH model. The predicted curves are derived with this variable included in a PH model. If observed and predicted curves are close, then the PH assumption is satisfied.

A second approach for assessing the PH assumption involves goodness-of-fit (GOF) tests. This approach provides large sample Z or chi-square statistics which can be computed for each variable in the model, adjusted for the other variables in the model.

EXAMPLE

Remission data

Column name	Coeff	StErr	...	P(PH)
log WBC	1.604	0.329		0.469
Rx	1.294	0.422		0.497

An example using the leukemia remission data described in previous chapters, is shown here. The last column of the printout contains p-values for GOF tests for the variables Rx and log WBC. Both test results are nonsignificant, which indicates that each variable satisfies the PH assumption.

Time-dependent covariates:

Extended Cox model:
Add product term involving some function of time.

When time-dependent variables are used to assess the PH assumption for a time-independent variable, the Cox model is extended to contain **product** (i.e., interaction) **terms** involving the time-independent variable being assessed and some function of time.

EXAMPLE

$h(t, X) = h_0(t) \exp[\beta\, G + \delta(G \times t)]$

where G denotes GENDER

H_0: $\delta = 0 \Rightarrow$ PH assumption satisfied

For example, if the PH assumption is being assessed for GENDER, a Cox model might be extended to include the variable "GENDER $\times t$" in addition to GENDER. If the coefficient of the product term turns out to be nonsignificant, we can conclude that the PH assumption is satisfied for GENDER.

GOF is more appealing:
Graphical: subjective
Time-dependent: computationally
                  cumbersome
GOF: global, may not detect specific
     departures from PH

The GOF approach is more appealing than the other two approaches in that it provides a single test statistic for each variable being assessed. This approach is not as subjective as the graphical approach nor as cumbersome computationally as the time-dependent variable approach. Nevertheless, a GOF test may be too "global" in that it may not detect specific departures from the PH assumption that may be observed from the other two approaches.

III. Graphical Approach 1: log–log plots

- log–log survival curves
- observed versus expected survival curves

$$\text{log–log } \hat{S} = \text{transformation of } \hat{S}$$
$$= -\ln(-\ln \hat{S})$$

- $\ln \hat{S}$ is negative $\Rightarrow -(\ln \hat{S})$ is positive.
- can't take log of $\ln \hat{S}$, but can take log of $(-\ln \hat{S})$.
- $-\ln(-\ln \hat{S})$ may be positive or negative.

The two graphical approaches for checking the PH assumption are comparing log–log survival curves and comparing observed versus expected survival curves. We first explain what a –ln–ln survival curve is and how it is used.

A log–log survival curve is simply a transformation of an estimated survival curve that results from taking the natural log of an estimated survival probability *twice*. Mathematically, we write a log–log curve as $-\ln(-\ln \hat{S})$. Note that the log of a probability such as $\hat{S}$ is always a negative number. Because we can only take logs of positive numbers, we need to negate the first log before taking the second log. The value for $-\ln(-\ln \hat{S})$ may be positive or negative, either of which is acceptable, because we are not taking a third log.[1]

EXAMPLE

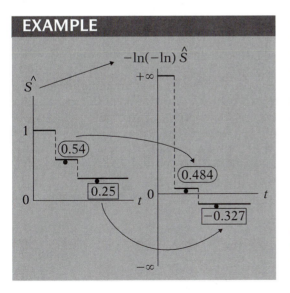

As an example, in the graph at left, the estimated survival probability of 0.54 is transformed to a log–log value of 0.484. Similarly, the point 0.25 on the survival curve is transformed to a –ln–ln value of –0.327.

Note that because the survival curve is usually plotted as a step function, so will the log–log curve be plotted as a step function.

---

[1]An equivalent way to write $-\ln(-\ln \hat{S})$ is $-\ln(\int_0^t h(u)du)$, where $\int_0^t h(u)du$ is called the "cumulative hazard" function. This result follows from the formula $\hat{S}(t) = \exp[-\int_0^t h(u)du]$, which relates the survivor function to the hazard function (see p. 14 in Chapter 1).

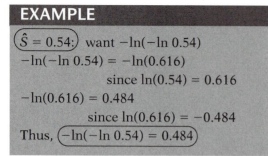

EXAMPLE

$(\hat{S} = 0.54:)$ want $-\ln(-\ln 0.54)$

$-\ln(-\ln 0.54) = -\ln(0.616)$

since $\ln(0.54) = 0.616$

$-\ln(0.616) = 0.484$

since $\ln(0.616) = -0.484$

Thus, $(-\ln(-\ln 0.54) = 0.484)$

To illustrate the computation of a log–log value, suppose we start with an estimated survival probability of 0.54. Then the log–log transformation of this value is $-\ln(-\ln 0.54)$, which is $-\ln(0.616)$, because $\ln(0.54)$ equals -0.616. Now, continuing further, $-\ln(0.616)$ equals 0.484, because $\ln(0.616)$ equals -0.484. Thus, the transformation $-\ln(-\ln 0.54)$ equals 0.484.

ANOTHER EXAMPLE

$(\hat{S} = 0.25:)$ want $-\ln(-\ln 0.25)$

$-\ln(-\ln 0.25) = -\ln(1.386) = -0.327$

Thus, $(-\ln(-\ln 0.25) = -0.327)$

As another example, if the estimated survival probability is 0.25, then $-\ln(-\ln 0.25)$ equals $-\ln(1.386)$, which equals -0.327.

y-axis scale:

$$
\begin{array}{cc}
1 & +\infty \\
\left.\begin{array}{c}\hat{S}\end{array}\right| & \left|\begin{array}{c}-\ln(-\ln)\,\hat{S}\end{array}\right. \\
0 & -\infty
\end{array}
$$

Note that the scale of the y-axis of an estimated survival curve ranges between 0 and 1, whereas the corresponding scale for a $-\ln(-\ln)$ curve ranges between $-\infty$ and $+\infty$.

log–log $\hat{S}$ for the Cox PH model:

We now show why the PH assumption can be assessed by evaluating whether or not log–log curves are parallel. To do this, we must first describe the log–log formula for the Cox PH model.

Cox PH hazard function:

$$h(t, \mathbf{X}) = h_0(t)\, e^{\sum_{j=1}^{p} \beta_j X_j}$$

↓ From math

Cox PH survival function:

$$S(t, \mathbf{X}) = \left[S_0(t)\right]^{e^{\sum_{j=1}^{p} \beta_j X_j}}$$

↗ Baseline survival function

We start with the formula for the survival curve that corresponds to the hazard function for the Cox PH model. Recall that there is a mathematical relationship between any hazard function and its corresponding survival function. We therefore can obtain the formula shown here for the survival curve for the Cox PH model. In this formula, the expression $S_0(t)$ denotes the baseline survival function that corresponds to the baseline hazard function $h_0(t)$.

log–log $\Rightarrow$ takes logs twice

log #1:

$$\ln S(t,\mathbf{X}) = e^{\sum\limits_{j=1}^{p}\beta_j X_j} \times \ln S_0(t)$$

$$0 \le S(t,\mathbf{X}) \le 1$$

ln(probability) = negative value,
so $S(t,\mathbf{X})$ and $\ln S_0(t)$ are negative.

But $-\ln S(t,\mathbf{X})$ is positive, which allows us to take logs again.

log #2:

$$\ln\left[-\ln S(t,\mathbf{X})\right] = \ln\left[-e^{\sum\limits_{j=1}^{p}\beta_j X_j} \times \ln S_0(t)\right]$$

$$= \ln\left[e^{\sum\limits_{j=1}^{p}\beta_j X_j}\right] + \ln\left[-\ln S_0(t)\right]$$

$$= \sum_{j=1}^{p}\beta_j X_j + \ln\left[-\ln S_0(t)\right]$$

$$-\ln\left[-\ln S(t,\mathbf{X})\right] = -\sum_{i=1}^{p}\beta_i X_i - \ln\left[-\ln S_0(t)\right]$$

Two individuals:
$\mathbf{X}_1 = (X_{11}, X_{12},..., X_{1p})$
$\mathbf{X}_2 = (X_{21}, X_{22},..., X_{2p})$

The log–log formula requires us to take logs of this survival function twice. The first time we take logs we get the expression shown here.

Now since $S(t,\mathbf{X})$ denotes a survival probability, its value for any t and any specification of the vector $\mathbf{X}$ will be some number between 0 and 1. It follows that the natural log of any number between 0 and 1 is a negative number, so that the log of $S(t,\mathbf{X})$ as well as the log of $S_0(t)$ are both negative numbers. This is why we have to put a minus sign in front of this expression before we can take logs a second time, because there is no such thing as the log of a negative number.

Thus, when taking the second log, we must obtain the log of $-\ln S(t,\mathbf{X})$, as shown here. After using some algebra, the expression on the right can be rewritten as the sum of two terms, one of which is the **linear sum of the $\beta_i X_i$** and the other is the **log of the negative log of the baseline survival function.**

This second log may be either positive or negative, and we aren't taking any more logs, so we actually don't have to take a second negative. However, for consistency's sake, the usual practice is to put a minus sign in front of the second log to obtain the $-\ln-\ln$ expression shown here.

Now suppose we consider two different specifications of the $\mathbf{X}$ vector, corresponding to two different individuals, $\mathbf{X}_1$ and $\mathbf{X}_2$.

$$-\ln\left[-\ln S(t,\mathbf{X}_1)\right] = -\sum_{j=1}^{p}\beta_j X_{1j} - \ln\left[-\ln S_0(t)\right]$$

$$-\ln\left[-\ln S(t,\mathbf{X}_2)\right] = -\sum_{j=1}^{p}\beta_j X_{2j} - \ln\left[-\ln S_0(t)\right]$$

$$-\ln\left[-\ln S(t,\mathbf{X}_1)\right] - \left(-\ln\left[-\ln S(t,\mathbf{X}_2)\right]\right)$$

$$= \sum_{j=1}^{p}\beta_j\left(X_{2j} - X_{1j}\right)$$

does not involve t

Then the corresponding log–log curves for these individuals are given as shown here, where we have simply substituted $\mathbf{X}_1$ and $\mathbf{X}_2$ for $\mathbf{X}$ in the previous expression for the log–log curve for any individual $\mathbf{X}$.

Subtracting the second log–log curve from the first yields the expression shown here. This expression is a linear sum of the differences in corresponding predictor values for the two individuals. Note that the baseline survival function has dropped out, so that the difference in log–log curves involves an expression that does not involve time t.

$$\boxed{-\ln\left[-\ln S(t,\mathbf{X}_1)\right] = -\ln\left[-\ln S(t,\mathbf{X}_2)\right] + \sum_{j=1}^{p}\beta_j\left(X_{2j} - X_{1j}\right)}$$

Alternatively, using algebra, we can write the above equation by expression the log–log survival curve for individual $\mathbf{X}_1$ as the log–log curve for individual $\mathbf{X}_2$ plus a linear sum term that is independent of t.

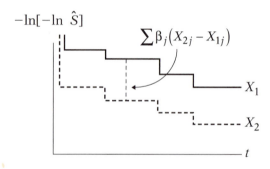

The above formula says that if we use a Cox PH model and we plot the estimated log–log survival curves for individuals on the same graph, the two plots would be approximately parallel. The distance between the two curves is the linear expression involving the differences in predictor values, which does not involve time.

The parallelism of log–log survival plots for the Cox PH model provides us with a graphical approach for assessing the PH assumption. That is, if a PH model is appropriate for a given set of predictors, one should expect that empirical plots of log–log survival curves for different individuals will be approximately parallel.

Graphical approach using log–log plots: PH model is appropriate if "empirical" plots of log–log survival curves are parallel. Empirical plots: use $-\ln[-\ln \hat{S}]$ where

1. $\hat{S}$ is a KM curve

2. $\hat{S}$ is an adjusted survival curve for predictors satisfying the PH assumption; predictor being assessed not included in model

By empirical plots, we mean plotting log–log survival curves based on Kaplan–Meier (KM) estimates that do not assume an underlying Cox model. Alternatively, one could plot log–log survival curves which have been adjusted for predictors already assumed to satisfy the PH assumption but have not included the predictor being assessed in a PH model.

<table>
<tr><td>

EXAMPLE

Clinical trial of leukemia patients:
T = weeks until patient goes out of
    remission

Predictors (X's):
Rx (= 1 if placebo, 0 if treatment)
log WBC

Cox PH model:
$h(t,\mathbf{X}) = h_0(t)e^{\beta_1 Rx + \beta_2 \log \text{WBC}}$

Assessing PH assumption:
compare log–log survival curves for
categories of Rx and log WBC

One-at-a-time strategy: Rx variable

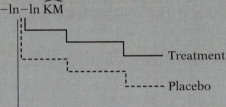

One-at-a-time strategy: log WBC

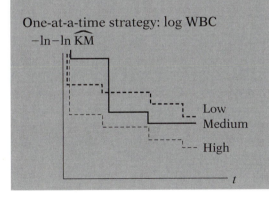

</td></tr>
</table>

As an example, suppose we consider the comparison of treatment and placebo groups in a clinical trial of leukemia patients, where survival time is time, in weeks, until a patient goes out of remission. Two predictors of interest in this study are treatment group status (1 = placebo, 0 = treatment), denoted as Rx, and log white blood cell count (log WBC), where the latter variable is being considered as a confounder.

A Cox PH model involving both these predictors would have the form shown at the left. To assess whether the PH assumption is satisfied for either or both of these variables, we would need to compare log–log survival curves involving categories of these variables.

One strategy to take here is to consider the variables one at a time. For the Rx variable, this amounts to plotting log–log KM curves for treatment and placebo groups and assessing parallelism. If the two curves are approximately parallel, as shown here, we would conclude that the PH assumption is satisfied for the variable Rx. If the two curves intersect or are not parallel in some other way, we would conclude that the PH assumption is not satisfied for this variable.

For the log WBC variable, we need to categorize this variable into categories—say, low, medium, and high—and then compare plots of log–log KM curves for each of the three categories. In this illustration, the three log–log Kaplan–Meier curves are clearly nonparallel, indicating that the PH assumption is not met for log WBC.

EXAMPLE: Computer (SPIDA) Results

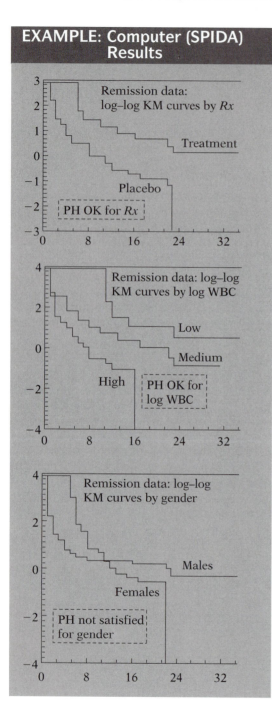

The above examples are sketches of some of the possibilities that could occur from comparisons of log–log curves. For the actual data set containing 42 leukemia patients, computer results using the SPIDA package are shown here for each variable separately. Similar output using SAS and BMDP packages is provided in Appendix A.

We first show the log–log KM curves by treatment, *Rx*. Notice that the two log–log curves are roughly parallel, indicating that the *Rx* variable satisfies the PH assumption when being considered by itself.

Here we show the log–log KM curves by log WBC, where we have divided this variable into low (below 2.3), medium (between 2.3 and 3), and high (above 3) values. Notice that there is some indication of nonparallelism below 8 days, but that overall the three curves are roughly parallel. Thus, these plots suggest that the PH assumption is more or less satisfied for the variable log WBC, when considered alone.

As a third example, we consider the log–log KM plots categorized by gender from the remission data. Notice that the two curves clearly intersect, and are therefore noticeably nonparallel. Thus, the variable, gender, when considered by itself, does not appear to satisfy the PH assumption and therefore should not be incorporated directly into a Cox PH model containing the other two variables, *Rx* and log WBC.

Problems with log–log survival curve approach:

How parallel is parallel?
Recommend:
- subjective decision
- conservative strategy: assume PH is OK unless strong evidence of nonparallelism

How to categorize a continuous variable?
- many categories ⇒ data "thins out"
- different categorizations may give different graphical pictures

Recommend:
- small # of categories (2 or 3)
- meaningful choice
- reasonable balance (e.g., terciles)

How to evaluate several variables simultaneously?

Strategy:
- categorize variables separately
- form combinations of categories
- compare log–log curves on same graph

Drawback:
- data "thins out"
- difficult to identify variables

The above examples suggest that there are some problems associated with this graphical approach for assessing the PH assumption. The main problem concerns how to decide "how parallel is parallel?" This decision can be quite subjective for a given data set, particularly if the study size is relatively small. We recommend that one should use a conservative strategy for this decision by assuming the PH assumption is satisfied unless there is **strong** evidence of nonparallelism of the log–log curves.

Another problem concerns how to categorize a continuous variable like log WBC. If many categories are chosen, the data "thins out" in each category, making it difficult to compare different curves. Also, one categorization into, say, three groups may give a different graphical picture from a categorization into three different groups.

In categorizing continuous variables, we recommend that the number of categories be kept reasonably small (e.g., two or three) if possible, and that the choice of categories be as meaningful as possible and also provide reasonable balance of numbers (e.g., as when using terciles).

In addition to the two problems just described, another problem with using log–log survival plots concerns how to evaluate the PH assumption for several variables simultaneously.

One strategy for simultaneous comparisons is to categorize all variables separately, form combinations of categories, and then compare log–log curves for all combinations on the same graph.

A drawback of this strategy is that the data will again tend to "thin out" as the number of combinations gets even moderately large. Also, even if there are sufficient numbers for each combined category, it is often difficult to determine which variables are responsible for any nonparallelism that might be found.

EXAMPLE

As an example of this strategy, suppose we use the remission data again and consider both Rx and log WBC together. Because we previously had two categories of Rx and three categories of log WBC, we get a total of six combined categories, consisting of treated subjects with low log WBC, placebo subjects with low log WBC, treated subjects with medium log WBC, and so on.

Remission Data

Rx \ log WBC	Low	Medium	High
Treatment	✔	✔	✔
Placebo	✔	✔	✔

Log–log $\widehat{\text{KM}}$ curves by six combinations of Rx by log WBC

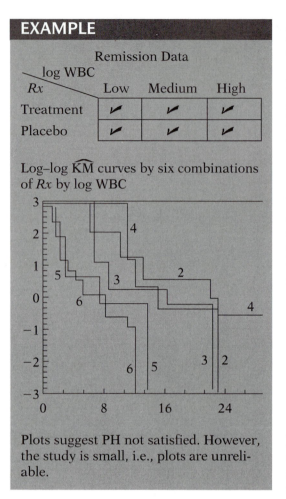

The computer results are shown here for the log–log curves corresponding to each of the six combinations of Rx with log WBC. Notice that there are several points of intersection among the six curves. Therefore, these results suggest that the PH assumption is not satisfied when considering Rx and log WBC together.

Plots suggest PH not satisfied. However, the study is small, i.e., plots are unreliable.

However, the sample sizes used to estimate these curves are quite small, ranging between four subjects for group 4 ($Rx = 1$, log WBC = low) to twelve subjects for group 6 ($Rx = 1$, log WBC = high), with the total study size being 42. Thus, for this small study, the use of six log–log curves provides unreliable information for assessing the PH assumption.

Alternative strategy:
Adjust for predictors already satisfying PH assumption, i.e., use adjusted log–log $\hat{S}$ curves

An alternative graphical strategy for considering several predictors together is to assess the PH assumption for one predictor adjusted for other predictors that are assumed to satisfy the PH assumption. Rather than using Kaplan–Meier curves, this involves a comparison of adjusted log–log survival curves.

Remission data:
- compare *Rx* categories adjusted for log WBC
- fit PH model for each *Rx* stratum
- obtain adjusted survival curves using overall mean of log WBC

Log–log $\hat{S}$ curves for *Rx* groups using PH model adjusted for log WBC

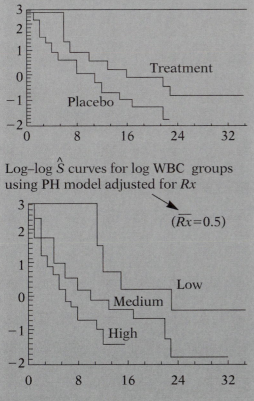

Log–log $\hat{S}$ curves for log WBC groups using PH model adjusted for *Rx*

As an example, again we consider the remission data and the predictors *Rx* and log WBC. To assess the PH assumption for *Rx* adjusted for log WBC, we would compare adjusted log–log survival curves for the two treatment categories, where each adjusted curve is derived from a PH model containing log WBC as a predictor. In computing the adjusted survival curve, we need to stratify the data by treatment, fit a PH model in each stratum, and then obtain adjusted survival probabilities using the overall mean log WBC in the estimated survival curve formula for each stratum.

For the remission data example, the estimated log–log survival curves for the two treatment groups adjusted for log WBC are shown here. Notice that these two curves are roughly parallel, indicating that the PH assumption is satisfied for treatment.

As another example, we consider adjusted log–log survival curves for three categories of log WBC, adjusted for the treatment status (*Rx*) variable. The adjusted survival probabilities in this case use the overall mean *Rx* score, i.e., 0.5, the proportion of the 42 total subjects that are in the placebo group (i.e., half the subjects have a score of *Rx* = 1).

The three log–log curves adjusted for treatment status are shown here. Although two of these curves intersect early in follow-up, they do not suggest a strong departure from parallelism overall, indicating that the PH assumption is satisfied for log WBC, after adjusting for treatment status.

EXAMPLE (continued)

Remission data:
Assess PH assumption for gender:
- use PH model containing Rx and log WBC
- use Rx and log WBC in survival probability formula

Log–log $\hat{S}$ curves for gender adjusted for Rx and log WBC

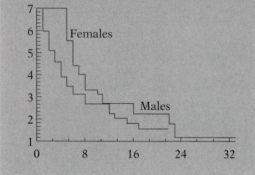

↙1.   log–log survival curves
 2.   observed versus expected survival curves

As a third example, again using the remission data, we assess the PH assumption for gender, adjusting for both treatment status and log WBC in the model. This involves obtaining log–log survival curves for males and females separately, using a PH model that contains both treatment status and log WBC. The adjustment requires using both the overall mean treatment score and the overall mean log WBC score in the formula for the estimated survival probability.

The estimated log–log survival curves for gender, adjusted for treatment and log WBC are shown here. These curves clearly cross, indicating that the PH assumption is not satisfied for gender, after adjusting for treatment and log WBC.

We have thus described and illustrated one of the two graphical approaches for checking the PH assumption, that is, using log–log survival plots. In the next section, we describe an alternative approach that compares "observed" with "expected" survival curves.

IV. Graphical Approach 2: Observed Versus Expected Plots

Graphical analog of GOF test

Both GOF test and plots use observed and expected survival probability estimates.

Two strategies:
1.   One-at-a-time: uses KM curves to obtain observed plots
2.   Adjusting for other variables: uses stratified Cox PH model to obtain observed plots (see Chapter 5)

The use of observed versus expected plots to assess the PH assumption is the graphical analog of the goodness-of-fit (GOF) testing approach to be described later, and is therefore a reasonable alternative to the log–log survival curve approach. In particular, the GOF test uses the same observed and expected survival probability estimates that are used to obtain observed and expected plots.

As with the log–log approach, the observed versus expected approach may be carried out using either or both of two strategies—(1) assessing the PH assumption for variables one-at-a-time, or (2) assessing the PH assumption after adjusting for other variables.

One-at-a-time:
- stratify data by categories of predictor
- obtain KM curves for each category

Here, we describe only the one-at-a-time strategy, which involves using KM curves to obtain observed plots. The strategy which adjusts for other variables uses a stratified Cox PH model to form observed plots, where the PH model contains the variables to be adjusted and the stratified variable is the predictor being assessed. The stratified Cox procedure is described in Chapter 5.

Using the one-at-a-time strategy, we first must stratify our data by categories of the predictor to be assessed. We then obtain observed plots by deriving the KM curves separately for each category.

As an example, for the remission data on 42 leukemia patients we have illustrated earlier, the KM plots for the treatment and placebo groups, with 21 subjects in each group, are shown here. These are the "observed" plots.

EXAMPLE: Remission Data

KM (Observed) Plots by *Rx* Group

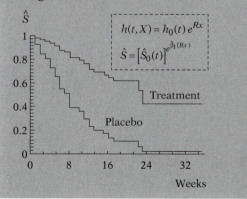

Expected Survival Plots by *Rx* Group
Using PH Model

$$h(t, X) = h_0(t)\, e^{Rx}$$

$$\hat{S} = \left[\hat{S}_0(t)\right]^{e^{\hat{\beta}_1 (Rx)}}$$

To obtain "expected" plots, we fit a Cox PH model containing the predictor being assessed. We obtain expected plots by separately substituting the value for each category of the predictor into the formula for the estimated survival curve, thereby obtaining a separate estimated survival curve for each category.

As an example, again using the remission data, we fit the Cox PH model with *Rx* as its only variable. Using the corresponding survival curve formula for this Cox model, as given in the box at the left, we then obtain separate expected plots by substituting the values of 0 (for treatment group) and 1 (for placebo group). The expected plots are shown here.

EXAMPLE (continued)

Observed Versus Expected Plots by *Rx*

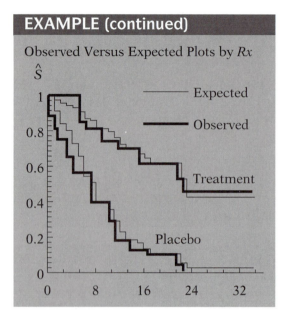

To compare observed with expected plots we then put both sets of plots on the same graph as shown here.

If observed and expected plots are:
- **close**, complies with PH assumption
- **discrepant**, PH assumption violated

If for each category of the predictor being assessed, the observed and expected plots are "close" to one another, we then can conclude that the PH assumption is satisfied. If, however, one or more categories show quite discrepant observed and expected plots, we conclude that the PH assumption is violated.

EXAMPLE: Remission Data (continued)

Observed and expected plots are close for each treatment group.

Conclude PH assumption not violated.

For the example shown above, observed and expected curves appear to be quite close for each treatment group. Thus, we would conclude using this graphical approach that the treatment variable satisfies the PH assumption.

Drawback: How close is close?

Recommend: PH not satisfied *only* when plots are strongly discrepant.

An obvious drawback to this graphical approach is deciding "how close is close" when comparing observed versus expected curves for a given category. This is analogous to deciding "how parallel is parallel" when comparing log–log survival curves. Here, we recommend that the PH assumption be considered as not satisfied only when observed and expected plots are strongly discrepant.

EXAMPLE: Remission Data

Observed Versus Expected Plots by Gender

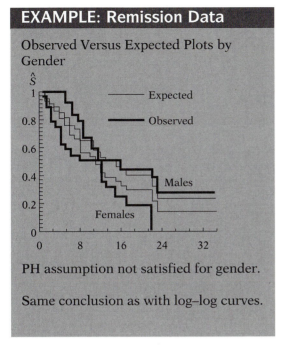

PH assumption not satisfied for gender.

Same conclusion as with log–log curves.

As another example, again using the remission data, we consider observed versus expected plots by gender, as shown here. Note that the observed plots for males and females, which are described by the thicker lines, cross at about 12 weeks, whereas the expected plots don't actually intersect, with the female plot lying below the male plot throughout follow-up. Moreover, for males and females separately, the observed and expected plots are quite different from one another.

Thus, the above plots suggest that the PH assumption is not satisfied for the variable gender. We came to the same conclusion when using log–log survival curves, which crossed one another and were therefore clearly nonparallel.

Continuous variable:
- form strata from categories
- observed plots are KM curves for each category

- two options for expected plots
  1. Use PH model with $k-1$ dummy variables X_i for k categories, i.e.,

$$h(t,\mathbf{X}) = h_0(t)\exp\left(\sum_{i=1}^{k-1}\beta_i X_i\right)$$

Obtain adjusted survival curve:

$$\hat{S}(t,\mathbf{X}_c) = \left[\hat{S}_0(t)\right]^{\exp\left(\sum\hat{\beta}_i X_{ci}\right)}$$

where $X_c = (X_{c1}, X_{c2},..., X_{c,k-1})$

gives values of dummy variables for category c.

When using observed versus expected plots to assess the PH assumption for a continuous variable, observed plots are derived, as for categorical variables, by forming strata from categories of the continuous variable and then obtaining KM curves for each category.

However, for continuous predictors, there are two options available for computing expected plots. One option is to use a Cox PH model which contains $k - 1$ dummy variables to indicate k categories. The expected plot for a given category is then obtained as an adjusted survival curve by substituting the values for the dummy variables that define the given category into the formula for the estimated survival curve, as shown here for category c.

Options for a continuous variable:

2.   Use PH model:

$$h(t, X) = h_0(t) \exp(\beta X)$$

Continuous

Obtain adjusted survival curve:

$$\hat{S}(t, \bar{X}_c) = [\hat{S}_0(t)]^{\exp(\hat{\beta}\bar{X}_c)}$$

where $\bar{X}_c$ denotes the mean value for the variable X within category c.

The second option is to use a Cox PH model containing the continuous predictor being assessed. Expected plots are then obtained as adjusted survival curves by specifying predictor values that distinguish categories, as, for example, when using mean predictor values for each category.

EXAMPLE: Remission Data

Observed (KM) Plots by log WBC Categories

Option 1:

$$h(t, \mathbf{X}) = h_0(t) \exp(\beta_1 X_1 + \beta_2 X_2)$$

where $X_1 = \begin{cases} 1 \text{ if high} \\ 0 \text{ if other} \end{cases}$ $X_2 = \begin{cases} 1 \text{ if medium} \\ 0 \text{ if other} \end{cases}$

so that

high = (1,0); medium = (0,1); low = (0,0)

Expected survival plots:

$X_1 = 1, X_2 = 0: \hat{S}(t, X_{\text{high}}) = [\hat{S}_0(t)]^{\exp(\hat{\beta}_1)}$

$X_1 = 0, X_2 = 1: \hat{S}(t, X_{\text{medium}}) = [\hat{S}_0(t)]^{\exp(\hat{\beta}_2)}$

$X_1 = 0, X_2 = 0: \hat{S}(t, X_{\text{low}}) = [\hat{S}_0(t)]$

As an example to illustrate both options, we consider the continuous variable log WBC from the remission data example. To assess the PH assumption for this variable, we would first stratify log WBC into, say, three categories—low, medium, and high. The observed plots would then be obtained as KM curves for each of the three strata, as shown here.

Using option 1, expected plots would be obtained by fitting a Cox PH model containing two dummy variables X_1 and X_2, as shown here, where X_1 takes the values 1 if high or 0 if other and X_2 takes the values 1 if medium or 0 if other. Thus, when log WBC is high, the values of X_1 and X_2 are 1 and 0, respectively; whereas when log WBC is medium, the values are 0 and 1, respectively; and when log WBC is low, the values are both 0.

The expected survival plots for high, medium, and low categories are then obtained by substituting each of the three specifications of X_1 and X_2 into the formula for the estimated survival curve, and then plotting the three curves.

EXAMPLE (continued)

Expected Plots for log WBC Using Option 1 (Dummy Variables)

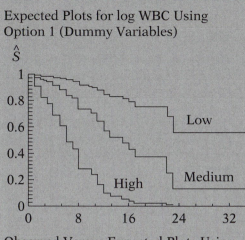

The expected plots using option 1 (the dummy variable approach) are shown here for the three categories of log WBC.

Observed Versus Expected Plots Using Option 1

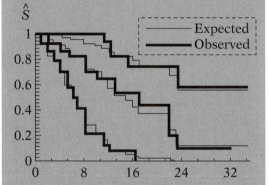

Here we put the observed and expected plots on the same graph. Although there are some discrepancies, particularly early in follow-up for the low log WBC category, these plots suggest overall that the PH assumption is satisfied for log WBC.

Option 2: Treat log WBC as continuous
$$h(t,X) = h_0(t)\exp[\beta(\log \text{WBC})]$$

$\overline{\log \text{WBC}}_{\text{high}} = 3.83$:

$$\hat{S}(t,X_{\text{high}}) = [\hat{S}_0(t)]^{\exp[3.83\hat{\beta}]}$$

$\overline{\log \text{WBC}}_{\text{med}} = 2.64$:

$$\hat{S}(t,X_{\text{med}}) = [\hat{S}_0(t)]^{\exp[2.64\hat{\beta}]}$$

$\overline{\log \text{WBC}}_{\text{low}} = 1.71$:

$$\hat{S}(t,X_{\text{low}}) = [\hat{S}_0(t)]^{\exp[1.71\hat{\beta}]}$$

Using option 2, expected plots would be obtained by first fitting a Cox PH model containing the continuous variable log WBC, as shown here.

Adjusted survival curves are then obtained for specified values of log WBC that summarize the three categories used to form observed curves. Here, we find that the mean log WBC scores for low, medium, and high categories are, respectively, 1.71, 2.64, and 3.83. These values are substituted into the estimated survival curve formula as shown here.

EXAMPLE (continued)

Observed Versus Expected Plots for log WBC Using Option 2

Here are the observed and expected plots using option 2. As with option 1, although there are some discrepancies within categories, overall, these plots indicate that the PH assumption is satisfied for the log WBC variable.

V. The Goodness-of-Fit (GOF) Testing Approach

GOF appealing:
- provides test statistic (or p-value);
- more clear-cut decision than when using graphical approaches.

Reference: Schonfeld (*Biometrika*, 1982)

SPIDA package Schonfeld's method

The GOF method:
- uses a χ^2 statistic with 1 df
- based on observed and expected survival probabilities

The GOF testing approach is appealing because it provides a test statistic or equivalent p-value for assessing the PH assumption for a given predictor of interest. Thus, the researcher can make a more clear-cut decision using a GOF test than is typically possible when using either of the two graphical approaches described above.

Although a number of different GOF tests for assessing the PH assumption have been proposed in the literature, a method originally proposed by Schonfeld (*Biometrika*, 1982) is incorporated into SPIDA's Cox procedure.

The GOF method uses a one-degree-of-freedom chi-square statistic based on observed and expected survival probabilities computed from the data.

SPIDA: gives p-value only, *P(PH)*

P(PH) small $\Rightarrow$ departure from PH
   (e.g., < 0.05)

The SPIDA package, which we have used here, provides the p-value only, without the test statistic. The notation used for this p-value is given as *P(PH)*. A small *P(PH)* value for any predictor indicates a departure from the PH assumption. Following statistical convention, values of *P(PH)* below 0.05 typically are considered to indicate departure from the assumption.

EXAMPLE: Remission Data

Column name	Coeff	StErr	$\cdots$	P(PH)
Rx	1.294	0.422		0.917
log WBC	1.604	0.329		0.944

Both variables satisfy PH assumption.

Note: *P(PH)* = 0.469 assesses PH for log WBC, assuming PH OK for *Rx*.

To illustrate the GOF approach, we again return to the remission data example. The printout shown here gives *P(PH)* values for treatment group and log WBC variables based on fitting a Cox PH model containing these two variables.

The *P(PH)* values for both variables are quite high, indicating that both variables satisfy the PH assumption. Note that each of these p-values tests the assumption for one variable given that the other variable belongs in the model. For example, the *P(PH)* of 0.944 assesses the PH assumption for log WBC, assuming that the PH assumption is satisfied for *Rx*.

EXAMPLE

Column name	Coeff	StErr	$\cdots$	P(PH)
Rx	1.391	0.457		0.935
log WBC	1.594	0.330		0.828
Sex	0.263	0.449		0.038

log WBC and *Rx* satisfy PH.

Sex does not satisfy PH.

(Same conclusions using graphical approaches).

As another example, consider the computer results shown here for a Cox PH model containing the variable, SEX, in addition to log WBC and treatment group. The *P(PH)* values for log WBC and treatment group are still nonsignificant. However, the *P(PH)* value for Sex is significant below the 0.05 level. This result indicates that log WBC and treatment group satisfy the PH assumption, whereas the Sex variable does not. We came to the same conclusions about these variables using the graphical procedures described earlier.

Drawbacks of GOF test:
- global test (i.e., summary statistic); may fail to detect a specific kind of departure from PH.

Although the GOF test we have just described is appealing, it nevertheless has some drawbacks. First, it is a global test, in that it is designed to detect departures from the PH assumption in an overall sense. That is, the test statistic uses all the observed and expected probabilities as a summary statistic. It is possible, however, that this test may fail to detect a specific kind of departure from the PH assumption that may get glossed over in the summary statistic.

Graphical approaches more suitable for detecting specific departures from PH.

The graphical approaches described earlier are more suitable for detecting specific kinds of departures from the PH assumption; the researcher can see what is going on from the graph. Consequently, we recommend that when assessing the PH assumption, the researcher use both graphical procedures and GOF tests before making a final decision.

Recommend: use both graphical and GOF tests.

Drawbacks (continued)
- several strategies to choose from:
  i.   one-at-a-time
  ii. all variables simultaneously
  iii. each variable adjusted for others

Another drawback of GOF tests, which is also a drawback of graphical approaches, concerns the strategy to be used with any of these approaches. One strategy previously described for graphical approaches involves considering predictors one-at-a-time. Another strategy considers all variables simultaneously. A third strategy considers each variable adjusted for other variables assumed to satisfy the PH assumption.

- No one strategy is clearly preferable; researcher may use more than one strategy

Each of these strategies has its own merits, but it has not been demonstrated in the statistical literature that any one strategy is clearly preferable over the others. Consequently, when using the GOF approach, the researcher needs to decide which of several strategies to use and perhaps should consider using more than one strategy.

VI. Assessing the PH Assumption Using Time-Dependent Covariates

When time-dependent variables are used to assess the PH assumption for a time-independent variable, the Cox model is extended to contain product (i.e., interaction) terms involving the time-independent variable being assessed and some function of time.

Extended Cox model:
contains product terms of the form $X \times g(t)$, where $g(t)$ is a function of time.

One-at-a-time model:

$$h(t,\mathbf{X}) = h_0(t) \exp[\beta X + \delta X \times g(t)]$$

When assessing predictors one-at-a-time, the extended Cox model takes the general form shown here for the predictor X.

Some choices for $g(t)$:
$$g(t) = t$$
$$g(t) = \log t$$
$$g(t) = \begin{cases} 1 & \text{if } t \geq t_0 \\ 0 & \text{if } t < t_0 \end{cases} \quad \text{(heaviside function)}$$

One choice for the function $g(t)$ is simply $g(t)$ equal to t, so that the product term takes the form $X \times t$. Other choices for $g(t)$ are also possible, for example, $\log t$.

$H_0: \delta = 0$
Under H_0, the model reduces to:

$h(t,\mathbf{X}) = h_0(t) \exp[\beta X]$

Using the above one-at-a-time model, we assess the PH assumption by testing for the significance of the product term. The null hypothesis is therefore "δ equal to zero." Note that if the null hypothesis is true, the model reduces to a Cox PH model containing the single variable X.

Use either Wald statistic or likelihood ratio statistic:
χ^2 with 1 df under H_0

The test can be carried out using either a Wald statistic or a likelihood ratio statistic. In either case, the test statistic has a chi-square distribution with one degree of freedom under the null hypothesis.

EXAMPLE

$h(t,\mathbf{X}) = h_0(t) \exp[\beta_1 G + \beta_2 (G \times t)]$

where G denotes GENDER

$H_0: \beta_2 = 0 \Rightarrow$ PH assumption satisfied

For example, if the PH assumption is being assessed for GENDER, a Cox model might be extended to include the variable GENDER $\times t$ in addition to GENDER. If the coefficient of the product term turns out to be nonsignificant, we can conclude that the PH assumption is satisfied for GENDER.[2]

Strategies for assessing PH:
- one-at-a-time
- several predictors simultaneously
- for a given predictor adjusted for other predictors

In addition to a one-at-a-time strategy, the extended Cox model can also be used to assess the PH assumption for several predictors simultaneously as well as for a given predictor adjusted for other predictors in the model.

Several predictors simultaneously:

$h(t,\mathbf{X}) = h_0(t) \exp\left(\sum_{i=1}^{p} [\beta_i X_i + \delta_i X_i \times g_i(t)] \right)$

$g(t) = $ function of time for ith predictor

To assess the PH assumption for several predictors simultaneously, the form of the extended model is shown here. This model contains the predictors being assessed as main effect terms and also as product terms with some function of time. Note that different predictors may require different functions of time; hence, the notation $g_i(t)$ is used to define the time function for the ith predictor.

$H_0: \delta_1 = \delta_2 = \ldots = \delta_p = 0$
$LR = -2 \ln \hat{L}_{\text{PH model}} - (-2 \ln \hat{L}_{\text{ext. Cox model}})$
$\dot{\sim} \chi_p^2$ under H_0

Cox PH (reduced) model:

$h(t,\mathbf{X}) = h_0(t) \exp\left(\sum_{i=1}^{p} \beta_i X_i \right)$

With the above model, we test for the PH assumption simultaneously by assessing the null hypothesis that all the δ_i coefficients are equal to zero. This requires a likelihood ratio chi-square statistic with p degrees of freedom, where p denotes the number of predictors being assessed. The LR statistic computes the difference between the log likelihood statistic— $-2 \ln L$ "hat"—for the PH model and the log likelihood statistic for the extended Cox model. Note that under the null hypothesis, the model reduces to the Cox PH model shown here.

---

[2]Actually, if the test for $H_0:\beta_2=0$ is nonsignificant, we can conclude only that the particular version of the extended Cox model being considered is not supported by the data.

EXAMPLE: Remission Data

$$h(t,\mathbf{X}) = h_0(t)\exp[\hat{\beta}_1 (Rx)$$
$$+ \beta_2 (\log WBC) + \beta_3 (gender)$$
$$+ \delta_1 (Rx) \times g(t) + \delta_2 (\log WBC)$$
$$\times g(t) + \delta_3 (gender) \times g(t)]$$

where $g(t) = \begin{cases} 1 & \text{if } t \geq 7 \\ 0 & \text{if } t < 7 \end{cases}$

$H_0: \delta_1 = \delta_2 = \delta_3 = 0$

$LR \sim \chi^2$ with 3 df

If test is significant, use backward elimination to find predictors not satisfying PH assumption.

As an example, we assess the PH assumption for the predictors Rx, log WBC, and gender from the remission data considered previously. The extended Cox model is given as shown here, where the functions $g_i(t)$ have been chosen to be the same "heavyside" function defined by $g(t)$ equals 1 if t is 7 weeks or more and $g(t)$ equals 0 if t is less than 7 weeks. The null hypothesis is that all three δ coefficients are equal to zero. The test statistic is a likelihood-ratio chi-square with 3 degrees of freedom.

If the above test is found to be significant, then we can conclude that the PH assumption is not satisfied for at least one of the predictors in the model. To determine which predictor(s) do not satisfy the PH assumption, we could proceed by backward elimination of nonsignificant product terms until a final model is attained.

Heavyside function: $g(t) = \begin{cases} 1 & \text{if } t \geq 7 \\ 0 & \text{if } t < 7 \end{cases}$

$h(t,\mathbf{X})$ differs for $t \geq 7$ and $t < 7$.

Properties of heavyside functions and numerical results are described in Chapter 6.

Assessing PH for a given predictor adjusted for other predictors:

$$h(t,\mathbf{X}) = h_0(t)\exp\left[\sum_{i=1}^{p-1}\beta_i X_i + \beta * X * + \delta * X * \times g(t)\right]$$

$X*$ = predictor of interest
$H_0: \delta* = 0$
Wald or LR statistic $\sim \chi^2$ with 1 df

Note that the use of a heavyside function for $g(t)$ in the above example yields different expressions for the hazard function depending on whether t is greater than or equal to 7 weeks or t is less than 7 weeks. Chapter 6 provides further details on the properties of heavyside functions, and also provides numerical results from fitting extended Cox models.

We show here an extended Cox model that can be used to evaluate the PH assumption for a given predictor **adjusted for predictors already satisfying the PH assumption.** The predictor of interest is denoted as $X*$, and the predictors considered to satisfy the PH assumption are denoted as X_i. The null hypothesis is that the coefficient $\delta*$ of the product term $X*g(t)$ is equal to zero. The test statistic can either be a Wald statistic or a likelihood ratio statistic, with either statistic having a chi-square distribution with 1 degree of freedom under the null hypothesis.

EXAMPLE: Remission Data

For gender, adjusted for Rx and log WBC:
$$h(t,\mathbf{X}) = h_0(t)\exp[\beta_1 (Rx)$$
$$+ \beta_2 (\log WBC) + \beta* (gender)$$
$$+ \delta* (gender) \times g(t)]$$

As an example, suppose, again considering the remission data, we assess the PH assumption for the variable, GENDER, adjusted for the variables Rx and log WBC, which we assume already satisfy the PH assumption. Then, the extended Cox model for this situation is shown here.

Two computer programs:
1.   Cox PH model
2.   extended Cox model

To carry out the computations for any of the likelihood ratio tests described above, two different types of models, a PH model and an extended Cox model, need to be fit. This essentially requires two different computer programs to fit these two models.

SAS: same procedure (PHREG) used for each model

SPIDA: different procedures (cox, scox, tcox) See Appendix A for computer examples on same dataset.

SAS's PHREG procedure allows the user to fit each type of model using the same procedure. However, other programs, like SPIDA, require different procedures. Appendix A illustrates SPIDA, SAS, and BMDP procedures for fitting extended Cox models to the same dataset.

Drawback: choice of $g_i(t)$

Different choices may lead to different conclusions about PH assumption.

The primary drawback of the use of an extended Cox model for assessing the PH assumption concerns the choice of the functions $g_i(t)$ for the time-dependent product terms in the model. This choice is typically not clear-cut, and it is possible that different choices, such as $g(t)$ equal to t versus log t versus a heavyside function, may result in different conclusions about whether the PH assumption is satisfied.

Chapter 6: Time-dependent covariables

Further discussion of the use of time-dependent covariables in an extended Cox model is provided in Chapter 6.

This presentation:
Three methods for assessing PH.
  i.   graphical
  ii. GOF
  iii. time-dependent covariates

Recommend using at least two methods.

This presentation is now complete. We have described and illustrated three methods for assessing the PH assumption: graphical, goodness-of-fit (GOF), and time-dependent covariate methods. Each of these methods has both advantages and drawbacks. We recommend that the research use at least two of these approaches when assessing the PH assumption.

Chapters

We suggest that the reader review this presentation using the detailed outline that follows. Then answer the practice exercises and the test that follow.

The next Chapter (5) is entitled "The Stratified Cox Procedure." There, we describe how to use a stratification procedure to fit a PH model when one or more of the predictors do not satisfy the PH assumption.

Detailed Outline

I. Background (pages 132–133)

A. The formula for the Cox PH model:

$$h(t, \mathbf{X}) = h_0(t) \exp\left[\sum_{i=1}^{p} \beta_i X_i \right]$$

B. Formula for hazard ratio comparing two individuals, $\mathbf{X^*} = (X_1^*, X_2^*, ..., Xp^*)$ and $\mathbf{X} = (X_1, X_2, ..., X_p)$:

$$\frac{h(t, \mathbf{X^*})}{h(t, \mathbf{X})} = \exp\left[\sum_{i=1}^{p} \beta_i \left(X_i^* - X_i \right) \right]$$

C. Adjusted survival curves using the Cox PH model:

$$S(t, \mathbf{X}) = \left[S_0(t) \right]^{e^{\sum \beta_i X_i}}$$

   i. To graph $S(t, \mathbf{X})$, must specify values for $\mathbf{X} = (X_1, X_2, ..., X_p)$.

   ii. To obtain "adjusted" survival curves, usually use overall mean values for the X's being adjusted.

D. The meaning of the PH assumption

   i. Hazard ratio formula shows that hazard ratio is independent of time:

$$\frac{\hat{h}(t, \mathbf{X^*})}{\hat{h}(t, \mathbf{X})} = \hat{\theta}$$

   ii. Hazard ratio for two X's are proportional: $\hat{h}(t, \mathbf{X^*}) = \hat{\theta}\, \hat{h}(t, \mathbf{X})$

II. Checking the PH assumption: Overview (pages 133–135)

A. Three methods for checking the PH assumption:

   i. Graphical: compare –ln–ln survival curves or observed versus predicted curves.

   ii. Goodness-of-fit test: use a large sample Z statistic.

   iii. Time-dependent covariates: use product (i.e., interaction) terms of the form $X \times g(t)$.

B. Abbreviated illustrations of each method are provided.

III. Graphical approach 1: log–log plots (pages 135–144)

A. A log–log curve is a transformation of an estimated survival curve, where the scale for a log–log curve is $-\infty$ to $+\infty$.

B. The log–log expression for the Cox model survival curve is given by

$$-\ln\left[-\ln S(t, \mathbf{X}) \right] = - \sum_{j=1}^{p} \beta_j X_j - \ln\left[-\ln S_0(t) \right]$$

C. For the Cox model, the log–log survival curve for individual $\mathbf{X}_1$ can be written as the log–log curve for individual $\mathbf{X}_2$ plus a linear sum term that is independent of time t. This formula is given by

$$-\ln\left[-\ln S(t,\mathbf{X}_1)\right] = -\ln\left[-\ln S(t,\mathbf{X}_2)\right] + \sum_{j=1}^{p}\beta_j\left(X_{2j}-X_{1j}\right)$$

D. The above log–log formula can be used to check the PH assumption as follows: the PH model is appropriate if "empirical" plots of log–log survival curves are parallel.

E. Two kinds of empirical plots for $-\ln$–$\ln$ $\hat{S}$:
   i. $\hat{S}$ is a KM curve
   ii. $\hat{S}$ is an adjusted survival curve where predictor being assessed is not included in the Cox regression model.

F. Several examples of log–log plots are provided using remission data from a clinical trial of leukemia patients.

G. Problems with log–log curves:
   i. How parallel is parallel?
   ii. How to categorize a continuous variable?
   iii. How to evaluate several variables simultaneously?

H. Recommendation about problems:
   i. Use small number of categories, meaningful choice, reasonable balance.
   ii. With several variables, two options:
      a. Compare log–log curves from combinations of categories.
      b. Adjust for predictors already satisfying PH assumption.

IV. **Graphical approach 2: observed versus expected plots** (pages 144–150)

A. Graphical analog of the GOF test.

B. Two strategies
   i. One-at-a-time: uses KM curves to obtain observed plots.
   ii. Adjusting for other variables: uses stratified Cox PH model to obtain observed plots.

C. Expected plots obtained by fitting a Cox model containing the predictor being assessed; substitute into the fitted model the value for each category of the predictor to obtain the expected value for each category.

D. If observed and expected plots are close, conclude PH assumption is satisfied.

E. Drawback: how close is close?

F.   Recommend: conclude PH not satisfied *only* if plots are strongly discrepant.

G.   Another drawback: what to do if assessing continuous variable.

H.   Recommend for continuous variable:
  i.   Form strata from categories.
  ii.   Observed plots are KM curves for each category.
  iii.   Two options for expected plots:
    a.   Use PH model with $k - 1$ dummy variables for k categories.
    b.   Use PH model with continuous predictor and specify predictor values that distinguish categories.

V.   **The goodness-of-fit (GOF) approach** (pages 150–152)
  A.   Appealing approach because
    i.   provides a test statistic (p-value).
    ii.   researcher can make clear-cut decision.
  B.   References
    i.   methodological: Schonfeld (*Biometrika*, 1982).
    ii.   computer package: SPIDA(COX).
  C.   The method:
    i.   uses a chi-square statistic with 1 df.
    ii.   based on observed and expected probabilities.
    iii.   SPIDA gives *P(PH)*: If *P* small, then departure from PH.
  D.   Examples using remission data.
  E.   Drawbacks:
    i.   global test: may fail to detect a specific kind of departure from PH; recommend using both graphical and GOF methods.
    ii.   several strategies to choose from, with no one strategy clearly preferable (one-at-a-time, all variables, each variable adjusted for others).

VI.   **Assessing the PH assumption (using time-dependent covariates)** (pages 152–155)
  A.   Use extended Cox model: contains product terms of form $X \times g(t)$, where $g(t)$ is function of time, e.g., $g(t) = t$, or log t, or heavyside function.
  B.   One-at-a-time model: $h(t,\mathbf{X}) = h_0(t) \exp[\beta X + \delta X g(t)]$.
       Test H_0: $\delta = 0$ using Wald or LR test (chi-square with 1 df).
  C.   Evaluating several predictors simultaneously:

$$h(t, \mathbf{X}) = h_0(t) \exp\left(\sum_{i=1}^{p} \left[\beta_i X_i + \delta_i X_i g_i(t)\right]\right)$$

where $g_i(t)$ is function of time for ith predictor. Test H_0: $\delta_1 = \delta_2 = \cdots = \delta_p = 0$ using LR (chi-square) test with p df.

D. Examples using remission data.

E. Two computer programs, required for test:

   i.   Cox PH model program—widely available.

   ii. Extended Cox model program—available in some packages.

F. Drawback: choice of $g(t)$ not always clear; different choices may lead to different conclusions about PH assumption.

Practice Exercises

The dataset "vets.dat" considers survival times in days for 137 patients from the Veteran's Administration Lung Cancer Trial cited by Kalbfleisch and Prentice in their text (*The Statistical Analysis of Survival Time Data*, Wiley, pp. 223–224, 1980). The exposure variable of interest is treatment status (standard = 1, test = 2). Other variables of interest as control variables are cell type (four types, defined by dummy variables), performance status, disease duration, age, and prior therapy status. Failure status is defined by the status variable (0 if censored, 1 if died). A complete list of the variables as stored in a SPIDA file is given below; the actual dataset is provided in Appendix B.

Column 1: Treatment (standard = 1, test = 2)
Column 2: Cell type 1 (large = 1, other = 0)
Column 3: Cell type 2 (adeno = 1, other = 0)
Column 4: Cell type 3 (small = 1, other = 0)
Column 5: Cell type 4 (squamous = 1, other = 0)
Column 6: Survival time (days)
Column 7: Performance status (0 = worst, $\cdots$, 100 = best)
Column 8: Disease duration (months)
Column 9: Age
Column 10: Prior therapy (none = 0, some = 10)
Column 11: Status (0 = censored, 1 = died)

1. State the hazard function form of the Cox PH model that describes the effect of the treatment variable and controls for the variables, cell type, performance status, disease duration, age, and prior therapy. In stating this model, make sure to incorporate the cell type variable using dummy variables, but do not consider possible interaction variables in your model.

2. State three general approaches that can be used to evaluate whether the PH assumption is satisfied for the variables included in the model you have given in question 1.

3. The following printout is obtained from fitting a Cox PH model to these data. Using the information provided, what can you conclude about whether the PH assumption is satisfied for the variables used in the model? Explain briefly.

Response: Surv. Time

Column name	Coeff	StErr	p-value	HR	0.95	CI	P(PH)
1 Treatment	0.290	0.207	0.162	1.336	0.890	2.006	0.629
2 Large cell	0.400	0.283	0.157	1.491	0.857	2.594	0.035
3 Adeno cell	1.188	0.301	0.000	3.281	1.820	5.915	0.083
4 Small cell	0.856	0.275	0.002	2.355	1.374	4.037	0.080
7 Performance status	−0.033	0.006	0.000	0.968	0.958	0.978	0.000
8 Disease duration	0.000	0.009	0.992	1.000	0.982	1.018	0.919
9 Age	−0.009	0.009	0.358	0.991	0.974	1.010	0.199
10 Prior therapy	0.007	0.023	0.755	1.007	0.962	1.054	0.147

4. For the variables used in the PH model in question 3, describe a strategy for evaluating the PH assumption using log–log survival curves for variables considered one-at-a-time.

5. Again considering the variables used in question 3, describe a strategy for evaluating the PH assumption using log–log survival curves that are adjusted for other variables in the model.

6. For the variable "performance status," describe how you would evaluate the PH assumption using observed versus expected survival plots?

7. For the variable "performance status," log–log plots which compare high (≥ 50) with low (< 50) are given by the following graph. Based on this graph, what do you conclude about the PH assumption with regard to this variable?

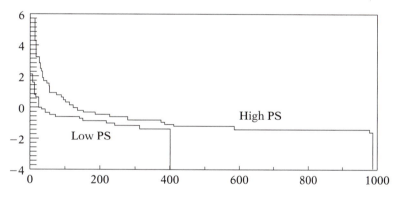

8. What are some of the drawbacks of using the log–log approach for assessing the PH assumption and what do you recommend to deal with these drawbacks?

9. For the variable "performance status," observed versus expected plots that compare high (≥ 50) with low (< 50) are given by the following graph. Based on this graph, what do you conclude about the PH assumption with regard to this variable?

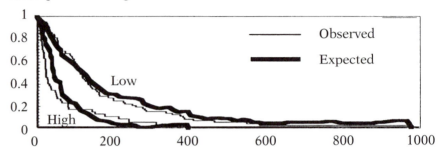

10. State the form of an extended Cox model that allows for the one-at-a-time assessment of the PH assumption for the variable "performance status," and describe how you would carry out a statistical test of the assumption for this variable.

11. State the form of an extended Cox model that allows for the simultaneous assessment of the PH assumption for the variables cell type, performance status, disease duration, age, and prior therapy. For this model, describe how you would carry out a statistical test of the PH assumption for these variables. Also, provide a strategy for assessing which of these variables satisfy the PH assumption and which do not using the extended Cox model approach.

12. Using any of the information provided above and any additional analyses that you perform with this dataset (see Appendix B for a listing), what do you conclude about which variables satisfy the PH assumption and which variables do not? In answering this question, summarize any additional analyses performed.

Test

The following questions consider a dataset from a study by Caplehorn et al. ("Methadone Dosage and Retention of Patients in Maintenance Treatment," *Med. J. Aust.*, 1991). These data comprise the times in days spent by heroin addicts from entry to departure from one of two methadone clinics. There are two additional covariates, namely, prison record and maximum methadone dose, believed to affect the survival times. The dataset name is **addicts.dat.** A listing of the data as stored in a SPIDA file is given in Appendix B. A listing of the variables is given below:

Column 1: Subject ID
Column 2: Clinic (1 or 2)
Column 3: Survival status (0 = censored, 1 = departed from clinic)
Column 4: Survival time in days
Column 5: Prison record (0 = none, 1 = any)
Column 6: Maximum methadone dose (mg/day)

1. The following printout was obtained from fitting a Cox PH model to these data:

    Cox Regression Analysis
    Response: days survival

Column name	Coeff	StErr	p-value	HR	0.95	CI	P(PH)
2 Clinic	–1.009	0.215	0.000	0.365	0.239	0.556	0.001
5 Prison	0.327	0.167	0.051	1.386	0.999	1.924	0.333
6 Dose	–0.035	0.006	0.000	0.965	0.953	0.977	0.348

    n: 238   %Cen: 36.975   –2 log *L*: 1346.805   #iter: 5

    Based on the information provided in this printout, what do you conclude about which variables satisfy the PH assumption and which do not? Explain briefly.

2. Suppose that for the model fit in question 1, log–log survival curves for each clinic adjusted for prison and dose are plotted on the same graph. Assume that these curves are obtained by substituting into the formula for the estimated survival curve the values for each clinic and the overall mean values for the prison and dose variables. Below, we show these two curves. Are they parallel? Explain your answer.

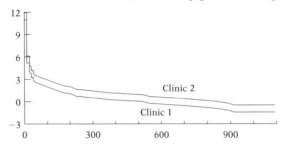

3. The following printout was obtained from fitting a stratified Cox PH model to these data, where the variable being stratified is clinic:

Stratified Cox Regression Analysis on Variable: clinic
Response: days survival

Column name	Coeff	StErr	p-value	HR	0.95	CI
5 Prison	0.389	0.169	0.021	1.475	1.059	2.054
6 Dose	−0.035	0.006	0.000	0.965	0.953	0.978
n: 238		%Cen: 36.975		−2 log L: 1195.428 #iter: 5		

Using the above fitted model, we can obtain the log–log curves below that compare the log–log survival for each clinic (i.e., stratified by clinic) adjusted for the variables prison and dose. Using these curves, what do you conclude about whether or not the clinic variable satisfies the PH assumption? Explain briefly.

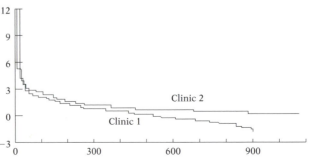

4. Consider the two plots of log–log curves below that compare the log–log survival for the prison variable ignoring other variables and adjusted for the clinic and dose variables. Using these curves, what do you conclude about whether or not the prison variable satisfies the PH assumption? Explain briefly.

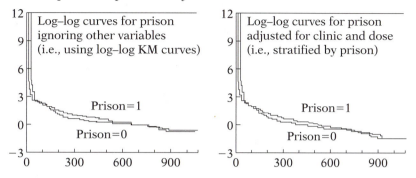

5. How do your conclusions from question 1 compare with your conclusions from question 4? If the conclusions differ, which conclusion do you prefer? Explain.

6. Describe briefly how you would evaluate the PH assumption for the variable maximum methadone dose using observed versus expected plots.

7. State an extended Cox model that would allow you to assess the PH assumption for the variables clinic, prison, and dose simultaneously. For this model, state the null hypothesis for the test of the PH assumption and describe how the likelihood ratio statistic would be obtained and what its degrees of freedom would be under the null hypothesis.

8. State at least one drawback to the use of the extended Cox model approach described in question 7.

9. State an extended Cox model that would allow you to assess the PH assumption for the variable clinic alone, assuming that the prison and dose variables already satisfy the PH assumption. For this model, state the null hypothesis for the test of the PH assumption, and describe how the likelihood ratio (LR) statistic would be obtained. What is the degrees of freedom of the LR test under the null hypothesis?

10. Consider the situation described in question 9, where you wish to use an extended Cox model that would allow you to assess the PH assumption for the variable clinic alone, assuming that the assumption is satisfied for the prison and dose variables. Suppose you use the following extend Cox model:

$h(t,\mathbf{X}) = h_0(t)\exp[\beta_1(\text{prison}) + \beta_2(\text{dose}) + \beta_3(\text{clinic}) + \delta(\text{clinic})g(t)]$

where $g(t)$ is defined as follows:

$$g(t) = \begin{cases} 1 & \text{if } t > 365 \text{ days} \\ 0 & \text{if } t \le 365 \text{ days} \end{cases}$$

For the above model, what is the formula for the hazard ratio that compares clinic 1 to clinic 2 when t is greater than 365 days? when t is less than or equal to 365 days? In terms of the hazard ratio formulae just described, what specific departure from the PH assumption is being tested when the null hypothesis is H_0: $\delta = 0$?

Answers to Practice Exercises

1. $h(t,\mathbf{X}) = h_0(t)\exp[\beta_1(\text{treatment}) + \beta_2(\text{CT1}) + \beta_3(\text{CT2}) + \beta_4(\text{CT3}) + \beta_7(\text{PS}) + \beta_8(\text{DD}) + \beta_9(\text{Age}) + \beta_{10}(\text{PT})]$

   where CTi denotes the cell type i dummy variable, PS denotes the performance status variable (#7), DD denotes the disease duration variable (#8), Age is variable #9, and PT denotes the prior therapy variable (#10).

2. The three general approaches for assessing the PH model for the above model are

   (a) graphical, using either log–log plots or observed versus expected plots;
   (b) goodness-of-fit test;
   (c) an extended Cox model containing product terms involving the variables being assessed with some function(s) of time.

3. The *P(PH)* values given in the printout provide goodness-of-fit tests for each variable in the fitted model adjusted for the other variables in the model. The *P(PH)* values shown indicate that the large cell type variables and the performance status variable do not satisfy the PH assumption, whereas the treatment, age, disease duration, and prior therapy variables satisfy the PH assumption, and the adeno and small cell type variable are of borderline significance.

4. A strategy for evaluating the PH assumption using log–log survival curves for variables considered one-at-a-time is given as follows:

    Obtain log–log Kaplan–Meier curves for each variable separately. For the cell type variable, this requires obtaining four log–log KM curves, one for each cell type. (Note that this is not the same as obtaining four separate plots of two log–log curves, where each plot corresponds to one of the dummy variables used in the model.) For the variables PS, DD, and Age, which are interval variables, each variable must be separately categorized into two or more groups—say, low versus high values—and KM plots are obtained for each group. For the variable PT, which is a dichotomous variable, two log–log plots are obtained which compare the "none" versus "some" groups.

    For each set of plots (i.e., one set for each variable), those plots that are noticeably nonparallel indicate variables which do not satisfy the PH assumption. The remaining variables are assumed to satisfy the PH assumption.

5. One strategy for evaluating the PH assumption for each variable adjusted for the others is to use adjusted log–log survival curves instead of KM curves separately for each of the variables in the model. That is, for each variable separately, a stratified Cox model is fit stratifying on the given variable while adjusting for the other variables. Those variables that yield adjusted log–log plots that are noticeably nonparallel are then to be considered as not satisfying the PH assumption. The remaining variables are assumed to satisfy the PH assumption.

    A variation of the above strategy uses adjusted log–log curves for only those variables *not satisfying* the PH assumption from a one-at-a-time approach, adjusting for those variables *satisfying* the PH assumption from the one-at-a-time approach. This second iteration would flag a subset of the one-at-a-time flagged variables for further iteration. At each new iteration, those variables found to satisfy the assumption get added to the list of variables previously determined to satisfy the assumption.

6.   For the performance status (PS) variable, **observed plots** are obtained by categorizing the variable into strata (say, two strata: low versus high) and then obtaining KM survival plots for each stratum. **Expected plots** can be obtained by fitting a Cox model containing the (continuous) PS variable and then obtaining estimated survival curves for values of the performance status (PS) variable that represent summary descriptive statistics for the strata previously identified. For example, if there are two strata, say, high (PS > 50) and low (PS ≤ 50), then the values of PS to be used could be the mean or median PS score for persons in the high stratum and the mean or median PS score for persons in the low stratum.

An alternative method for obtaining expected plots involves first dichotomizing the PS variable—say, into high and low groups—and then fitting a Cox model containing the dichotomized PS variable instead of the original continuous variable. The expected survival plots for each group are estimated survival curves obtained for each value of the dichotomized PS variable.

Once observed and expected plots are obtained for each stratum of the PS variable, they are then compared on the same graph to determine whether or not corresponding observed and expected plots are "close." If it is determined that, overall, comparisons for each stratum are close, then it is concluded that the PH assumption is satisfied for the PH variable. In determining how close is close, the researcher should look for noticeably discrepant observed versus expected plots.

7.   The log–log plots that compare high versus low PS groups (ignoring other variables) are *arguably* parallel early in follow-up, and are not comparable later because survival times for the two groups do not overlap after 400 days. These plots do not strongly indicate that the PH assumption is violated for the variable PS. This contradicts the conclusion previously obtained for the PS variable using the *P(PH)* results.

8.   Drawbacks of the log–log approach are:

- How parallel is parallel?
- How to categorize a continuous variable?
- How to evaluate several variables simultaneously?

Recommendations about problems:

- Look for noticeable nonparallelism; otherwise PH assumption is OK.
- For continuous variables, use a small number of categories, a meaningful choice of categories, and a reasonable balance in sample size for categories.

- With several variables, there are two options:

  i. Compare log–log curves from combinations of categories.
  ii. Adjust for predictors already satisfying PH assumption.

9. The observed and expected plots are relatively close for low and high groups separately, although there is somewhat more discrepancy for the high group than for the low group. Deciding how close is close is quite subjective for these plots. Nevertheless, because there are no major discrepancies for either low or high groups, we consider the PH assumption satisfied for this variable.

10. $h(t,\mathbf{X}) = h_0(t)\exp[\beta_1(PS) + \delta(PS)g(t)]$

    where $g(t)$ is a function of t, such as $g(t) = t$, or $g(t) = \log t$, or a heavyside function. The PH assumption is tested using a 1 df Wald or LR statistic for H_0: $\delta = 0$.

11. $h(t,\mathbf{X}) = h_0(t)\exp[\beta_1(\text{treatment}) + \beta_2(CT1) + \beta_3(CT2) + \beta_4(CT3) + \beta_5(PS) + \beta_6(DD) + \beta_7(Age) + \beta_8(PT) + \delta_1(\text{treatment}) \times g(t) + \delta_2(CT1) \times g(t) + \delta_3(CT2) \times g(t) + \delta_4(CT3) \times g(t) + \delta_5(PS) \times g(t) + \delta_6(DD) \times g(t) + \delta_7(Age) \times g(t) + \delta_8(PT) \times g(t)]$

    where $g(t)$ is some function of time, such as $g(t) = t$, or $g(t) = \log t$, or a heavyside function. To test the PH assumption simultaneously for all variables, the null hypothesis is stated as H_0: $\delta_1 = \delta_2 = \ldots = \delta_8 = 0$. The test statistic is a likelihood-ratio statistic of the form

    $$LR = -2 \ln \hat{L}_R - (-2 \ln \hat{L}_F)$$

    where R denotes the reduced (PH) model obtained when all δ's are 0, and F denotes the full model given above. Under H_0, the LR statistic is approximately chi-square with 8 df.

12. The question here is somewhat open-ended, leaving the reader the option to explore additional graphical, GOF, or extended Cox model approaches for evaluating the PH assumption for the variables in the model. The conclusions from the GOF statistics provided in question 1 are likely to hold up under further scrutiny, so that a reasonable conclusion is that cell type and performance status variables do not satisfy the PH assumption, with the remaining variables satisfying the assumption. The only other variable that is questionable (from the GOF results) is the prior therapy variable, because its $P(PH)$ value of 0.07 is close to significance. A graphical look at this variable (using log–log or observed versus expected plots) would provide further information about the PH assumption for this variable.

5

The Stratified Cox Procedure

■ **Contents**

Introduction

We begin with an example of the use of the stratified Cox procedure for a single predictor that does not satisfy the PH assumption. We then describe the general approach for fitting a stratified Cox model, including the form of the (partial) likelihood function used to estimate model parameters.

We also describe the assumption of no interaction that is typically incorporated into most computer programs that carry out the stratified Cox procedure. We show how the no-interaction assumption can be tested, and what can be done if interaction is found.

We conclude with a second example of the stratified Cox procedure in which more than one variable is stratified.

Abbreviated Outline

The outline below gives the user a preview of the material to be covered by the presentation. A detailed outline for review purposes follows the presentation.

Objectives

Upon completing the module, the learner should be able to:

1. Recognize a computer printout for a stratified Cox procedure.
2. State the hazard form of a stratified Cox model for a given survival analysis scenario and/or a given set of computer results for such a model.
3. Evaluate the effect of a predictor of interest based on computer results from a stratified Cox procedure.
4. For a given survival analysis scenario and/or a given set of computer results involving a stratified Cox model,
   - state the no-interaction assumption for the given model;
   - describe and/or carry out a test of the no-interaction assumption;
   - describe and/or carry out an analysis when the no-interaction assumption is not satisfied.

I. Preview

Stratified Cox model:
- modification of Cox PH model
- Stratification of predictor not satisfying PH
- includes predictors satisfying PH

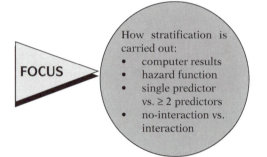

FOCUS

How stratification is carried out:
- computer results
- hazard function
- single predictor vs. ≥ 2 predictors
- no-interaction vs. interaction

The "stratified Cox model" is a modification of the Cox proportional hazards (PH) model that allows for control by "stratification" of a predictor that does not satisfy the PH assumption. Predictors that are assumed to satisfy the PH assumption are included in the model, whereas the predictor being stratified is not included.

In this presentation, we focus on how stratification is carried out by describing the analysis of computer results and the form of the hazard function for a stratified Cox model. We first consider stratifying on a single predictor and then later consider stratifying on two or more predictors. Further, we distinguish between the use of a "no-interaction" version of the stratified Cox model and an alternative approach that allows interaction.

II. An Example

EXAMPLE

Clinical trial: 42 leukemia patients
Response-days in remission

Column name	Coeff	StErr	P(PH)
log WBC	1.594	0.330	0.828
Rx	1.391	0.457	0.935
Sex	0.263	0.449	0.038

- log WBC and *Rx* satisfy PH
- Sex does not satisfy PH

(Same conclusions using graphical approaches)

Stratified Cox (SC):
- control for sex (stratified);
- simultaneously include log WBC and *Rx* in the model

Consider the computer results shown here for a Cox PH model containing the three variables, log WBC, treatment group (*Rx*), and SEX. These results derive from a clinical trial of 42 leukemia patients, where the response of interest is days in remission. The computer package used here is SPIDA; see Appendix A for examples of SAS and BMDP procedures.

From the printout, the *P(PH)* values for log WBC and treatment group are nonsignificant. However, the *P(PH)* values for SEX is significant below the .05 level and almost at the .01 level. These results indicate that log WBC and treatment group satisfy the PH assumption, whereas the SEX variable does not. The same conclusions regarding the PH assumption about these variables would also be made using the graphical procedures described earlier.

Because we have a situation where one of the predictors does not satisfy the PH assumption, we carry out a stratified Cox (SC) procedure for the analysis. Using SC, we can control for the SEX variable—which does not satisfy the PH assumption—by stratification while simultaneously including in the model the log WBC and treatment variables—which do satisfy the PH assumption.

EXAMPLE (continued)

SPIDA OUTPUT USING SC:
Stratified Cox Regression Analysis on
Variable: (sex)
Response: Surv

Column

Name	Coeff	StErr	p-value	*HR*	0.95	CI
4 log WBC	1.390	0.338	0.000	4.016	2.072	7.783
5 Rx	(0.931)	0.472	0.048	(2.537)	1.006	6.396

n:42   %Cen: 28.571   –2 log *L*: (115.119)   # iter:6

Appendix A illustrates SC procedures using SPIDA, SAS, and BMDP.

- Log WBC and *Rx* are included in SC model.
- SC model is stratified by SEX variable.

Effect of *Rx* adjusted for log WBC and SEX:
- Hazard ratio: $2.537 = e^{0.931}$
- Interpretation: Placebo group (*Rx* = 1) has 2.5 times the hazard as the treatment group (Rx = 0)

Stratified Cox Regression Analysis on
Variable: sex
Response: Surv

Column

name	Coeff	StErr	p-value	*HR*	0.95	CI
4 log WBC	1.390	0.338	0.000	1.016	2.072	7.783
5 Rx	(0.931	0.472)	0.048	2.537	(1.006	6.396)

n:42   %Cen: 28.571   – 2log *L*: (115.119)   # iter:6

95% CI for *Rx* (1.006, 6.396) indicates considerable variability.

CI formula: $\exp(0.931 \pm 1.96 \times 0.472)$

The computer results from a SC procedure are shown here. These results come from the SPIDA package. Other packages, like SAS and BMD, also have SC procedures; their output provides essentially the same information as SPIDA, although the layout of results may vary somewhat from SPIDA's layout. In Appendix A, we illustrate SC procedures applied to the same data set using SPIDA, SAS, and BMDP packages.

The computer results show that the log WBC and *Rx* variables are included in the model listing, whereas the sex variable is not included; rather, the model stratifies on the SEX variable, as indicated at the top of the output. Note that the SEX variable is being adjusted by stratification, whereas log WBC is being adjusted by its inclusion in the model along with *Rx*.

In the above output, we have also circled some key information that can be used to assess the effect of the *Rx* variable adjusted for both log WBC and SEX. In particular, we can see that the hazard ratio for the effect of *Rx* adjusted for log WBC and SEX is given by the value 2.537. This value can be obtained by exponentiating the coefficient 0.931 of the *Rx* variable. The hazard ratio value can be interpreted to mean that the placebo group (for which *Rx* = 1) has 2.5 times the hazard for going out of remission as the treatment group (for which *Rx* = 0).

Also, we can see from the output that a 95% confidence interval for the effect of the *Rx* variable is given by the limits 1.006 to 6.396. This is a fairly wide range, thus indicating considerable variability in the 2.537 hazard ratio point estimate. Note that these confidence limits can be obtained by exponentiating the quantity 0.931 plus or minus 1.96 times the standard error 0.472.

EXAMPLE (continued)

Wald test: P = 0.048 (two-tailed), significant at the 0.05 level.

LR test: Output for reduced model
Stratified Cox Regression Analysis on Variable: sex
Response: Surv

Column name	Coeff	StErr	p-value	HR	0.95	CI
4 log WBC	1.456	0.320	0	4.289	2.291	8.03

n:42   %Cen: 28.571   −2 log *L*: (119.297) # iter: 5

LR = 119.297 − 115.119 = 4.178 (*P* < 0.05)

LR and Wald give same conclusion.

Hazard function for stratified Cox model:

$$h_g(t,\mathbf{X}) = h_{0g}(t)\exp[\beta_1 Rx + \beta_2 \log WBC]$$
$$g = 1,2;$$
g denotes stratum #.

SC model for males and females:
Females ($g = 1$):
$$h_1(t,\mathbf{X}) = h_{01}(t)\exp[\beta_1 Rx + \beta_2 \log WBC]$$
Males ($g = 2$):
$$h_2(t,\mathbf{X}) = h_{02}(t)\exp[\beta_1 Rx + \beta_2 \log WBC]$$

Rx and log WBC in the model
Sex *not* in the model (stratified)

From the above output, a test for the significance of the *Rx* variable adjusted for log WBC and SEX is given by the Wald statistic P value of 0.048. This is a two-tailed P-value, and the test is just significant at the 0.05 level.

An alternative test involves a likelihood ratio (*LR*) statistic that compares the above (full model) with a reduced model that does not contain the *Rx* variable. The output for the reduced model is shown here. The log-likelihood statistic for the reduced model is 119.297, which is to be compared with the log-likelihood statistic of 115.119 for the full model.

The *LR* statistic is therefore 119.297 minus 115.119, which equals 4.178. This statistic has a chi-square distribution with one degree of freedom and is significant at the 0.05 level. Thus, the *LR* and Wald tests give the same conclusion.

So far, we have illustrated the results from a stratified Cox procedure without actually describing the model form being used. For the remission data example, we now present the hazard function form for the stratified Cox model, as shown here. This hazard function formula contains a subscript g that indicates the gth stratum.

Thus, in our remission data example, where we have stratified on SEX, g takes on one of two values, so that we have a different hazard function for males and females.

Notice that the hazard function formula contains the variables *Rx* and log WBC, but does not contain the variable SEX. SEX is not included in the model because it doesn't satisfy the PH assumption. So, instead, the SEX variable is controlled by stratification.

$\widehat{HR}$ for effect of Rx adjusted for log WBC and sex:

$e^{\hat{\beta}_1}$

where β_1 is the coefficient of Rx.

Cannot estimate HR for SEX variable (SEX doesn't satisfy PH).

Different baseline hazard functions: $h_{01}(t)$ for females and $h_{02}(t)$ for males.

Same coefficients β_1 and β_2 for both female and male models.

Different baselines $\begin{cases} h_{01}(t) \Rightarrow \text{Survival curve} \\ \qquad\quad \text{for females} \\ h_{02}(t) \Rightarrow \text{Survival curve} \\ \qquad\quad \text{for males} \end{cases}$

Female and males:
same β_1 and $\beta_2 \Rightarrow$ same $\widehat{HR}$'s, e.g., $e^{\hat{\beta}_1}$

No interaction assumption
(see Section IV)

Because the variables Rx and log WBC are included in the model, we can estimate the effect of each variable adjusted for the other variable and the SEX variable using standard exponential hazard ratio expressions. For example, the estimated hazard ratio for the effect of Rx, adjusted for log WBC and SEX, is given by e to the β_1 "hat," where β_1 is the coefficient of the Rx variable.

Nevertheless, because the SEX variable is not included in the model, it is not possible to obtain a hazard ratio value for the effect of SEX adjusted for the other two variables. This is the price to be paid for stratification on the SEX variable. Note that a single value for the hazard ratio for SEX is not appropriate if SEX doesn't satisfy the PH assumption, because the hazard ratio must then vary with time.

Notice also that the hazard functions for males and females differ only insofar as they have different baseline hazard functions, namely, $h_{01}(t)$ for females and $h_{02}(t)$ for males. However, the coefficients β_1 and β_2 are the same for both female and male models.

Because there are different baseline hazard functions, the fitted stratified Cox model will yield different estimated survival curves for females and males. These curves will be described shortly.

Note, however, that because the coefficients of Rx and log WBC are the same for females and males, estimates of hazard ratios, such as e to the β_1 "hat," are the same for both females and males. This feature of the stratified Cox model is called the "no-interaction" assumption. It is possible to evaluate whether this assumption is tenable and to modify the analysis if not tenable. We will discuss this assumption further in Section IV.

EXAMPLE (continued)

Estimates of β_1 and β_2:
Maximize partial likelihood (L),
where $L = L_1 \times L_2$
L_1 is the likelihood for females derived from $h_1(t)$,
and L_2 is the likelihood for males derived from $h_2(t)$.

Adjusted Survival Curves for Rx
from Stratified Cox Model
(adjusted for log WBC)

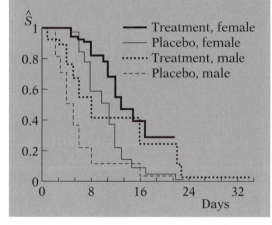

To obtain estimates of β_1 and β_2, a (partial) likelihood function (L) is formed from the model and the data; this function is then maximized using computer iteration. The likelihood function (L) for the stratified Cox (SC) model is different from the nonstratified Cox model. For the SC model, L is obtained by multiplying together likelihood functions for each stratum. Thus, L is equal to the product of L_1 and L_2, where L_1 and L_2 denote the female and male likelihood functions, respectively, which are derived from their respective hazard functions $h_1(t)$ and $h_2(t)$.

As mentioned above, adjusted survival curves can be obtained for each stratum as shown here. Here we have shown *four* survival curves because we want to compare the survival for two treatment groups over each of two strata.

If we compare treatment and placebo group separately by sex, we can see that the treatment group has consistently better survival prognosis than the placebo group for females and males separately. This supports our findings about the hazard ratio for the treatment effect derived earlier from the computer results for the stratified Cox model.

III. The General Stratified Cox (SC) Model

Example: one binary predictor
↓
General: several predictors, several strata

$Z_1, Z_2, ..., Z_k$, do not satisfy PH

$X_1, X_2, ..., X_p$, satisfy PH

In the previous example, we illustrated the SC model for one binary predictor not satisfying the PH assumption. We now describe the general form of the SC model that allows for stratification of several predictors over several strata.

We assume that we have k variables not satisfying the PH assumption and p variables satisfying the PH assumption. The variables not satisfying the PH assumption we denote as $Z_1, Z_2, \ldots, Z_k$; the variables satisfying the PH assumption we denote as $X_1, X_2, \ldots, X_p$.

Define a single new variable Z^*:
1. categorize each Z_i
2. form combinations of categories (strata)
3. the strata are the categories of Z^*

To perform the stratified Cox procedure, we define a single new variable, which we call Z^*, from the Z's to be used for stratification. We do this by forming categories of each Z_i, including those Z_i that are interval variables. We then form combinations of categories, and these combinations are our strata. These strata are the categories of the new variable Z^*.

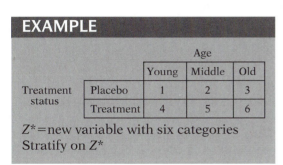

EXAMPLE

		Age		
		Young	Middle	Old
Treatment status	Placebo	1	2	3
	Treatment	4	5	6

Z^*=new variable with six categories
Stratify on Z^*

For example, suppose k is 2, and the two Z's are age (an interval variable) and treatment status (a binary variable). Then we categorize age into, say, three age groups—young, middle, and old. We then form six age group–by–treatment-status combinations, as shown here. These six combinations represent the different categories of a single new variable that we stratify for our stratified Cox model. We call this new variable Z^*.

Z^* has k^* categories where $k^* =$ total # of combinations (strata), e.g., $k^* = 6$ in above example.

In general, the stratification variable Z^* will have k^* categories, where k^* is the total number of combinations (or strata) formed after categorizing each of the Z's. In the above example, k^* is equal to 6.

The general SC model:
$h_g(t,\mathbf{X}) = h_{0g}(t)\exp[\beta_1 X_1 + \beta_2 X_2 + \cdots + \beta_p X_p]$
$g = 1, 2, ..., k^*$, strata defined from Z^*

We now present the general hazard function form for the stratified Cox model, as shown here. This formula contains a subscript g which indicates the gth stratum. The strata are defined as the different categories of the stratification variable Z^*, and the number of strata equals k^*.

Z^* not included in the model

$X_1, X_2, ..., X_p$ included in the model

Note that the variable Z^* is not explicitly included in the model but that the X's, which are assumed to satisfy the PH assumption, are included in the model.

Different baseline hazard functions:
$h_{0g}(t), g = 1, 2, ..., k^*$
Same coefficients: $\beta_1, \beta_2, ..., \beta_p$

Note also that the baseline hazard function $h_{0g}(t)$ is allowed to be different for each stratum. However, the coefficients $\beta_1, \beta_2, \ldots, \beta_p$ are the same for each stratum.

Different baselines
$$\begin{cases} \hat{h}_{01}(t) \Rightarrow \hat{S}_1(t) \\ \hat{h}_{02}(t) \Rightarrow \hat{S}_2(t) \\ \vdots \\ \hat{h}_{0k}(t) \Rightarrow \hat{S}_k(t) \end{cases} \text{Different survival curves}$$

As previously described by example, the fitted SC model will yield different estimated survival curves for each stratum because the baseline hazard functions are different for each stratum.

$\widehat{HR}$ same for each stratum

(no-interaction assumption, Section IV)

(Partial) likelihood function:
$$L = L_1 \times L_2, \times \cdots \times L_{k*}$$

Strata:	1	2	...	$k*$
Likelihood:	L_1	L_2	...	L_k
Hazard:	$h_1(t,\mathbf{X})$	$h_2(t,\mathbf{X})$	...	$h_{k*}(t,\mathbf{X})$

However, because the coefficients of the X's are the same for each stratum, estimates of hazard ratios are the same for each stratum. This latter feature of the SC model is what we previously have called the "no-interaction" assumption to be discussed further in Section IV.

To obtain estimates of the regression coefficients β_1, $\beta_2, \ldots, \beta_p$, we maximize a (partial) likelihood function L that is obtained by multiplying together likelihood functions for each stratum, as shown here. Thus, L is equal to the product of L_1 times L_2, and so on, up until L_{k*}, where the subscripted L's denote the likelihood function for different strata, with each of these L's being derived from its corresponding hazard function.

IV. The No-Interaction Assumption and How to Test It

Stratified Cox model
$$h_g(t,\mathbf{X}) = h_{0g}(t)\exp[\beta_1 X_1 + \beta_2 X_2 + \cdots + \beta_p X_p]$$

β coefficients do not vary over strata
(no-interaction assumption)
- how to evaluate
- what to do if violated

We previously pointed out that the SC model contains regression coefficients, denoted as β's, that do not vary over the strata. We have called this property of the model the "no-interaction assumption." In this section, we explain what this assumption means. We also describe how to evaluate the assumption and what to do if the assumption is violated.

EXAMPLE

No-interaction SC model:
Stratified Cox Regression Analysis on
Variable: sex
Response: Surv

Column name	Coeff	StErr	p-value	HR	0.95	CI
4 log WBC	1.390	0.338	0.000	4.016	2.072	7.783
5 Rx	0.931	0.472	0.048	2.537	1.006	6.396
n:42	%Cen: 28.571		−2 log L:	115.119	# iter: 6	

We return to the SC output previously illustrated. Notice that only one set of coefficients, namely, 1.390 for log WBC and 0.931 for Rx, are provided, even though there are two strata, one for females and one for males. These results assume no interaction of the sex variable with either log WBC or Rx.

EXAMPLE (continued)

Interaction by fitting separate models:
Cox Regression Analysis (Females)
Response: Surv

Column name	Coeff	StErr	p-value	HR	0.95	CI	P(PH)
4 log WBC	1.639	0.519	0.002	5.150	1.862	14.242	0.114
5 Rx	1.859	0.729	0.011	6.418	1.537	26.790	0.291

n: 20   %Cen: 30.000   −2 log L: 44.199   # iter:6

Cox Regression Analysis (Males)
Response: Surv

Column name	Coeff	StErr	p-value	HR	0.95	CI	P(PH)
4 log WBC	1.170	0.499	0.019	3.222	1.213	8.562	0.329
5 Rx	0.267	0.566	0.637	1.306	0.431	3.959	0.278

n: 22   %Cen: 27.273   −2 Log L   67.471   # iter:5

Which model is more appropriate statistically?

Interaction model:
($\blacklozenge$) $h_g(t, \mathbf{X})$
$= h_{0g}(t)\exp[\beta_{1g} \log \text{WBC} + \beta_{2g} Rx]$
where $g = 1$ (females), $g = 2$ (males)

No-interaction model:
$h_g(t, \mathbf{X}) = h_{0g}(t)\exp[\beta_1 \log \text{WBC} + \beta_2 Rx]$
where $g = 1$ (females), $g = 2$ (males)

Alternative interaction model:
($\star$) $h_g(t, \mathbf{X}) = h_{0g}(t)\exp[\beta_1^* \log \text{WBC} + \beta_2^* Rx + \beta_3^* (\text{SEX} \times \log \text{WBC}) + \beta_4^* \times (\text{SEX} \times Rx)]$

where $\text{SEX} = \begin{cases} 1 \text{ if female} \\ 0 \text{ if male} \end{cases}$

$h_{0g}(t)$ are different for $g = 1, 2$
β^* coefficients do not involve g

If we allow for interaction, then we would expect to obtain different coefficients for each of the (SEX) strata. This would happen if we fit separate hazard models to the female and male data, with each model containing the log WBC and Rx variables. The computer results from fitting separate models are shown here.

Notice that the coefficient of log WBC is 1.639 for females but is 1.170 for males. Also, the coefficient for *Rx* is 1.859 for females but 0.267 for males. These results show different coefficients for females than for males, particularly for the *Rx* variable.

But are corresponding coefficients statistically different? That is, which model is more appropriate statistically, the no-interaction model or the interaction model? To answer this question, we must first look at the hazard function model for the interaction situation.

One way to state the hazard model formula when there is interaction is shown here ($\blacklozenge$). Notice that each variable in this model has a different coefficient for females than for males, as indicated by the subscript g in the coefficients β_{1g} and β_{2g}.

In contrast, in the no-interaction model, the coefficient (β_1) of log WBC is the same for females and for males; also, the coefficient (β_2) of *Rx* is the same for females and for males.

An alternative way to write the interaction model is shown here (*). This alternative form contains two product terms—SEX × log WBC and SEX × *Rx*—as well as the main effects of log WBC and *Rx*. We have coded the SEX so that 1 denotes female and 0 denotes male.

In this alternative model, note that although the baseline hazards $h_{0g}(t)$ are different for each sex, the β^* coefficients do not involve the subscript g and therefore are the same for each sex.

EXAMPLE (continued)

Equivalence of models ($\blacklozenge$) and ($\star$):
$g = 1$ (females), so that sex = 1:

$h_1(t,\mathbf{X}) = h_{01}(t)\exp[\beta_1^* \log \text{WBC} + \beta_2^* Rx$
$\qquad + \beta_3^* (1 \times \log \text{WBC}) + \beta_4^* (1 \times Rx)]$

$= h_{01}(t)\exp[\,(\beta_1^* + \beta_3^*)\, \log \text{WBC}$
$\qquad + (\beta_2^* + \beta_4^*)\, Rx]$

$g = 2$ (males), so that sex = 0:

$h_2(t,\mathbf{X}) = h_{02}(t)\exp[\beta_1^* \log \text{WBC} + \beta_2^* Rx +$
$\qquad\quad \beta_3^* (0 \times \log \text{WBC}) + \beta_4^* (0 \bullet Rx)]$

$\qquad = h_{02}(t)\exp[\,\beta_1^*\,\log \text{WBC} + \beta_2^* Rx]$

Interaction models in same format:

Females ($g = 1$): $h_1(t,\mathbf{X})$
$(\blacklozenge) = h_{01}(t)\exp[\beta_{11}\log \text{WBC} + \beta_{21}Rx]$
$(\star) = h_{01}(t)\exp[(\beta_1^* + \beta_3^*) \log \text{WBC}$
$\qquad + (\beta_2^* + \beta_4^*)Rx]$

Males ($g=2$): $h_2(t,\mathbf{X})$
$(\blacklozenge) = h_{02}(t)\exp[\beta_{12}\log \text{WBC} + \beta_{22}Rx]$
$(\star) = h_{02}(t)\exp[\beta_1^*\log \text{WBC} + \beta_2^* Rx]$

$$\qquad\qquad\qquad (\blacklozenge) \qquad (\star)$$
Females ($g = 1$): $\beta_{11} = \beta_1^* + \beta_3^*$
$\qquad\qquad\qquad\quad \beta_{21} = \beta_2^* + \beta_4^*$

$$\qquad\qquad\qquad (\blacklozenge) \quad (\star)$$
Males ($g = 2$): $\beta_{12} = \beta_1^*$
$\qquad\qquad\qquad\quad \beta_{22} = \beta_2^*$

Nevertheless, this alternative formula (*) is equivalent to the interaction formula ($\blacklozenge$) above. We show this by specifying the form that the model takes for $g = 1$ (females) and $g = 2$ (males).

Notice that the coefficients of log WBC are different in each formula, namely, $(\beta_1^* + \beta_3^*)$ for females versus β_1^* for males.

Similarly, the coefficients of Rx are different, namely, $(\beta_2^* + \beta_4^*)$ for females versus β_2^* for males.

The preceding formulae indicate that two seemingly different formulae for the interaction model—($\blacklozenge$) versus (*), shown earlier—can be written in the same format. We show these formulae here separately for females and males.

Notice that for females, the coefficient β_{11} in model ($\blacklozenge$) must be equivalent to $(\beta_1^* + \beta_3^*)$ in model (*) because both models have the same format, and both β_{11} and $(\beta_1^* + \beta_3^*)$ are coefficients of the same variable, log WBC. Similarly, β_{21} in model ($\blacklozenge$) is equivalent to $(\beta_2^* + \beta_4^*)$ in model (*) because both are coefficients of the same variable, Rx.

For males, it follows in an analogous way, that the coefficient β_{12} is equivalent to β_1^*, and, similarly, β_{22} equals β_2^*.

EXAMPLE (continued)

Stratified Cox Regression Analysis on Variable: sex
Response: Surv

Column name	Coeff	StErr	p-value	HR	0.95	CI
4 log WBC	1.170	0.499	0.019	3.222	1.213	8.562
5 Rx	0.267	0.566	0.637	1.306	0.431	3.959
7 sex × log WBC	0.469	0.720	0.515	1.598	0.390	6.549
8 sex × Rx	1.592	0.923	0.084	4.915	0.805	30.003

n:42   %Cen: 28.571 $-2 \log L$: 111.670   # iter:6

Females:

$$\log WBC \begin{cases} \beta_{11} = \boxed{1.639} \\ \hat{\beta}_1^* + \hat{\beta}_3^* = 1.170 + 0.469 = 1.\boxed{639} \end{cases}$$

$$Rx \begin{cases} \beta_{21} = \boxed{1.859} \\ \hat{\beta}_2^* + \hat{\beta}_4^* = 0.267 + 1.592 + 1.\boxed{859} \end{cases}$$

Males:

$$\log WBC \; \hat{\beta}_{12} = \boxed{1.170} = \hat{\beta}_1^*$$
$$Rx \qquad \hat{\beta}_{22} = \boxed{0.267} = \hat{\beta}_2^*$$

Interaction model:

$$h_g(t, \mathbf{X}) = h_{0g}(t) \exp[\beta_1^* \log WBC + \beta_2^* Rx + \beta_3^* (SEX \bullet \log WBC) + \beta_4^* (SEX \bullet Rx)]$$

Testing the no-interaction assumption:

$$LR = -2 \ln \hat{L}_R - (-2 \ln \hat{L}_F)$$
R = reduced (no-interaction) model
F = full (interaction) model

Here we provide computer results obtained from fitting the alternative interaction model. The estimated regression coefficients $\hat{\beta}_1^*$, $\hat{\beta}_2^*$, $\hat{\beta}_3^*$, and $\hat{\beta}_4^*$, respectively, are circled.

We have shown above that the sums $\hat{\beta}_1^* + \hat{\beta}_3^*$ and $\hat{\beta}_2^* + \hat{\beta}_4^*$ are equal to the coefficients $\hat{\beta}_{11}$ and $\hat{\beta}_{21}$, respectively, in the original interaction model for females.

Also, we have shown that $\hat{\beta}_1^*$ and $\hat{\beta}_2^*$ are equal to the coefficients $\hat{\beta}_{12}$ and $\hat{\beta}_{22}$, respectively, in the original interaction model for the males. The numerical equivalences are shown here. Note again that the coefficients of log WBC and Rx for females are different from males, as is to be expected if sex interacts with each variable.

We have thus seen that the interaction model can be written in a format that contains product terms involving the variable being stratified—SEX—being multiplied by each of the predictors not being stratified. We show this model involving product terms again here. We will use this model to describe a test of the no-interaction assumption.

The test is a likelihood ratio (LR) test which compares log-likelihood statistics for the interaction model and the no-interaction model. That is, the LR test statistic is of the form $-2 \ln L_R$ "hat" minus $-2 \ln L_F$ "hat," where R denotes the reduced model, which in this case is the no-interaction model, and F denotes the full model, which is the interaction model.

EXAMPLE (continued)

$LR \sim \chi^2_{2df}$ under H_0: no interaction (2 df because two product terms tested in interaction model)

No interaction (reduced model):
Output: $-2 \log L$: 115.119
$\quad\quad -2 \ln \hat{L}_R$

Interaction (full model):
Output: $-2 \log L$: 111.670
$\quad\quad -2 \ln \hat{L}_F$

$LR = 115.119 - 111.670 = 3.44$
($P > 0.05$ not significant).
Thus, the no-interaction model is acceptable.

This LR test statistic has approximately a chi-square distribution with 2 degrees of freedom under the null hypothesis that the no-interaction model is correct. The degrees of freedom here is 2 because there are two product terms being tested in the interaction model.

The log-likelihood statistic for the reduced model comes from the computer output for the no-interaction model and is equal to 115.119.

The log-likelihood statistic for the full model comes from the computer results for the interaction model and is equal to 111.670.

The LR statistic is therefore 115.119 minus 111.670, which equals 3.44. This value is not significant at the 0.05 level for 2 degrees of freedom. Thus, it appears that despite the numerical difference between corresponding coefficients in the female and male models, there is no statistically significant difference. We can therefore conclude for these data that the no-interaction model is acceptable (at least at the 0.05 level).

Remission data example:
- described no-interaction assumption
- evaluated assumption using LR test
- provided interaction model if needed

Now, we generalize this process.

Using the remission data example, we have described the no-interaction assumption, have shown how to evaluate this assumption using a likelihood ratio test, and have provided the form of an interaction model that should be used in case the no-interaction assumption does not hold. We now describe this process more generally for any stratified Cox analysis.

No-interaction SC model:

$$h_g(t,\mathbf{X}) = h_{0g}(t)\exp[\beta_1 X_1 + \beta_2 X_2 + \cdots + \beta_p X_p]$$
$g = 1, 2, \ldots, k^*$, strata defined from Z^*

Recall that the general form of the no-interaction model for the stratified Cox procedure is given as shown here. This model allows for several variables being stratified through the use of a newly defined variable called Z^*, whose strata consist of combinations of categories of the variables being stratified.

SC model allowing interaction:

$$h_g(t,\mathbf{X}) = h_{0g}(t)\exp[\beta_{1g} X_1 + \beta_{2g} X_2 + \cdots + \beta_{pg} X_p]$$
$g = 1, 2, \ldots, k^*$, strata defined from Z^*

If, in contrast, we allow for interaction of the Z^* variable with the X's in the model, we can write the model as shown here. Notice that in this interaction model, each regression coefficient has the subscript g, which denotes the gth stratum and indicates that the regression coefficients are different for different strata of Z^*.

Alternative SC interaction model:
- uses product terms involving Z^*
- define $k^* - 1$ dummy variables $Z_1^*, Z_2^*, \cdots, Z_{k^*-1}^*$, from Z^*
- products of the form $Z_1^* \times X_j$, where $i = 1, \ldots, k$ and $j = 1, \ldots, p$.

An alternative way to write the interaction model uses product terms involving the variable Z^* with each of the predictors. However, to write this model correctly, we need to use $k^* - 1$ dummy variables to distinguish the k^* categories of Z^*; also, each of these dummy variables, which we denote as $Z_1^*, Z_2^*, \ldots, Z_{k^*-1}^*$, needs to be involved in a product term with each of the X's.

$$h_g(t,\mathbf{X}) = h_{0g}(t)\exp[\beta_1 X_1 + \cdots + \beta_p X_p$$
$$+ \beta_{11}(Z_1^* \times X_1) + \cdots + \beta_{p1}(Z_1^* \times X_p)$$
$$+ \beta_{12}(Z_2^* \times X_1) + \cdots + \beta_{p2}(Z_2^* \times X_p)$$
$$+ \cdots$$
$$+ \beta_{1,k^*-1}(Z_{k^*-1}^* \times X_1) + \cdots$$
$$+ \beta_{p,k^*-1}(Z_{k^*-1}^* \times X_p)]$$
$$g = 1, 2, \ldots, k^*, \text{ strata defined from } Z^*$$

The hazard model formula alternative model is shown here. Notice that the first line of the formula contains the X's by themselves, the next line contains products of each X_j with Z_1^*, the third line contains the products with Z_2^*, and the last line contains products with $Z_{k^*-1}^*$. Note also that the subscript g occurs only with the baseline hazard function $h_{0g}(t)$, and is not explicitly used in the β coefficients.

EXAMPLE (Remission Data)

$Z^* = $ sex, $k^* = 2$,
$Z_1^* = $ sex$(0,1)$,
$X_1 = \log$ WBC, $X_2 = Rx$ $(p = 2)$
$$h_g(t,\mathbf{X}) = h_{0g}(t)\exp[\beta_1 X_1 + \beta_2 X_2$$
$$+ \beta_{11}(Z_1^* \times X_1)$$
$$+ \beta_{21}(Z_1^* \times X_2)]$$
$$= h_{0g}(t)\exp[\beta_1^* \log \text{WBC}$$
$$+ \beta_2^* Rx + \beta_3^*(\text{sex} \times \log \text{WBC})$$
$$+ \beta_4^*(\text{sex} \times Rx)]$$
$g = 1, 2$
$\beta_1 = \beta_1^*, \beta_2 = \beta_2^*, \beta_{11} = \beta_3^*, \text{ and } \beta_{21} = \beta_4^*$

In our previous example involving the remission data, the stratification variable (Z^*) was the variable, sex, and k^* was equal to 2; thus, we have only one dummy variable Z_1^*, which uses a $(0,1)$ coding to indicate sex, and we have only (p equal to) two predictors—X_1 equal to log WBC and X_2 equal to Rx. The interaction model is then written in either of the forms shown here.

The latter version of the interaction model is what we previously presented for the remission data example. Because the two versions presented here are equivalent, it follows that $\beta_1^* = \beta_1$, $\beta_2 = \beta_2^*$, $\beta_{11} = \beta_3^*$, and $\beta_{21} = \beta_4^*$.

Stratified Cox interaction model:
$$h_g(t,\mathbf{X}) = h_{0g}(t)\exp[\beta_1 X_1 + \cdots + \beta_p X_p$$
$$+ \beta_{11}(Z_1^* \times X_1) + \cdots + \beta_{p1}(Z_1^* \times X_p)$$
$$+ \beta_{12}(Z_2^* \times X_1) + \cdots + \beta_{p2}(Z_2^* \times X_p)$$
$$\vdots$$
$$+ \beta_{1,k^*-1}(Z_{k^*-1}^* \times X_1)$$
$$+ \cdots + \beta_{p,k^*-1}(Z_{k^*-1}^* \times X_p)]$$
$$g = 1, 2, \cdots, k^*, \text{ strata defined from } Z^*$$

We have thus seen that the interaction model can be written in a format that contains product terms involving dummy variables (i.e., Z_i) for the variable being stratified being multiplied by each of the predictors (i.e., X_i) not being stratified. We show this model involving product terms again here. We will use this model to describe a test of the no-interaction assumption.

Testing the no-interaction assumption:

$$LR = -2 \ln \hat{L}_R - (-2 \ln \hat{L}_F)$$

R = reduced (no-interaction) model
F = full (interaction) model contains product terms

$$H_0: \begin{cases} \beta_{11} = \cdots = \beta_{p1} = 0 \\ \beta_{12} = \cdots = \beta_{p2} = 0 \\ \vdots \\ \beta_{1,k^*-1} = \cdots = \beta_{p,k^*-1} = 0 \end{cases}$$

$$\boxed{LR \sim \chi^2_{p(k^*-1)\text{df}} \text{ under } H_0: \text{ no interaction}}$$

$p(k^*-1)$ gives number of product terms being tested in interaction model

The test is a likelihood ratio (LR) test which compares log likelihood statistics for the interaction model and the no-interaction model. That is, the LR test statistic is of the form $-2 \ln L_R$ "hat" minus $-2 \ln L_F$ "hat," where R denotes the reduced model, which in this case is the no-interaction model, and F denotes the full model, which is the interaction model.

The no-interaction model differs from the interaction model in that the latter contains additional product terms. Thus, one way to state the null hypothesis of no interaction is that the coefficients of each of these product terms are all zero.

The LR test statistic has approximately a chi-square distribution with $p(k^*-1)$ degrees of freedom under the null hypothesis. The degrees of freedom here is $p(k^*-1)$ because this value gives the number of product terms that are being tested in the interaction model.

EXAMPLE (Remission Data)

Z^* = sex, k^* = 2,
Z_1^* = sex(0,1),
X_1 = log WBC, X_2 = Rx ($p = 2$)
$p(k^* - 1) = 2$, so
$LR \sim \chi^2_{2\text{df}}$ under H_0: no interaction

Returning to the remission data example, for which $p=2$ and $k^*=2$, the value of $p(k^*-1)$ is equal to two times $(2-1)$, which equals two. Thus, to test whether the sex variable interacts with the log WBC and Rx predictors, the degrees of freedom for the LR statistic is two, as previously described.

V. A Second Example Involving Several Stratification Variables

The dataset "vets.dat" considers survival times in days for 137 patients from the Veteran's Administration Lung Cancer Trial cited by Kalbfleisch and Prentice in their text (*The Statistical Analysis of Survival Time Data*, Wiley, pp. 223–224, 1980). The exposure variable of interest is treatment status. Other variables of interest as control variables are cell type (four types, defined in terms of dummy variables), performance status, disease duration, age, and prior therapy status. Failure status is defined by the status variable. A complete list of the variables as stored in a SPIDA file is shown here and continues to the top of the next page. The actual data set is provided in Appendix B.

EXAMPLE

vets.dat: survival time in days, $n = 137$

Veteran's Administration Lung Cancer Trial
Column 1: Treatment (standard = 1, test = 2)
Column 2: Cell type 1 (large = 1, other = 0)
Column 3: Cell type 2 (adeno = 1, other = 0)
Column 4: Cell type 3 (small = 1, other = 0)
Column 5: Cell type 4 (squamous = 1, other = 0)

EXAMPLE (continued)

Column   6: Survival time (days)
Column   7: Performance status (0 = worst, ...,
                100 = best)
Column   8: Disease duration (months)
Column   9: Age
Column 10: Prior therapy (none = 0, some = 10)
Column 11: Status (0 = censored, 1 = died)

Cox Regression Analysis
Response: Surv. Time

Column name	Coeff	StErr	p-value	HR	0.95	CI	P(PH)
1 Treatment	0.290	0.207	0.162	1.336	0.890	2.006	0.629
2 Large cell	0.400	0.283	0.157	1.491	0.857	2.594	0.035
3 Adeno cell	1.188	0.301	0.000	3.281	1.820	5.915	0.083
4 Small cell	0.856	0.275	0.002	2.355	1.374	4.037	0.080
7 Perf. Stat	−0.033	0.006	0.000	0.968	0.958	0.978	0.000
8 Dis. Durat.	0.000	0.009	0.992	1.000	0.982	1.018	0.919
9 Age	−0.009	0.009	0.358	0.991	0.974	1.010	0.199
10 Pr. Therapy	0.007	0.023	0.755	1.007	0.962	1.054	0.147

n:137   %Cen: 6.569   −2 log L: 950.359   # iter:5

Variables not satisfying PH:
- cell type (3 dummy variables)
- performance status
- prior therapy (possibly)

SC model: stratifies on cell type and performance status

Z^* given by combinations of categories:
- cell type (four categories)
- performance status (interval) change to
- PSbin (two categories)

Z^* has $k^* = 4 \times 2 = 8$ categories

Here we provide computer output obtained from fitting a Cox PH model to these data. Using the $P(PH)$ information in the last column, we can see that at least four of the variables listed have $P(PH)$ values below the 0.010 level. These four variables are labeled in the output as large cell (0.080), adeno cell (0.083), small cell (0.033), and Perf. Stat (0.000). Notice that the three variables, large cell, adeno cell, and small cell, are dummy variables that distinguish the four categories of cell type.

Thus, it appears from the $P(PH)$ results that the variables cell type (defined using dummy variables) and performance status do not satisfy the PH assumption.

Based on the conclusions just made about the PH assumption, we now describe a stratified Cox analysis that stratifies on the variables, cell type and performance status.

Because we are stratifying on two variables, we need to form a single new categorical variable Z^* whose categories represent combinations of categories of the two variables. The cell type variable has four categories by definition. The performance status variable, however, is an interval variable ranging between 0 for worst to 100 for best, so it needs to be categorized. We categorize this variable into two groups using a cutpoint of 60, and we denote this binary variable as PSbin. Thus, the number of categories for our Z^* variable is 4×2, or 8; that is, $k^* = 8$.

EXAMPLE (continued)

Four other variables considered as X's:
- treatment status
- disease duration
- age
- prior therapy

In addition to the two stratification variables, cell type and performance status, there are four other variables to be considered as predictors in the stratified Cox model. These are treatment status, disease duration, age, and prior therapy.

Here, we use treatment status and age as X's

For illustrative purposes here, we use only treatment status and age as predictors. The other two variables, disease duration and prior therapy, are considered in exercises following this presentation.

Stratified Cox Regression Analysis on Variable: Z^*
Response: Surv. Time

Here we show computer output from fitting a stratified Cox model that stratifies on cell type and performance status using the eight-category stratification variable Z^*. This model also includes treatment and age as predictors. These results consider a no-interaction model, because only one regression coefficient is provided for the treatment and age predictors. Notice that the estimated hazard ratio is 1.134 for the effect of the treatment variable adjusted for age and Z^*, the latter being adjusted by stratification. The p-value for this adjusted treatment effect is 0.548, which is highly nonsignificant.

Column name	Coeff	StErr	p-value	HR	0.95	CI
1 Treatment	0.125	0.208	0.548	1.134	0.753	1.706
9 Age	−0.001	0.010	0.897	0.999	0.979	1.019
n:137		%Cen: 6.569	−2 log L: 524.039	# iter:4		

No-interaction model

$\widehat{HR} = 1.134 \ (P = 0.548)$

Treatment effect (adjusted for age and Z^*) is nonsignificant

No-interaction model:
$$h_g(t,\mathbf{X})$$
$$= h_{0g}(t)\exp[\beta_1 \text{ Treatment} + \beta_2 \text{ Age}]$$
$$g = 1, 2, \ldots, 8 \ (= \text{\# of strata defined from } Z^*)$$

The no-interaction model we have just described has the hazard function formula shown here.

Interaction model:
$$h_g(t,\mathbf{X})$$
$$= h_{0g}(t)\exp[\beta_{1g} \text{ Treatment} + \beta_{2g} \text{ Age}]$$
$$g = 1, 2, \ldots, 8$$

To evaluate whether the no-interaction model is appropriate, we need to define an interaction model that allows different regression coefficients for different strata. One way to write this interaction model is shown here.

EXAMPLE (continued)

Alternative interaction model:

$h_g(t,\mathbf{X})$

$= h_{0g}(t)\exp[\beta_1 \text{ Treatment}$

$\quad + \beta_2 \text{ Age}$

$+ \beta_{11}(Z_1^* \times \text{Treatment}) + \cdots$

$\quad + \beta_{17}(Z_7^* \times \text{Treatment})$

$+ \beta_{21}(Z_1^* \times \text{Age}) + \cdots + \beta_{27}(Z_7^* \times \text{Age})]$

$g = 1, 2, \ldots, 8$

Another version of interaction model:
Replace $Z_1^*, \ldots, Z_7^*$ by

$Z_1^* = \text{large cell (binary)}$

$Z_2^* = \text{adeno cell (binary)}$

$Z_3^* = \text{small cell (binary)}$

$Z_4^* = \text{PSbin (binary)}$

$Z_5^* = Z_1^* \times Z_4^*$

$Z_6^* = Z_2^* \times Z_4^*$

$Z_7^* = Z_3^* \times Z_4^*$

$h_g(t,\mathbf{X}) = h_{0g}(t)\exp[\beta_1 \text{ Treatment}$

$\quad\quad + \beta_2 \text{ Age}$

An alternative version of this interaction model that involves product terms is shown here. This version uses seven dummy variables denoted as Z_1^*, Z_2^* up through Z_7^* to distinguish the eight categories of the stratification variable Z^*. The model contains the main effects of treatment and age plus interaction terms involving products of each of the seven dummy variables with each of the two predictors.

Yet another version of the interaction model is to replace the seven dummy variables Z_1^* to Z_7^* by the seven variables listed here. These variables are three of the binary variables making up the cell type variable, the binary variable for performance status, plus three product terms involving each of the cell type dummy variables multiplied by the PSbin dummy variable (Z_4^*).

The latter interaction model is shown here. In this model, the variable tr Z_1^* denotes the product of treatment status with the large cell dummy Z_1^*, the variable tr Z_2^* denotes the product of treatment status with the adeno cell variable Z_2^*, and so on. Also, the tr variable $Z_1^* Z_4^*$ denotes the triple product of treatment status times the large cell variable Z_1^* times the PSbin variable Z_4^*, and so on, for the other triple product terms involving treatment. Similarly, for the terms involving age, the variable Age Z_1^* denotes the product of age with Z_1^*, and the variable Age $Z_1^* Z_4^*$ denotes the triple product of age times Z_1^* times Z_4^*.

EXAMPLE (continued)

Stratified Cox Regression Analysis on Variable: Z^*
Response: Surv. Time

Column name	Coeff	StErr	p-value	HR	0.95	CI
Treatment	0.286	0.664	0.667	1.331	0.362	4.893
Age	0.000	0.030	0.978	0.999	0.942	1.060
tr Z_1^*	2.351	1.772	0.184	10.495	0.326	337.989
tr Z_2^*	−1.158	0.957	0.226	0.314	0.048	2.047
tr Z_3^*	0.582	0.855	0.496	1.790	0.335	9.562
tr Z_4^*	−1.033	0.868	0.234	0.356	0.065	1.950
tr $Z_1^*Z_4^*$	−0.794	1.980	0.688	0.452	0.009	21.882
tr $Z_2^*Z_4^*$	2.785	1.316	0.034	16.204	1.229	213.589
tr $Z_3^*Z_4^*$	0.462	1.130	0.683	1.587	0.173	14.534
Age Z_1^*	0.078	0.064	0.223	1.081	0.954	1.225
Age Z_2^*	−0.047	0.045	0.295	0.954	0.873	1.042
Age Z_3^*	−0.059	0.042	0.162	0.943	0.868	1.024
Age Z_4^*	0.051	0.048	0.287	1.053	0.958	1.157
Age $Z_1^*Z_4^*$	−0.167	0.082	0.042	0.847	0.721	0.994
Age $Z_2^*Z_4^*$	−0.045	0.068	0.511	0.956	0.838	1.092
Age $Z_3^*Z_4^*$	0.041	0.061	0.499	1.042	0.924	1.175

n:137   %Cen: 6.569   −2 log L: 499.944   # iter:7

Eight possible combinations of Z_1^* to Z_4^*:

$g = 1$: $Z_1^* = Z_2^* = Z_3^* = Z_4^* = 0$

$g = 2$: $Z_1^* = 1, Z_2^* = Z_3^* = Z_4^* = 0$

$g = 3$: $Z_2^* = 1, Z_1^* = Z_3^* = Z_4^* = 0$

$g = 4$: $Z_3^* = 1, Z_1^* = Z_2^* = Z_4^* = 0$

$g = 5$: $Z_1^* = Z_2^* = Z_3^* = 0, Z_4^* = 1$

$g = 6$: $Z_1^* = 1, Z_2^* = Z_3^* = 0, Z_4^* = 1$

$g = 7$: $Z_2^* = 1, Z_1^* = Z_3^* = 0, Z_4^* = 1$

$g = 8$: $Z_3^* = 1, Z_1^* = Z_2^* = 0, Z_4^* = 1$

$g=1$: $Z_1^*=Z_2^*=Z_3^*=Z_4^*=0$
(Squamous cell type and PSbin=0)

All product terms are zero:

$h_1(t,\mathbf{X})$

$= h_{01}(t)\exp[\beta_1 \text{ Treatment} +$
    $\beta_2 \text{ Age}]$,

where $\hat{\beta}_1 = 0.286$,

$\hat{\beta}_2 = 0.000$, so that

$\hat{h}_1(t,\mathbf{X}) = \hat{h}_{01}(t)\exp[(0.286)\text{Treatment}]$

Here we provide the computer results from fitting the interaction model just described. Notice that the first two variables listed are the main effects of treatment status and age. The next seven variables are product terms involving the interaction of treatment status with the seven categories of Z^*. The final seven variables are product terms involving the interaction of age with the seven categories of Z^*. As defined on the previous page, the seven variables used to define Z^* consist of three dummy variables Z_1^*, Z_2^* and Z_3^* for cell type, a binary variable Z_4^* for performance status and products of Z_4^* with each of Z_1^*, Z_2^*, and Z_3^*. Note that once the variables Z_1^*, Z_2^*, Z_3^*, and Z_4^* are specified, the values of the three product terms are automatically determined.

We can use these results to show that the interaction model being fit yields different regression coefficients for each of the eight categories defined by the subscript g for the stratification variable Z^*. These eight categories represent the possible combinations of the four variables Z_1^* to Z_4^*, as shown here.

Consider the hazard function when the variables Z_1^* through Z_4^* are all equal to zero. This stratum is defined by the combination of squamous cell type and a binary performance status value of 0. In this case, all product terms are equal to zero and the hazard model contains only the main effect terms treatment and age. The estimated hazard function for this stratum uses the coefficients 0.286 for treatment and 0.000 for age, yielding the expression shown here. Note that age drops out of the expression because its coefficient is zero to three decimal places.

EXAMPLE (continued)

$g = 2: Z_1^* = 1, Z_2^* = Z_3^* = Z_4^* = 0$
(Large cell type and PSbin = 0)

Nonzero product terms	Coefficients
Age Z_1^* = Age	β_{21}
tr Z_1^* = Treatment	β_{11}

$$h_2(t,\mathbf{X}) = h_{02}(t)\exp[(\beta_1 + \beta_{11})\text{Treatment} + (\beta_2 + \beta_{21})\,\text{Age}]$$
$$\hat{\beta}_1 = 0.286, \hat{\beta}_2 = 0.000$$
$$\hat{\beta}_{11} = 2.351, \hat{\beta}_{21} = 0.078$$

Hazard functions for interaction model:
$g = 1: (Z_1^* = Z_2^* = Z_3^* = Z_4^* = 0):$
$$\hat{h}_1(t,\mathbf{X}) = \hat{h}_{01}(t)\exp[(0.286)\text{Treatment}]$$
$g = 2: (Z_1^* = 1, Z_2^* = Z_3^* = Z_4^* = 0):$
$$\hat{h}_2(t,\mathbf{X}) = \hat{h}_{02}(t)\exp[(2.637)\text{Treatment} + (0.078)\text{Age}]$$
$g = 3: (Z_2^* = 1, Z_1^* = Z_3^* = Z_4^* = 0):$
$$\hat{h}_3(t,\mathbf{X}) = \hat{h}_{03}(t)\exp[(-0.872)\text{Treatment} + (-0.047)\text{Age}]$$
$g = 4: (Z_3^* = 1, Z_1^* = Z_2^* = Z_4^* = 0):$
$$\hat{h}_4(t,\mathbf{X}) = \hat{h}_{04}(t)\exp[(0.868)\text{Treatment} + (-0.059)\text{Age}]$$
$g = 5: (Z_1^* = Z_2^* = Z_3^* = 0, Z_4^* = 1):$
$$\hat{h}_5(t,\mathbf{X}) = \hat{h}_{05}(t)\exp[(-0.747)\text{Treatment} + (0.051)\text{Age}]$$
$g = 6: (Z_1^* = 1, Z_2^* = Z_3^* = 0, Z_4^* = 1):$
$$\hat{h}_6(t,\mathbf{X}) = \hat{h}_{06}(t)\exp[(0.810)\text{Treatment} + (-0.038)\text{Age}]$$
$g = 7: (Z_2^* = 1, Z_1^* = Z_3^* = 0, Z_4^* = 1):$
$$\hat{h}_7(t,\mathbf{X}) = \hat{h}_{07}(t)\exp[(0.880)\text{Treatment} + (-0.041)\text{Age}]$$
$g = 8: (Z_3^* = 1, Z_1^* = Z_2^* = 0, Z_4^* = 1):$
$$\hat{h}_8(t,\mathbf{X}) = \hat{h}_{08}(t)\exp[(0.297)\text{Treatment} + (0.033)\text{Age}]$$

Now consider the hazard function when the variable Z_1^* equals 1 and Z_2^* through Z_4^* are equal to zero. This stratum is defined by the combination of large cell type and a PSbin value of 0. In this case, the only nonzero product terms are Age Z_1^* and tr Z_1^*, whose coefficients are β_{21} and β_{11}, respectively.

The hazard function for this second stratum is shown here. Notice that the coefficients of the treatment and age variables are $(\beta_1 + \beta_{11})$ and $(\beta_2 + \beta_{21})$, respectively. The estimated values of each of these coefficients are given here.

The corresponding *estimated* hazard function for the second stratum (i.e., $g=2$) is shown here. For comparison, we repeat the estimated hazard function for the first stratum.

The estimated hazard functions for the remaining strata are provided here. We leave it up to the reader to verify these formulae. Notice that the coefficients of treatment are all different in the eight strata, and the coefficients of age also are all different in the eight strata.

EXAMPLE (continued)

LR test to compare no-interaction model with interaction model:

H_0: no-interaction model acceptable, i.e.,
Treatment: $\beta_{11} = \beta_{21} = \cdots = \beta_{71} = 0$
and Age: $\beta_{12} = \beta_{22} = \cdots = \beta_{72} = 0$

14 coefficients $\Rightarrow$ df=14

$LR = -2 \ln \hat{L}_R - (2 \ln \hat{L}_F)$

R = reduced (no-interaction) model

F = full (interaction) model

$LR \overset{\cdot}{\sim} \chi^2_{14df}$ under H_0: no interaction

$LR = 524.039 - 499.944 = 24.095$
 $P = 0.045$ (significant at 0.05)
Conclusion:
Reject H_0: interaction model is preferred.

Might use further testing to simplify interaction model, e.g., test for seven products involving treatment or test for seven products involving age.

We have presented computer results for both the no-interaction and the interaction models. To evaluate whether the no-interaction assumption is satisfied, we need to carry out a likelihood ratio test to compare these two models.

The null hypothesis being tested is that the no-interaction model is acceptable. Equivalently, this null hypothesis can be stated by setting the coefficients of all product terms in the interaction model to be zero. That is, the seven coefficients of product terms involving treatment and the seven coefficients of the product terms involving age are set equal to zero as shown here.

Because the null hypothesis involves 14 coefficients, the degrees of freedom of the LR chi-square statistic is 14. The test statistic takes the usual form involving the difference between log-likelihood statistics for the reduced and full models, where the reduced model is the no-interaction model and the full model is the interaction model.

Thus, under the null hypothesis, the *LR* statistic is approximately chi-square with 14 degrees of freedom.

The computer results for the no-interaction and interaction models give log-likelihood values of 524.039 and 499.944, respectively. The difference is 24.095. A chi-square value of 24.095 with 14 degrees of freedom yields a p-value of 0.045, so that the test gives a significant result at the 0.05 level. This indicates that the no-interaction model is not acceptable and the interaction model is preferred.

Note, however, that it may be possible from further statistical testing to simplify the interaction model to have fewer than 14 product terms. For example, one might test for only the seven product terms involving treatment or only the seven product terms involving age.

VI. Summary

We now summarize the most important features of the stratified Cox (SC) model described in this presentation.

Stratified Cox (SC) model:
- stratification of predictors not satisfying PH assumption
- includes predictors satisfying PH
- does not include stratified variables

The SC model is a modification of the Cox PH model to allow for control by "stratification" of predictors not satisfying the PH assumption. Variables that are assumed to satisfy the assumption are included in the model as predictors; the stratified variables are not included in the model.

Computer Results
Stratified Cox Regression Analysis on
Variable: (sex)
Response: Surv

Column name	Coeff	StErr	p-value	HR	0.95	CI
4 log WBC	1.390	0.338	0.000	4.016	2.072	7.783
5 Rx	0.931	0.472	0.048	2.537	1.006	6.396
n:42		%Cen: 28.571		−2 log L: 115.119		# iter: 6

The computer results for a SC model provides essentially the same information as provided for a Cox PH model without stratification. An example of SC output using the remission data is shown here. The variables included as predictors in the model are listed in the first column followed by their estimated coefficients, standard errors, p-values, hazard ratio values, and 95% confidence limits. Such information cannot be provided for the variables being stratified, because these latter variables are not explicitly included in the model.

Hazard function for stratified Cox model:
$$h_g(t,\mathbf{X}) = h_{0g}(t)\exp[\beta_1 X_1 + \beta_2 X_2 + \cdots + \beta_p X_p]$$
$g = 1, 2, ..., k^*$, strata defined from Z^*
Z^* has k^* categories
$X_1, X_2, ..., X_p$ satisfy PH

The general hazard function form for the stratified Cox model is shown here. This formula contains a subscript g that indicates the gth stratum, where the strata are different categories of the stratification variable Z^* and the number of strata equals k^*. Notice that the baseline hazard functions are different in each stratum.

Stratification variable Z^*:
- identify $Z_1, Z_2, ..., Z_k$ not satisfying PH
- categorize each Z
- form combinations of categories (strata)
- each combination is a stratum of Z^*

The variable Z^* is defined by first identifying the Z_i variables not satisfying the PH assumption. We then categorize each Z and form combinations of categories of each of the Z's. Each combination represents a different stratum making up the variable Z^*.

No-interaction model:
Same coefficients $\beta_1, \beta_2, ..., \beta_p$ for each g, i.e., Z^* does not interact with the X's.

The above model is designated as a "no-interaction" model because the β's in the model are the same for each subscript g. The no-interaction assumption means that the variables being stratified are assumed *not* to interact with the X's in the model.

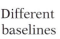

Different baselines
$$\left\{\begin{array}{l} h_{01}(t) \Rightarrow \hat{S}_1(t) \\ h_{02}(t) \Rightarrow \hat{S}_2(t) \\ \vdots \\ h_{0k}(t) \Rightarrow \hat{S}_{k^*}(t) \end{array}\right\}$$
Different survival curves

For the no-interaction model, the fitted SC model will yield different estimated survival curves for each stratum because the baseline hazard functions are different for each stratum.

$\widehat{HR}$ same for each stratum

However, because the coefficients of the X's are the same for each stratum, estimates of hazard ratios are the same for each stratum.

(Partial) likelihood function:
$$L = L_1 \times L_2 \times \cdots \times L_{k*}$$

Regression coefficients in the SC model are estimated by maximizing a partial likelihood function that is obtained by multiplying likelihood functions for each stratum.

Stratified Cox model allowing interaction:
$$h_g(t,\mathbf{X}) = h_{0g}(t)\exp[\beta_{1g}X_1 + \beta_{2g}X_2 + \cdots + \beta_{pg}X_p]$$
$g = 1, 2, ..., k*$, strata defined from $Z*$.

In order to evaluate the no-interaction assumption, we must define an interaction model for comparison. One version of the interaction model is shown here. This version shows regression coefficients with different subscripts in different strata; that is, each β coefficient has a subscript g.

Alternative stratified Cox interaction model:
- uses product terms involving $Z*$
- define $k* - 1$ dummy variables from $Z*$
- products of the form $Z_i^* \bullet X_j$

An alternative way to write the interaction model uses product terms involving the $Z*$ variable with each predictor. This model uses $k*-1$ dummy variables to distinguish the $k*$ categories of $Z*$. Each of these dummy variables is included as a product term with each of the X's.

Testing the no-interaction assumption:
$$LR = -2 \ln \hat{L}_R - (2 \ln \hat{L}_F)$$
R = reduced (no-interaction) model
F = full (interaction) model contains product terms
$LR \sim \chi^2_{p(k*-1)\mathrm{df}}$ under H_0: no interaction

To evaluate the no-interaction assumption, we can perform a likelihood ratio test that compares the no-interaction model to the (full) interaction model. The null hypothesis is that the no-interaction assumption is satisfied. The test statistic is given by the difference between the log-likelihood statistics for the no-interaction and interaction models. This statistic is approximately chi-square under the null hypothesis. The degrees of freedom is $p(k*-1)$ where p denotes the number of X's and $k*$ is the number of categories making up $Z*$.

PRESENTATION COMPLETE!

Chapters

1. Introduction to Survival Analysis
2. Kaplan–Meier Survival Curves and the Log–Rank Test
3. The Cox Proportional Hazards Model and Its Characteristics
4. Evaluating the Proportional Hazards Assumption

✓ 5. The Stratified Cox Procedure

Next:

6. Extension of the Cox Proportional Hazards Model for Time-Dependent Variables

This presentation is now complete. We suggest that the reader review this presentation using the detailed outline that follows. Then answer the practice exercises and the test that follow.

The next Chapter (6) is entitled "Extension of the Cox PH Model for Time-Dependent Variables." There we show how an "extended" Cox model can be used as an alternative to the stratified Cox model when one or more predictors do not satisfy the PH assumption. We also discuss more generally what is a time-dependent variable, and show how such a variable can be evaluated using an extended Cox model.

Detailed Outline

I. **Preview** (page 174)

Focus on how stratified Cox (SC) procedure is carried out:

- analysis of computer results from SC procedure;
- hazard function for SC model;
- stratifying on a single predictor versus two or more predictors;
- no-interaction versus interaction models.

II. **An Example** (pages 174–178)

A. Cox PH results for remission data yield $P(PH) = 0.038$ for SEX.

B. SC model used: control for SEX (stratified); include log WBC and Rx in model.

C. Analysis of Rx effect from stratified Cox results:
$\widehat{HR} = 2.537$; 95% CI: (1.006,6.396); LR and Wald tests: $P < 0.05$.

D. Hazard model: $h_g(t,\mathbf{X}) = h_{0g}(t) \exp [\beta_1 \log \text{WBC} + \beta_2 Rx], g = 1,2$

- different baseline hazard functions and survival curves for females and males;
- same coefficients β_1 and β_2 for both females and males (no-interaction assumption);
- obtain estimates by maximizing partial likelihood $L = L_1 \times L_2$.

E. Graph of four adjusted survival curves for Rx (adjusted for log WBC).

III. **The General Stratified Cox (SC) Model** (pages 178–180)

A. $\boxed{h_g(t,\mathbf{X}) = h_{0g}(t) \exp [\beta_1 X_1 + \beta_2 X_2 + \cdots + \beta_p X_p], g=1,2, \cdots ,k^*}$,
where the strata are defined from the stratification variable Z^*.

B. Z^* defined from $Z_1, Z_2, \ldots , Z_k$ variables that do not satisfy PH:

- categorize each Z_i
- form combinations of categories
- each combination is a stratum of Z^*

C. Different baseline hazard functions and survival curves for each stratum.

D. Assumes no interaction: same coefficients $\beta_1, \beta_2, \ldots , \beta_p$ for each g; i.e., Z^* does not interact with the X's; i.e., estimated HR is same for each stratum.

E. Obtain estimates by maximizing partial likelihood $L = L_1 \times L_2 \times \cdots \times L_{k^*}$, where L_i is likelihood for ith stratum.

IV. **The No-Interaction Assumption and How to Test It** (pages 180–186)

A. Assumes same coefficients $\beta_1, \beta_2, \ldots , \beta_p$ for each g.

B. Interaction model:

$$h_g(t,\mathbf{X}) = h_{0g}(t) \, \mathbf{exp} \, [\beta_{1g}X_1 + \beta_{2g}X_2 + \cdots + \beta_{pg}X_p] \, ,$$

$g = 1, 2, \ldots, k^*$ strata defined from Z^*.

C. Alternative stratified Cox interaction model:
   - uses product terms involving Z^*
   - define k^*-1 dummy variables $Z_1^*, Z_2^*, \ldots, Z_{k^*-1}^*$ from Z^*
   - products of the form $Z_i^* \times X_j$, where $i = 1, \ldots, k^*-1$; $j = 1, \ldots, p$
   - hazard function: $g = 1, 2, \ldots, k^*$ strata defined from Z^*

$$h_g(t,\mathbf{X}) = h_{0g}t)\mathbf{exp}[\beta_1 X_1 + \cdots + \beta_p X_p + \beta_{11}(Z_1^* \times X_1)$$
$$+ \cdots + \beta_{p1}(Z_1^* \times X_p) + \beta_{12}(Z_2^* \times X_1) + \cdots + \beta_{p2}(Z_2^* \times X_p)$$
$$+ \cdots + \beta_{1,k^*-1}(Z_{k^*-1}^* \times X_1) + \cdots + \beta_{p,k^*-1}(Z_{k^*-1}^* \times X_p)]$$

D. Testing the no-interaction assumption: use LR statistic given by
$$LR = -2 \ln \hat{L}_R - (-2 \ln \hat{L}_F)$$
where R = reduced (no interaction) model and F = full (interaction) model

$LR \overset{\sim}{\cdot} \chi^2_{p(k^*-1) \, df}$ under H_0: no interaction,

i.e., $\beta_{11} = \beta_{21} = \ldots = \beta_{p, \, k^*-1} = 0$

V. A Second Example Involving Several Stratification Variables
(pages 186–192)

A. Dataset "vets.dat" (SPIDA file) from Veteran's Administration Lung Cancer Trial; $n=137$; survival time in days.

B. Variables are: treatment status, cell type (four types), performance status, disease duration, age, and prior therapy status.

C. Cox PH results indicate [using $P(PH)$] that cell type and performance status do not satisfy PH assumption.

D. Example stratifies on cell type and performance status using four categories of cell type and two categories of performance status, so that Z^* has $k^* = 8$ strata.

E. X's considered in model are treatment status and age.

F. Computer results for no-interaction model: estimated HR for effect of treatment adjusted for age and Z^* is 1.134 ($P=0.548$); not significant.

G. Hazard function for no-interaction model:
$$h_g(t,\mathbf{X}) = h_{0g}(t)\mathbf{exp} \, [\beta_1 \, \text{Treatment} + \beta_2 \, \text{Age}], \, g = 1,2,\ldots,8$$

H. Hazard function for interaction model:
$$h_g(t,\mathbf{X}) = h_{0g}(t)\mathbf{exp} \, [\beta_{1g} \, \text{Treatment} + \beta_{2g} \, \text{Age}], \, g = 1,2,\ldots,8$$

I. Alternative version of interaction model:

$$h_g(t,\mathbf{X}) = h_{0g}(t)\mathbf{exp}[\beta_1 \text{ treatment} + \beta_2 \text{ Age} + \beta_{11}(Z_1^* \times \text{Treatment})$$
$$+ \cdots + \beta_{17}(Z_7^* \times \text{Treatment}) + \beta_{21}(Z_1^* \times \text{Age}) + \cdots + \beta_{27}(Z_7^* \times \text{Age})],$$
$$g = 1,2,\ldots,8$$

where $Z_1^* =$ large cell (binary), $Z_2^* =$ adeno cell (binary), $Z_3^* =$ small cell (binary), $Z_4^* =$ PSbin (binary), $Z_5^* = Z_1^* \times Z_4^*$, $Z_6^* = Z_2^* \times Z_4^*$, $Z_7^* = Z_3^* \times Z_4^*$

J. Demonstration that alternative interaction version (in item I) is equivalent to original interaction formulation (in item H) using computer results for the alternative version.

K. Test of no-interaction assumption:

- null hypothesis: $\beta_{11} = \beta_{21} = \ldots = \beta_{71} = 0$ and $\beta_{12} = \beta_{22} = \ldots = \beta_{72} = 0$
- $LR \sim \chi_{14 \text{ df}}^2$ under H_0: no interaction
- $LR = 524.039 - 499.944 = 24.095$ ($P=0.045$)

Conclusion: Reject null hypothesis; interaction model is preferred.

VI. **Summary** (pages 193–194)

Practice Exercises

The following questions derive from the dataset **vets.dat** concerning the Veteran's Administration Lung Cancer Trial that we previously considered in the presentation on the stratified Cox model. Recall that survival times are in days and that the study size contains 137 patients. The exposure variable of interest is treatment status (standard = 1, test = 2). Other variables of interest as control variables are cell type (four types, defined in terms of dummy variables), performance status, disease duration, age, and prior therapy status. Failure status is defined by the status variable (0 = censored, 1 = died).

1. Consider the following two printouts obtained from fitting a Cox PH model to these data.

Response: Surv. Time
Column

name	Coeff	StErr	p-value	HR	0.95	CI	P(PH)
1 Treatment	0.290	0.207	0.162	1.336	0.890	2.006	0.629
2 Large cell	0.400	0.283	0.157	1.491	0.857	2.594	0.035
3 Adeno cell	1.188	0.301	0.000	3.281	1.820	5.915	0.083
4 Small cell	0.856	0.275	0.002	2.355	1.374	4.037	0.080
7 Perf.Stat	−0.033	0.006	0.000	0.968	0.958	0.978	0.000
8 Dis.Durat.	0.000	0.009	0.992	1.000	0.982	1.018	0.919
9 Age	−0.009	0.009	0.358	0.991	0.974	1.010	0.199
10 Pr.Therapy	0.007	0.023	0.755	1.007	0.962	1.054	0.147

n:137   %Cen: 6.569   −2 log L: 950.359   #iter:5

Cox Regression Analysis:
Response: Surv.Time
Column

name	Coeff	StErr	p-value	HR	0.95	CI	P(PH)
1 Treatment	0.298	0.197	0.130	1.347	0.916	1.981	0.739
4 Small cell	0.392	0.210	0.062	1.481	0.981	2.235	0.383
7 Perf.Stat	−0.033	0.005	0.000	0.968	0.958	0.978	0.000
8 Dis.Durat.	−0.001	0.009	0.887	0.999	0.981	1.017	0.926
9 Age	−0.006	0.009	0.511	0.994	0.976	1.012	0.213
10 Pr.Therapy	−0.003	0.023	0.884	0.997	0.954	1.042	0.147

n:137   %Cen: 6.569   −2 log L: 965.540   #iter:5

How do the printouts differ in terms of what the $P(PH)$ information says about which variables do not satisfy the PH assumption?

2. Based on the above information, if you were going to stratify on the cell type variable, how would you define the strata? Explain.

3. Consider a stratified analysis that stratifies on the variables Z_1 = "small cell" and Z_2 = "performance status." The small cell variable is one of the dummy variables for cell type defined above. The performance status variable is dichotomized into high (60 or above) and low (below 60) and is denoted as PSbin. The stratification variable which combines categories from Z_1 and Z_2 is denoted as SZ^* and consists of four categories. The predictors included (but not stratified) in the analysis are treatment status, disease duration, age, and prior therapy. The computer results are as follows:

Stratified Cox Regression Analysis on Variable: SZ^*
Response: Surv.Time

Column name	Coeff	StErr	p-value	HR	0.95	CI
1 Treatment	0.090	0.197	0.647	1.095	0.744	1.611
8 Dis.Durat.	0.000	0.010	0.964	1.000	0.982	1.019
9 Age	0.002	0.010	0.873	1.002	0.983	1.021
10 Pr.Therapy	−0.010	0.023	0.656	0.990	0.947	1.035

n:137　　%Cen: 6.569　　−2 log L: 689.696 #iter:4

Based on these results, describe the point and interval estimates for the hazard ratio for the treatment effect adjusted for the other variables, including SZ^*. Is this hazard ratio meaningfully and/or statistically significant? Explain.

4. State the form of the hazard function for the model being fit in question 3. Why does this model assume no interaction between the stratified variables and the predictors in the model?

5. State two alternative ways to write the hazard function for an "interaction model" that allows for the interaction of the stratified variables with the treatment status variable, but assumes no other type of interaction.

6. State two alternative versions of the hazard function for an interaction model that allows for the interaction of the stratified variables (cell type and performance status) with each of the predictors treatment status, disease duration, age, and prior therapy.

7. For the interaction model described in question 6, what is the formula for the hazard ratio for the effect of treatment adjusted for the other variables? Does this formula give a different hazard ratio for different strata? Explain.

8. State two alternative versions of the null hypothesis for testing whether the no-interaction assumption is satisfied for the stratified Cox model. Note that one of these versions should involve a set of regression coefficients being set equal to zero.

9. State the form of the likelihood ratio statistic for evaluating the no-interaction assumption. How is this statistic distributed under the null hypothesis, and with what degrees of freedom?

10. Provided below are computer results for fitting the interaction model described in question 6. In this printout the variable Z3* denotes the small cell variable and the variable Z4* denotes the PSbin variable. The variable DDZ3* denotes the product of Z3* with disease duration, and other product terms are defined similarly.

Stratified Cox Regression Analysis on Variable: SZ^*
Response: Surv.Time

Column name	Coeff	StErr	p-value	HR	0.95	CI
1 Treatment	0.381	0.428	0.374	1.464	0.632	3.389
8 Dis.Durat.	0.015	0.021	0.469	1.015	0.975	1.057
9 Age	0.000	0.017	0.994	1.000	0.968	1.033
10 Pr.Therapy	0.023	0.041	0.571	1.023	0.944	1.109
17 DDZ_3^*	−0.029	0.024	0.234	0.971	0.926	1.019
20 $AgeZ_3^*$	−0.055	0.037	0.135	0.946	0.880	1.018
23 PTZ_3^*	0.043	0.075	0.564	1.044	0.901	1.211
24 DDZ_4^*	0.025	0.032	0.425	1.026	0.964	1.092
25 $AgeZ_4^*$	0.001	0.024	0.956	1.001	0.956	1.049
26 PTZ_4^*	−0.078	0.054	0.152	0.925	0.831	1.029
29 $DDZ_3Z_4^*$	−0.071	0.059	0.225	0.931	0.830	1.045
32 $AgeZ_3Z_4^*$	0.084	0.049	0.084	1.088	0.989	1.196
35 $PTZ_3Z_4^*$	−0.005	0.117	0.963	0.995	0.791	1.250
38 tr Z_3^*	0.560	0.732	0.444	1.751	0.417	7.351
39 tr Z_4^*	−0.591	0.523	0.258	0.554	0.199	1.543
42 tr $Z_3Z_4^*$	−0.324	0.942	0.731	0.723	0.114	4.583

n:137 %Cen: 6.569 −2 log L: 671.181 #iter:6

Use the above computer results to state the form of the **estimated** hazard model for each of the four strata of the stratification variable SZ^*. Also, for each strata, compute the hazard ratio for the treatment effect adjusted for disease duration, age, and prior therapy.

11. Carry out the likelihood ratio test to evaluate the no-interaction model described in question 4. In carrying out this test, make sure to state the null hypothesis in terms of regression coefficients being set equal to zero in the interaction model fitted in question 10. Also, determine the p-value for this test and state your conclusions about significance as well as which model you prefer, the no-interaction model or the interaction model.

12. The adjusted log–log survival curves for each of the four strata defined by the stratification variable *SZ** (adjusted for treatment status, disease duration, age, and prior therapy) are presented below.

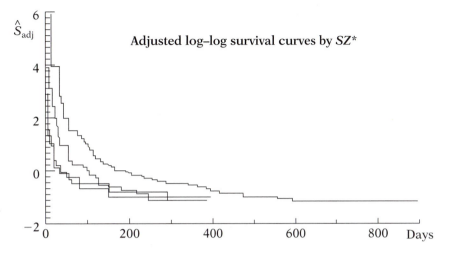

Using this graph, what can you conclude about whether the PH assumption is satisfied for the variables, small cell type and PSbin?

13. Comment on what you think can be learned by graphing adjusted survival curves that compare the two treatment groups for each of the four strata of *SZ**.

Test

The following questions consider a dataset from a study by Caplehorn et al. ("Methadone Dosage and Retention of Patients in Maintenance Treatment," *Med. J. Aust.*, 1991). These data comprise the times in days spent by heroin addicts from entry to departure from one of two methadone clinics. Two other covariates, namely, prison record and maximum methadone dose, are believed to affect the survival times. The dataset name is **addicts.dat.** A listing of the data as stored in a SPIDA file is given in Appendix B. A listing of the variables is given below:

Column 1: Subject ID
Column 2: Clinic (1 or 2)
Column 3: Survival status (0=censored, 1=departed from clinic)

Column 4: Survival time in days
Column 5: Prison record (0=none, 1=any)
Column 6: Maximum methadone dose (mg/day)

1. The following printout was obtained from fitting a Cox PH model to these data:

Cox Regression Analysis
Response: days survival

Column name	Coeff	StErr	p-value	HR	0.95	CI	P(PH)
2 clinic	−1.009	0.215	0.000	0.365	0.239	0.556	0.001
5 prison	0.327	0.167	0.051	1.386	0.999	1.924	0.333
6 dose	−0.035	0.006	0.000	0.965	0.953	0.977	0.348

n:238   %Cen: 36.975   −2 log L: 1346.805   #iter:5

Based on the P(PH) information in the above printout, it appears that clinic does not satisfy the PH assumption; this conclusion is also supported by comparing log–log curves for the two clinics and noticing strong nonparallelism. What might we learn from fitting a stratified Cox (SC) model stratifying on the clinic variable? What is a drawback to using a SC procedure that stratifies on the clinic variable?

2. The following printout was obtained from fitting a SC PH model to these data, where the variable being stratified is clinic:

Stratified Cox Regression Analysis on Variable: clinic
Response: days survival

Column name	Coeff	StErr	p-value	HR	0.95	CI
5 Prison	0.389	0.169	0.021	1.475	1.059	2.054
6 Dose	−0.035	0.006	0.000	0.965	0.953	0.978

n:238   %Cen: 36.975   −2 log L: 1195.428   #iter:5

Using the above fitted model, we can obtain the adjusted curves below that compare the adjusted survival probabilities for each clinic (i.e., stratified by clinic) adjusted for the variables, prison and maximum methadone dose.

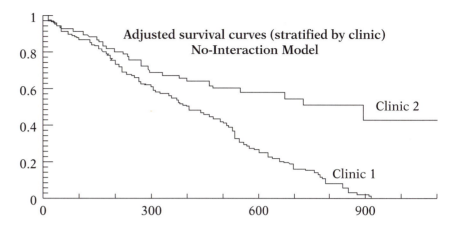

Based on these adjusted survival curves, what conclusions can you draw about whether the survival experience is different between the two clinics? Explain.

3. State the hazard function model being estimated in the above computer results. Why is this model a no-interaction model?

4. Using the above computer results, provide point and interval estimates for the effect of prison adjusted for clinic and dose. Is this adjusted prison effect significant? Explain.

5. The following computer results consider a SC model that allows for interaction of the stratified variable clinic with each of the predictors, prison and dose. Product terms in the model are denoted as clinpr = clinic × prison and clindos = clinic × dose.

Stratified Cox Regression Analysis on Variable: clinic
Response: days survival

Column name	Coeff	StErr	p-value	*HR*	0.95	CI
5 prison	1.087	0.539	0.044	2.966	1.032	8.523
6 dose	−0.035	0.020	0.079	0.966	0.929	1.004
7 clinpr	−0.585	0.428	0.172	0.557	0.241	1.290
8 clindos	−0.001	0.015	0.942	0.999	0.971	1.028

n:238   %Cen: 36.975   −2 log *L*: 1193.558   #iter:6

State two alternative versions of the interaction model being estimated by the above printout, where one of these versions should involve the product terms used in the above printout.

6. Using the computer results above, determine the estimated hazard models for each clinic. (Note that the clinics are coded as 1 or 2.)

7. Below are the adjusted survival curves for each clinic based on the interaction model results above. These curves are adjusted for the prison and dose variables.

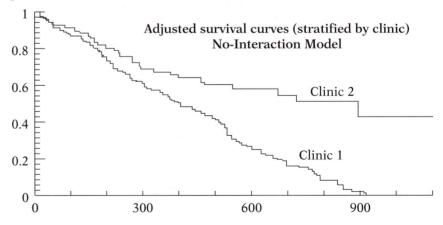

What do these curves say about the effect of clinic on survival time? What information is missing?

8. Compare the survival curves by clinic obtained for the interaction model with the corresponding curves previously shown for the no-interaction model. Do both curves indicate the similar conclusions about the clinic effect? Explain.

9. Carry out a likelihood ratio test to determine whether the no-interaction model is appropriate. In doing so, make use of the computer information described above, state the null and alternative hypotheses, state the form of the likelihood statistic and its distribution under the null hypothesis, and compute the value of the likelihood statistic and evaluate its significance. What are your conclusions?

Answers to Practice Exercises

1. The first printout indicates that the variables large cell, adeno cell, small cell, and performance status do not satisfy the PH assumption at the 0.10 level. The second printout considers a different model that does not contain the large cell and adeno cell variables. This latter printout indicates that small cell satisfies the PH assumption, in contrast to the first printout. The performance status variable, however, does not satisfy the PH assumption as in the first printout.

2. The cell type variable is defined to have four categories, as represented by the three dummy variables in the first printout. The "small cell" variable dichotomizes the cell type variable into the categories small cell type versus the rest. From the second printout, the small cell variable does not appear by itself to violate the PH assumption. This result conflicts with the results of the first printout, for which the cell type variable considered in four categories does not satisfy the PH assumption at the 0.10 level of significance. We therefore think it is more appropriate to use a SC procedure only if four strata are to be used. A drawback to using four strata, however, is that the number of survival curves to be plotted is larger than for two strata; consequently, a large number of curves is more difficult to interpret graphically than when there are only two curves. Thus, for convenience of interpretation, we may choose to dichotomize the cell type variable instead of considering four strata. We may also consider dichotomies other than those defined by the small cell variable. For instance, we might consider dichotomizing on either the adeno or large cell variables instead of the small cell variable. Alternatively, we may combine categories so as to compare, say, large and adeno cell types with small and squamous types.

3. $\widehat{HR}_{adj} = 1.095$, 95% CI: (0.744,1.611), two-tailed P-value is 0.647, not significant. The estimated hazard ratio for treatment is neither meaningfully or statistically significant. The point estimate is essentially 1, which says that there is no meaningful effect of treatment adjusted for the predictors in the model and for the stratified predictor SZ^*.

4. $h_g(t,\mathbf{X}) = h_{0g}(t)\exp[\beta_1 \text{ Treatment} + \beta_2 DD + \beta_3 \text{ Age} + \beta_4 PT], g = 1,\ldots,4$, where the strata are defined from the stratification variable SZ^*, DD = disease duration, and PT = prior therapy. This model assumes no interaction because the coefficient of each predictor in the model is not subscripted by g, i.e., the regression coefficients are the same for each stratum.

5. Version 1: $h_g(t,\mathbf{X}) = h_{0g}(t)\exp[\beta_{1g}\text{Treatment} + \beta_2 DD + \beta_3 \text{ Age} + \beta_4 PT], g=1,\ldots,4$.

   Version 2: $h_g(t,\mathbf{X}) = h_{0g}(t)\exp[\beta_1 \text{ Treatment} + \beta_2 DD + \beta_3 \text{ Age} + \beta_4 PT + \beta_5(Z_1^* \times \text{Treatment}) + \beta_6(Z_2^* \times \text{Treatment}) + \beta_7(Z_1^* \times Z_2^* \times \text{Treatment})]$, where Z_1^* = small cell type (0,1), Z_2^* = PSbin (0,1), and $g=1,\ldots,4$.

6. Version 1: $h_g(t,\mathbf{X}) = h_{0g}(t)\exp[\beta_{1g} \text{ Treatment} + \beta_{2g} DD + \beta_{3g} \text{ Age} + \beta_{4g} PT], g = 1,\ldots,4$.

   Version 2: $h_g(t,\mathbf{X}) = h_{0g}(t)\exp[\beta_1 \text{ Treatment} + \beta_2 DD + \beta_3 \text{ Age} + \beta_4 PT + \beta_5(Z_1^* \times \text{Treatment}) + \beta_6(Z_1^* \times DD) + \beta_7(Z_1^* \times \text{Age}) + \beta_8(Z_1^* \times PT) + \beta_9(Z_2^* \times \text{Treatment}) + \beta_{10}(Z_2^* \times DD) + \beta_{11}(Z_2^* \times \text{Age}) + \beta_{12}(Z_2^* \times PT) + \beta_{13}(Z_1^* \times Z_2^* \times \text{treatment}) + \beta_{14}(Z_1^* \times Z_2^* \times DD) + \beta_{15}(Z_1^* \times Z_2^* \times \text{Age}) + \beta_{16}(Z_1^* \times Z_2^* \times PT)], g = 1,\ldots,4$.

7. $HR_g = \exp^{(\beta_{1g})}$, using version 1 model form. Yes, this formula gives different hazard ratios for different strata because the value of the hazard ratio changes with the subscript g.

8. H_0: No interaction assumption is satisfied.

   H_0: $\beta_{11} = \beta_{12} = \beta_{13} = \beta_{14}, \beta_{21} = \beta_{22} = \beta_{23} = \beta_{24}, \beta_{31} = \beta_{32} = \beta_{33} = \beta_{34}, \beta_{41} = \beta_{42} = \beta_{43} = \beta_{44}$ from version 1.

   H_0: $\beta_5 = \beta_6 = \beta_7 = \beta_8 = \beta_9 = \beta_{10} = \beta_{11} = \beta_{12} = \beta_{13} = \beta_{14} = \beta_{15} = \beta_{16} = 0$ from version 2.

9. $LR = -2 \ln \hat{L}_R - (-2 \ln \hat{L}_F)$, where R denotes the reduced (no-interaction) model and F denotes the full (interaction) model. Under the null hypothesis, LR is approximately a chi-square with 12 degrees of freedom.

10. Estimated hazard models for each stratum:

$g = 1; Z_1^* = Z_2^* = 0$:

$\hat{h}_1(t,\mathbf{X}) = \hat{h}_{01}(t)\exp[(0.381)\text{Treatment} + (0.015)DD + (0.000)\text{Age} + (0.023)PT]$ $g = 2; Z_1^* = 1, Z_2^* = 0$:

$\hat{h}_2(t,\mathbf{X}) = \hat{h}_{02}(t)\exp[(0.941)\text{Treatment} + (-0.014)DD + (-0.055)\text{Age} + (0.066)PT]$ $g = 3; Z_1^* = 0, Z_2^* = 1$:

$\hat{h}_3(t,\mathbf{X}) = \hat{h}_{03}(t)\exp[(-0.210)\text{Treatment} + (0.040)DD + (0.001)\text{Age} + (-0.055)PT]$ $g = 3; Z_1^* = 1, Z_2^* = 1$:

$\hat{h}_4(t,\mathbf{X}) = \hat{h}_{04}(t)\exp[(0.026)\text{Treatment} + (-0.060)DD + (0.030)\text{Age} + (-0.017)PT]$

Estimated hazard ratios for treatment effect adjusted for DD, Age, and PT:

$g = 1: \widehat{HR}_1 = \exp(0.381) = 1.464$

$g = 2: \widehat{HR}_2 = \exp(0.941) = 2.563$

$g = 3: \widehat{HR}_3 = \exp(-0.210) = 0.811$

$g = 4: \widehat{HR}_4 = \exp(0.026) = 1.026$

11. $H_0: \beta_5 = \beta_6 = \beta_7 = \beta_8 = \beta_9 = \beta_{10} = \beta_{11} = \beta_{12} = \beta_{13} = \beta_{14} = \beta_{15} = \beta_{16} = 0$

$LR = 689.696 - 671.181 = 18.515$, which is approximately chi-square with 12 df.

$P = 0.101$, which is not significant below the .05 level.
Conclusion: Accept the null hypothesis and conclude that the no-interaction model is preferable to the interaction model.

12. The three curves at the bottom of the graph appear to be quite non-parallel. Thus, the PH assumption is not satisfied for one or both of the variables, small cell type and **PSbin**. Note, however, that because both these variables have been stratified together, it is not clear from the graph whether only one of these variables fails to satisfy the PH assumption.

13. If we graph adjusted survival curves that compare the two treatment groups for each of the four strata, we will be able to see graphically how the treatment effect, if any, varies over time within each strata. The difficulty with this approach, however, is that eight adjusted survival curves will be produced, so that if all eight curves are put on the same graph, it may be difficult to see what is going on.

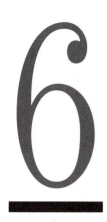

6

Extension of the Cox Proportional Hazards Model for Time-Dependent Variables

■ Contents

Introduction

We begin by defining a time-dependent variable and providing some examples of such a variable. We also state the general formula for a Cox model that is extended to allow time dependent variables, followed by a discussion of the characteristics of this model, including a description of the hazard ratio.

In the remainder of the presentation, we give examples of models with time-dependent variables, including models that allow for checking the PH assumption about time-independent variables. In particular, we describe a method that uses "heavyside functions" to evaluate the PH assumption for time-independent variables. We also describe two computer applications of the extended Cox model, one concerning a study on the treatment of heroin addiction and the other concerning the Stanford heart transplant study.

Abbreviated Outline

The outline below gives the user a preview of the material to be covered by the presentation. A detailed outline for review purposes follows the presentation.

Objectives

Upon completing the module, the learner should be able to:

1. State or recognize the general form of the Cox model extended for time-dependent variables.

2. State the specific form of an extended Cox model appropriate for the analysis, given a survival analysis scenario involving one or more time-dependent variables.

3. State the formula for a designated hazard ratio of interest, given a scenario describing a survival analysis using an extended Cox model.

4. State the formula for an extended Cox model that provides a method for checking the PH assumption for one more of the time-independent variables in the model, given a scenario describing a survival analysis involving time-independent variables.

5. State the formula for an extended Cox model that uses one or more heavyside functions to check the PH assumption for one more of the time-independent variables in the model, given a scenario describing a survival analysis involving time-independent variables.

6. State the formula for the hazard ratio during different time interval categories specified by the heavyside function(s), for a model involving heavyside function(s).

7. Carry out an appropriate analysis of the data to evaluate the effect of one or more of the explanatory variables in the model(s) being used, given computer results for a survival analysis involving time-dependent variables. Such an analysis will involve:
   - computing and interpreting any hazard ratio(s) of interest;
   - carrying out and interpreting appropriate test(s) of hypotheses for effects of interest;
   - obtaining confidence intervals for hazard ratios of interest;
   - evaluating interaction and confounding involving one or more covariates.

Presentation

I. Preview

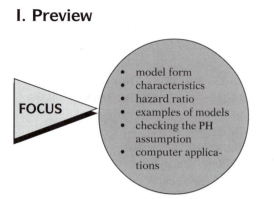

FOCUS

- model form
- characteristics
- hazard ratio
- examples of models
- checking the PH assumption
- computer applications

This presentation describes how the Cox proportional hazards (PH) model can be extended to allow time-dependent variables as predictors. Here, we focus on the model form, characteristics of this model, the formula for and interpretation of the hazard ratio, and examples of the extended Cox model. We also show how the extended Cox model can be used to check the PH assumption for time-independent variables, and we provide computer applications to illustrate different types of time-dependent variables.

II. Review of the Cox PH Model

$$h(t, \mathbf{X}) = h_0(t) \exp\left[\sum_{i=1}^{p} \beta_i X_i\right]$$

$\mathbf{X} = (X_1, X_2, ..., X_p)$

Explanatory/predictor variables

The general form of the Cox PH model is shown here. This model gives an expression for the hazard at time t for an individual with a given specification of a set of explanatory variables denoted by the bold $\mathbf{X}$. That is, the bold $\mathbf{X}$ represents a collection (sometimes called a "vector") of predictor variables that is being modeled to predict an individual's hazard.

$$h_0(t) \times \exp\left[\sum_{i=1}^{p} \beta_i X_i\right]$$

Baseline hazard	Exponential
Involves t but not X's	Involves X's but not t (X's are time-independent)

The Cox model formula says that the hazard at time t is the product of two quantities. The first of these, $h_0(t)$, is called the **baseline hazard** function. The second quantity is the exponential expression e to the linear sum of $\beta_i X_i$, where the sum is over the p explanatory X variables.

An important feature of this formula, which concerns the proportional hazards (PH) assumption, is that the baseline hazard is a function of t but does not involve the X's, whereas the exponential expression involves the X's but does not involve t. The X's here are called **time-independent** X's.

X's involving t: time dependent

Requires extended Cox model (no PH)

It is possible, nevertheless, to consider X's that do involve t. Such X's are called **time-dependent** variables. If time-dependent variables are considered, the Cox model form may still be used, but such a model no longer satisfies the PH assumption and is called the **extended Cox model.** We will discuss time-dependent variables and the corresponding extended Cox model beginning in the next section.

Hazard ratio formula:

$$\widehat{HR} = \exp\left[\sum_{i=1}^{p}\hat{\beta}_i\left(X_i^* - X_i\right)\right]$$

where $\mathbf{X^*} = (X_1^*, X_2^*, ..., X_p^*)$ and $\mathbf{X} = (X_1, X_2, ..., X_p)$ denote the two sets of X's.

From the Cox PH model, we can obtain a general formula, shown here, for estimating a hazard ratio that compared two specifications of the X's, defined as $\mathbf{X^*}$ and $\mathbf{X}$.

PH assumption:

$$\frac{\hat{h}(t, \mathbf{X}^*)}{\hat{h}(t, \mathbf{X})} = \hat{\theta} \text{ (a constant over } t\text{)}$$

i.e., $\hat{h}(t, \mathbf{X}^*) = \hat{\theta}\,\hat{h}(t, \mathbf{X})$

The (PH) assumption underlying the Cox PH model is that the hazard ratio comparing any two specifications of $\mathbf{X}$ predictors is constant over time. Equivalently, this means that the hazard for one individual is proportional to the hazard for any other individual, where the proportionality constant is independent of time.

Hazards cross $\Rightarrow$ PH not met

Hazards don't cross $\not\Rightarrow$ PH met

An example of when the PH assumption is not met is given by any study situation in which the hazards for two or more groups cross when graphed against time. However, even if the hazard functions do not cross, it is possible that the PH assumption is not met.

Three approaches:
- graphical
- time-dependent variables
- goodness-of-fit test

As described in more detail in Chapter 4, there are three general approaches for assessing the PH assumption. These are

- a graphical approach;
- the use of time-dependent variables in an extended Cox model; and
- the use of a goodness-of-fit test.

Time-dependent covariates:

Extend Cox model: add product term(s) involving some function of time

When time-dependent variables are used to assess the PH assumption for a time-independent variable, the Cox model is extended to contain **product** (i.e., interaction) **terms** involving the time-independent variable being assessed and some function of time.

EXAMPLE

$h(t, \mathbf{X}) = h_0(t) \exp[\beta_1 G + \beta_2 (G \times t)]$

where G denotes GENDER

$H_0 : \beta_2 = 0 \Rightarrow$ PH assumption satisfied

For example, if the PH assumption is being assessed for gender, a Cox model might be extended to include the variable GENDER $\times t$ in addition to GENDER. If the coefficient of the product term turns out to be non-significant, we can conclude that the PH assumption is satisfied for GENDER provided that the variable $G \times t$ is an appropriate choice of time-dependent variable.

Options when PH assumption not satisfied:
- Use a stratified Cox (SC) model.
- Use time-dependent variables.

There are two options to consider if the PH assumption is not satisfied for one or more of the predictors in the model. In Chapter 5, we described the option of using a stratified Cox (SC) model, which stratifies on the predictor(s) not satisfying the PH assumption, while keeping in the model those predictors that satisfy the PH assumption. In this chapter, we describe the other option, which involves using time-dependent variables.

Time-dependent variables may be:
- inherently time-dependent
- defined to analyze a time-independent predictor not satisfying the PH assumption.

Note that a given study may consider predictors that are inherently defined as time-dependent, as we will illustrate in the next section. Thus, in addition to considering time-dependent variables as an option for analyzing a time-independent variable not satisfying the PH assumption, we also discuss predictors which are inherently defined as time-dependent.

III. Definition and Examples of Time-Dependent Variables

Definition:

Time-dependent	Time-independent
Value of variable differs over time	Value of variable is constant over time

Example:

(Race $\times t$) | (Race)

A time-dependent variable is defined as any variable whose value for a given subject may differ over time (t). In contrast, a time-independent variable is a variable whose value for a given subject remains constant over time.

As a simple example, the variable RACE is a time-independent variable, whereas the variable RACE $\times$ time is a time-dependent variable.

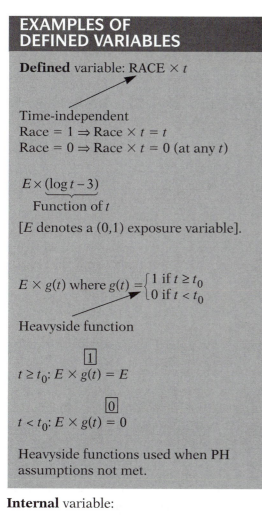

EXAMPLES OF DEFINED VARIABLES

Defined variable: RACE $\times t$

Time-independent
Race $= 1 \Rightarrow$ Race $\times t = t$
Race $= 0 \Rightarrow$ Race $\times t = 0$ (at any t)

$E \times \underbrace{(\log t - 3)}_{\text{Function of } t}$

[E denotes a (0,1) exposure variable].

$E \times g(t)$ where $g(t) = \begin{cases} 1 \text{ if } t \geq t_0 \\ 0 \text{ if } t < t_0 \end{cases}$

Heavyside function

$\boxed{1}$
$t \geq t_0: E \times g(t) = E$

$\boxed{0}$
$t < t_0: E \times g(t) = 0$

Heavyside functions used when PH assumptions not met.

Internal variable:

EXAMPLES OF INTERNAL VARIABLES

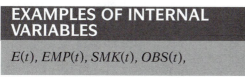

$E(t), EMP(t), SMK(t), OBS(t),$

Values change because of "internal" characteristics or behavior of the individual.

The variable RACE $\times$ time is an example of what is called a "defined" time-dependent variable. Most defined variables are of the form of the product of a time-independent variable (e.g., RACE) multiplied by time or some function of time. Note that after RACE is determined for a given subject, all the values of the RACE $\times$ time variable are completely defined over a specified time interval of study.

A second example of a defined variable is given by $E \times (\log t - 3)$, where E denotes, say, a (0,1) exposure status variable determined at one's entry into the study. Notice that here we have used a function of time—that is, $\log t - 3$—rather than time alone.

Yet another example of a defined variable, which also involves a function of time, is given by $E \times g(t)$, where $g(t)$ is defined to take on the value 1 if t is greater than or equal to some specified value of t, called t_0, and takes on the value 0 if t is less than t_0.

The function $g(t)$ is called a "heavyside" function. Note that whenever t is greater than or equal to t_0, $g(t)$ equals 1, so $E \times g(t) = E$; however, whenever t is less than t_0, $g(t) = 0$, so the value of $E \times g(t)$ is always 0. We will later return to illustrate how heavyside functions may be used as one method for the analysis when a time-independent variable like E does not satisfy the proportional hazards assumption.

Another type of time-dependent variable is called an "internal" variable. Examples of such a variable include exposure level E at time t, employment status (EMP) at time t, smoking status (SMK) at time t, and obesity level (OBS) at time t.

All these examples consider variables whose values may change over time for any subject under study; moreover, for internal variables, the reason for a change in value depends on "internal" characteristics or behavior specific to the individual.

"Ancillary" variable:
Values change because of "external" characteristics.

EXAMPLES OF ANCILLARY VARIABLES

Air pollution index at time t; $EMP(t)$

ANOTHER EXAMPLE

Heart transplant status at time t:

$$HT(t) = \begin{cases} 1 & \text{if received transplant at some time } t_0 \leq t \\ 0 & \text{if did not receive transplant by time } t \end{cases}$$

Transplant $HT(t): 0000...0\,111111111$
$$\underset{t \rightarrow \qquad t_0}{}$$

$HT(t)$:
No transplant $HT(t): 0000...00000$
$$\underset{t \rightarrow}{}$$

Heart transplant status $= HT(t)$

Internal:
Status determined from individual traits

Ancillary:
Status determined from external availability of a donor

In contrast, a variable is called an "ancillary" variable if its values change primarily because of "external" characteristics of the environment that may affect several individuals simultaneously. An example of an ancillary variable is air pollution index at time t for a particular geographical area. Another example is employment status (EMP) at time t, if the primary reason for whether someone is employed or not depends more on general economic circumstances than on individual characteristics.

As another example, which may be part internal and part ancillary, we consider heart transplant status (HT) at time t for a person identified to have a serious heart condition, making him or her eligible for a transplant. The value of this variable HT at time t is 1 if the person has already received a transplant at some time, say t_0, prior to time t. The value of HT is 0 at time t if the person has not yet received a transplant by time t.

Note that once a person receives a transplant, at time t_0, the value of HT remains at 1 for all subsequent times. Thus, for a person receiving a transplant, the value of HT is 0 up to the time of transplant, and then remains at 1 thereafter. In contrast, a person who never receives a transplant has HT equal to 0 for all times during the period he or she is in the study.

The variable "heart transplant status," $HT(t)$, can be considered essentially an internal variable, because individual traits of an eligible transplant recipient are important determinants of the decision to carry out transplant surgery. Nevertheless, the availability of a donor heart prior to tissue and other matching with an eligible recipient can be considered an "ancillary" characteristic external to the recipient.

Computer commands differ for defined vs. internal vs. ancillary.

But, the form of extended Cox model and procedures for analysis are the same regardless of variable type.

The primary reason for distinguishing among defined, internal, or ancillary variables is that the computer commands required to define the variables for use in an extended Cox model are somewhat different for the different variable types, depending on the computer program used. Nevertheless, the form of the extended Cox model is the same regardless of variable type, and the procedures for obtaining estimates of regression coefficients and other parameters, as well as for carrying out statistical inferences, are also the same.

IV. The Extended Cox Model for Time-Dependent Variables

$$h(t, \mathbf{X}(t)) = h_0(t) \exp\left[\sum_{i=1}^{p_1} \beta_i X_i + \sum_{j=1}^{p_2} \delta_j X_j(t)\right]$$

$$\mathbf{X}(t) = \underbrace{\left(X_1, X_2, \ldots X_{p_1}\right.}_{\text{Time-independent}}, \underbrace{\left. X_1(t), X_2(t), \ldots X_{p_2}(t)\right)}_{\text{Time-dependent}}$$

Given a survival analysis situation involving both time-independent and time-dependent predictor variables, we can write the extended Cox model that incorporates both types as shown here at the left. As with the Cox PH model, the extended model contains a baseline hazards function $h_0(t)$ which is multiplied by an exponential function. However, in the extended model, the exponential part contains both time-independent predictors, as denoted by the X_i variables, and time-dependent predictors, as denoted by the $X_j(t)$ variables. The entire collection of predictors at time t is denoted by the bold $\mathbf{X}(t)$.

EXAMPLE

$h(t, \mathbf{X}(t)) = h_0(t) \exp[\beta E + \delta(E \times t)]$,
$p_1 = 1, p_2 = 1$,
$\mathbf{X}(t) = (X_1 = E, X_1(t) = E \times t)$

As a simple example of an extended Cox model, we show here a model with one time-independent variable and one time-dependent variable. The time-independent variable is exposure status E, say a $(0,1)$ variable, and the time-dependent variable is the product term $E \times t$.

Estimating regression coefficients:
ML procedure:
Maximize (partial) L.
Risk sets more complicated than for PH model.

As with the simpler Cox PH model, the regression coefficients in the extended Cox model are estimated using a maximum likelihood (ML) procedure. ML estimates are obtained by maximizing a (partial) likelihood function L. However, the computations for the extended Cox model are more complicated than for the Cox PH model, because the risk sets used to form the likelihood function are more complicated with time-dependent variables.

Computer programs for the extended Cox model:

$$\left.\begin{array}{l} \text{SPIDA(TCOX)} \\ \text{SAS (PHREG)} \\ \text{BMDP (2PL)} \\ \text{EGRET} \end{array}\right\} \text{Appendix A}$$

Computer packages that include programs for fitting the extended Cox model include SPIDA(TCOX), SAS (PHREG), BMDP(2PL), and EGRET. See Appendix A at the end of this text for a comparison of the SPIDA, SAS, and BMDP procedures applied to the same dataset.

Statistical inferences:

Wald and/or *LR* tests

Large sample confidence intervals

Methods for making statistical inferences are essentially the same as for the PH model. That is, one can use Wald and/or likelihood ratio (*LR*) tests and large sample confidence interval methods.

Assumption of the model:

The hazard at time *t* depends on the value of $X_j(t)$ at that same time.

An important assumption of the extended Cox model is that the effect of a time-dependent variable $X_j(t)$ on the survival probability at time *t* depends on the value of this variable at that *same* time *t*, and not on the value at an earlier or later time.

$$h(t, \mathbf{X}(t)) = h_0(t) \exp\left[\sum_{i=1}^{p_1} \beta_i X_i + \sum_{j=1}^{p_2} \delta_j X_j(t)\right]$$

One coefficient for $X_j(t)$

Note that even though the values of the variable $X_j(t)$ may change over time, the hazard model provides only one coefficient for each time-dependent variable in the model. Thus, at time *t*, there is only one value of the variable $X_j(t)$ that has an effect on the hazard, that value being measured at time *t*.

Can modify for lag-time effect

It is possible, nevertheless, to modify the definition of the time-dependent variable to allow for a "lag-time" effect.

Lag-time effect:

EXAMPLE

$EMP(t)$ = employment status at week *t*

Model without lag-time:
$$h(t, \mathbf{X}(t)) = h_0(t) \exp[\delta EMP(t)]$$

Same week

Model with 1-week lag-time:
$$h(t, \mathbf{X}(t)) = h_0(t) \exp[\delta^* EMP(t - 1)]$$

One-week earlier

To illustrate the idea of a lag-time effect, suppose, for example, that employment status, measured weekly and denoted as $EMP(t)$, is the time-dependent variable being considered. Then, an extended Cox model that does *not* consider lag-time assumes that the effect of employment status on the probability of survival at week *t* depends on the observed value of this variable at the same week *t*, and not, for example, at an earlier week.

However, to allow for, say, a time-lag of one week, the employment status variable may be modified so that the hazard model at time *t* is predicted by the employment status at week *t* – 1. Thus, the variable $EMP(t)$ is replaced in the model by the variable $EMP(t - 1)$.

General lag-time extended model:

$$h\big(t, \mathbf{X}(t)\big) = h_0(t) \exp\left[\sum_{i=1}^{p_1} \beta_i X_i + \sum_{j=1}^{p_2} \delta_j X_j\big(t - L_j\big) \right]$$

$X_j(t - L_j)$ replaces $X_j(t)$

More generally, the extended Cox model may be alternatively written to allow for a lag-time modification of any time-dependent variable of interest. If we let L_j denote the lag-time specified for time-dependent variable j, then the general "lag-time extended model" can be written as shown here. Note that the variable $X_j(t)$ in the earlier version of the extended model is now replaced by the variable $X_j(t - L_j)$.

V. The Hazard Ratio Formula for the Extended Cox Model

PH assumption is not satisfied for the extended Cox model.

$$\widehat{HR}(t) = \frac{\hat{h}(t, \mathbf{X}^*(t))}{\hat{h}(t, \mathbf{X}(t))}$$

$$= \exp\left[\sum_{i=1}^{p_1} \hat{\beta}_i \Big[X_i^* - X_i \Big] + \sum_{j=1}^{p_2} \delta_j \Big[X_j^*(t) - X_j(t) \Big] \right]$$

Two sets of predictors:
$$\mathbf{X}^*(t) = (X_1^*, X_2^*, ..., X_{p_1}^*, X_1^*(t), X_2^*(t), ..., X_{p_2}^*(t))$$

$$\mathbf{X}(t) = (X_1, X_2, ..., X_{p_1}, X_1(t), X_2(t), ..., X_{p_2}(t))$$

We now describe the formula for the hazard ratio that derives from the extended Cox model. The most important feature of this formula is that the proportional hazards assumption is no longer satisfied when using the extended Cox model.

The general hazard ratio formula for the extended Cox model is shown here. This formula describes the ratio of hazards at a particular time t, and requires the specification of two sets of predictors at time t. These two sets are denoted as bold $\mathbf{X}^*(t)$ and bold $\mathbf{X}(t)$.

The two sets of predictors, $\mathbf{X}^*(t)$ and $\mathbf{X}(t)$, identify two specifications at time t for the combined set of predictors containing both time-independent and time-dependent variables. The individual components for each set of predictors are shown here.

EXAMPLE

$$h(t, \mathbf{X}(t) = h_0(t) \exp[\beta E + \delta(E \times t)]$$

$$E = \begin{cases} 1 & \text{if exposed} \\ 0 & \text{if unexposed} \end{cases}$$

$$\mathbf{X}^*(t) = (E = 1, E \times t = t)$$
$$\mathbf{X}(t) = (E = 0, E \times t = 0)$$

$$\widehat{HR}(t) = \frac{\hat{h}(t, E = 1)}{\hat{h}(t, E = 0)}$$

$$= \exp\big[\hat{\beta}(1 - 0) + \hat{\delta}(1 \times t) - (0 \times t)\big]$$

$$= \exp\big[\hat{\beta} + \hat{\delta}t\big]$$

$\hat{\delta} > 0 \Rightarrow \widehat{HR}(t) \uparrow$ as $t \uparrow$
PH assumption *not* satisfied

As a simple example, suppose the model contains only one time-independent predictor, namely, exposure status E, a (0,1) variable, and one time-dependent predictor, namely, $E \times t$. Then, to compare exposed persons, for whom $E = 1$, with unexposed persons, for whom $E = 0$, at time t, the bold $\mathbf{X}^*(t)$ set of predictors has as its two components $E = 1$ and $E \times t = t$; the bold $\mathbf{X}(t)$ set has as its two components, $E = 0$ and $E \times t = 0$.

If we now calculate the estimated hazard ratio that compares exposed to unexposed persons at time t, we obtain the formula shown here; that is, HR "hat" equals the exponential of β "hat" plus δ "hat" times t. This formula says that the hazard ratio is a function of time; in particular, if δ "hat" is positive, then the hazard ratio increases with increasing time. Thus, the hazard ratio in this example is certainly not constant, so that the PH assumption is not satisfied for this model.

$$\widehat{HR}(t) = \exp\left[\sum_{i=1}^{p_1} \hat{\beta}_i \left[X_i^* - X_i\right] + \sum_{j=1}^{p_2} \hat{\delta}_j \boxed{\left[X_j^*(t) - X_j(t)\right]}\right]$$

A function of time

In general, PH assumption not satisfied for extended Cox model.

$\hat{\delta}_j$ is not time-dependent.

$\hat{\delta}_j$ represents "overall" effect of $X_i(t)$.

More generally, because the general hazard ratio formula involves differences in the values of the time-dependent variables at time t, this hazard ratio is a function of time. Thus, in general, the extended Cox model does not satisfy the PH assumption if any δ_j is not equal to zero.

Note that, in the hazard ratio formula, the coefficient δ_j "hat" of the difference in values of the jth time-dependent variable is itself not time-dependent. Thus, this coefficient represents the "overall" effect of the corresponding time-dependent variable, considering all times at which this variable has been measured in the study.

EXAMPLE

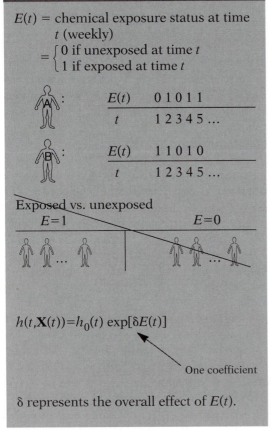

$E(t)$ = chemical exposure status at time
t (weekly)
$= \begin{cases} 0 \text{ if unexposed at time } t \\ 1 \text{ if exposed at time } t \end{cases}$

A: $E(t)$ 0 1 0 1 1
     ─────────────────
     t 1 2 3 4 5 …

B: $E(t)$ 1 1 0 1 0
     ─────────────────
     t 1 2 3 4 5 …

Exposed vs. unexposed
   $E=1$ $E=0$

$h(t, \mathbf{X}(t)) = h_0(t) \exp[\delta E(t)]$

One coefficient

δ represents the overall effect of $E(t)$.

As another example to illustrate the formula for the hazard ratio, consider an extended Cox model containing only one variable, say a weekly measure of chemical exposure status at time t. Suppose this variable, denoted as $E(t)$, can take one of two values, 0 or 1, depending on whether a person is unexposed or exposed, respectively, at a given weekly measurement.

As defined, the variable $E(t)$ can take on different patterns of values for different subjects. For example, for a five-week period, subject A's values may be 01011, whereas subject B's values may be 11010.

Note that in this example, we do not consider two separate groups of subjects, with one group always exposed and the other group always unexposed throughout the study. This latter situation would require a (0,1) time-independent variable for exposure, whereas our example involves a time-dependent exposure variable.

The extended Cox model that includes only the variable $E(t)$ is shown here. In this model, the values of the exposure variable may change over time for different subjects, but there is only one coefficient, δ, corresponding to the one variable in the model. Thus, δ represents the overall effect on survival time of the time-dependent variable $E(t)$.

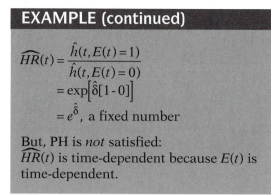

EXAMPLE (continued)

$$\widehat{HR}(t) = \frac{\hat{h}(t, E(t) = 1)}{\hat{h}(t, E(t) = 0)}$$
$$= \exp\left[\hat{\delta}[1 - 0]\right]$$
$$= e^{\hat{\delta}}, \text{ a fixed number}$$

But, PH is *not* satisfied:
$\widehat{HR}(t)$ is time-dependent because $E(t)$ is time-dependent.

Notice, also, that the hazard ratio formula, which compares an exposed person to an unexposed person at time t, yields the expression e to the δ "hat."

Although this result is a fixed number, the PH assumption is not satisfied. The fixed number gives the hazard ratio at a given time, assuming that the exposure status at that time is 1 in the numerator and is 0 denominator. Thus, the hazard ratio is time-dependent, because exposure status is time-dependent, even though the formula yields a single fixed number.

VI. Assessing Time-Independent Variables That Do Not Satisfy the PH Assumption

Use an extended Cox model to
- check PH assumption;
- assess effect of variable not satisfying PH assumption.

We now discuss how to use an extended Cox model to check the PH assumption for time-independent variables and to assess the effect of a variable that does not satisfy the PH assumption.

Three methods for checkng PH assumption:
1. graphical
2. (extended Cox model)
3. GOF test

As described previously (see Chapter 4), there are three methods commonly used to assess the PH assumption: (1) graphical, using, say, log–log survival curves; (2) using an extended Cox model; and (3) using a goodness-of-fit (GOF) test. We have previously (in Chapter 4) discussed items 1 and 3, but only briefly described item 2, which we focus on here.

Cox PH model for p time-independent X's:

$$h(t, \mathbf{X}) = h_0(t) \exp\left[\sum_{i=1}^{p} \beta_i X_i\right]$$

If the dataset for our study contains several, say p, time-independent variables, we might wish to fit a Cox PH model containing each of these variables, as shown here.

Extended Cox model:
Add product terms of the form:
$X_i \times g_i(t)$

However, to assess whether such a PH model is appropriate, we can extend this model by defining several product terms involving each time-independent variable with some function of time. That is, if the ith time-independent variable is denoted as X_i, then we can define the ith product term as $X_i \times g_i(t)$ where $g_i(t)$ is some function of time for the ith variable.

$$h(t, \mathbf{X}(t)) = h_0(t) \exp\left[\sum_{i=1}^{p_1} \beta_i X_i + \sum_{i=1}^{p} \delta_i X_i g_i(t)\right]$$

The extended Cox model that simultaneously considers all time-independent variables of interest is shown here.

EXAMPLE

$g_i(t) = 0$ for all i implies no time-dependent variable involving X_i, i.e.,

$$h(t, \mathbf{X}(t)) = h_0(t) \exp\left[\sum_{i=1}^{p} \beta_i X_i\right].$$

In using this extended model, the crucial decision is the form that the functions $g_i(t)$ should take. The simplest form for $g_i(t)$ is that all $g_i(t)$ are identically 0 at any time; this is another way of stating the original PH model, containing no time-dependent terms.

EXAMPLE 2

$g_i(t) = t \Rightarrow X_i g_i(t) = X_i \times t$

$$h(t, \mathbf{X}(t)) = h_0(t) \exp\left[\sum_{i=1}^{p} \beta_i X_i + \sum_{i=1}^{p} \delta_i (X_i \times t)\right]$$

Another choice for the $g_i(t)$ is to let $g_i(t) = t$. This implies that for each X_i in the model as a main effect, there is a corresponding time-dependent variable in the model of the form $X_i \times t$. The extended Cox model in this case takes the form shown here.

EXAMPLE 3: one variable at a time

X_L only $\Rightarrow \begin{cases} g_L(t) = t, \\ g_i(t) = 0 \text{ for other } i \end{cases}$

$$h(t, \mathbf{X}(t)) = h_0(t) \exp\left[\sum_{i=1}^{p} \beta_i X_i + \delta_L (X_L \times t)\right]$$

Suppose, however, we wish to focus on a particular time-independent variable, say, variable X_L. Then $g_i(t) = t$ for $i = L$, but equals 0 for all other i. The corresponding extended Cox model would then contain only one product term $X_L \times t$, as shown here.

EXAMPLE 4

$g_i(t) = \log t \Rightarrow X_i g_i(t) = X_i \times \ln t$

$$h(t, \mathbf{X}(t)) = h_0(t) \exp\left[\sum_{i=1}^{p} \beta_i X_i + \sum_{i=1}^{p} \delta_i (X_i \times \ln t)\right]$$

Another choice for the $g_i(t)$ is the log of t, rather than simply t, so that the corresponding time-dependent variables will be of the form $X_i \times \log t$.

EXAMPLE 5: Heaviside Function

$g_i(t) = \begin{cases} 0 & \text{if } t \geq t_0 \\ 1 & \text{if } t < t_0 \end{cases}$

And yet another choice would be to let $g_i(t)$ be a "heavyside function" of the form $g_i(t) = 1$ when t is at or above some specified time, say t_0, and $g_i(t) = 0$ when t is below t_0. We will discuss this choice in more detail shortly.

Extend Cox model:

$$h(t, \mathbf{X}(t)) = h_0(t) \exp\left[\sum_{i=1}^{p} \beta_i X_i + \sum_{i=1}^{p} \delta_i X_i g_i(t)\right]$$

- Check PH assumption.
- Obtain hazard ratio when PH assumption not satisfied.

$$H_0 : \delta_1 = \delta_2 = \cdots = \delta_p = 0$$

Given a particular choice of the $g_i(t)$, the corresponding extended Cox model, shown here again in general form, may then be used to check the PH assumption for the time-independent variables in the model. Also, we can use this extended Cox model to obtain a hazard ratio formula that considers the effects of variables not satisfying the PH assumption.

To check the PH assumption using a statistical test, we consider the null hypothesis that all the δ terms, which are coefficients of the $X_i g_i(t)$ product terms in the model, are zero.

Under H_0, the model reduces to PH model:

$$h(t, \mathbf{X}) = h_0(t) \exp\left[\sum_{i=1}^{p_1} \beta_i X_i\right]$$

$$LR = -2 \ln \hat{L}_{\text{PH model}} - (-2 \ln L_{\text{ext. Cox model}})$$

$$\sim \chi_p^2 \text{ under } H_0$$

Under this null hypothesis, the model reduces to the PH model.

This test can be carried out using a likelihood ratio (LR) test which computes the difference between the log likelihood statistic, $-2 \ln L$ "hat," for the PH model and the log likelihood statistic for the extended Cox model. The test statistic thus obtained has approximately a chi-square distribution with p degrees of freedom under the null hypothesis, where p denotes the number of parameters being set equal to zero under H_0.

EXAMPLE

$h(t, \mathbf{X}(t)) = h_0(t) \exp[\beta E + \delta(E \times t)]$
$H_0 : \delta = 0$ (i.e., PH assumption is satisfied)

Reduced model:
$h(t, \mathbf{X}) = h_0(t) \exp[\beta E]$

$LR = -2 \ln \hat{L}_R - (-2 \ln \hat{L}_F)$
$\sim \chi^2 \text{ with 1 df under } H_0$

$F = \text{full (extended)}, R = \text{reduced (PH)}$

As an example of this test, suppose we again consider an extended Cox model that contains the product term $E \times t$ in addition to the main effect of E, where E denotes a $(0,1)$ time-independent exposure variable.

For this model, a test for whether or not the PH assumption is satisfied is equivalent to testing the null hypothesis that $\delta = 0$. Under this hypothesis, the reduced model is given by the PH model containing the main effect E only. The likelihood ratio statistic, shown here as the difference between log-likelihood statistics for the full (i.e., extended model) and the reduced (i.e., PH) model, will have an approximate chi-square distribution with one degree of freedom in large samples.

Note: This test requires two different computer programs:

SAS: **PHREG** fits both PH and extended Cox models.

SPIDA: cox for PH model, **tcox** for extended Cox model.

Note that to carry out the computations for this test, two different types of models, a PH model and an extended Cox model, need to be fit. This essentially requires two different computer programs to fit these two models. SAS's PHREG procedure allows the user to fit each type of model using the same procedure. However, other programs, like SPIDA, require different procedures.

If PH test significant: Extended Cox model is preferred; HR is time-dependent.

If the result of the test for the PH assumption is significant, then the extended Cox model is preferred to the PH model. Thus, the hazard ratio expression obtained for the effect of an exposure variable of interest is time-dependent. That is, the effect of the exposure on the outcome cannot be summarized by a single HR value, but can only be expressed as a function of time.

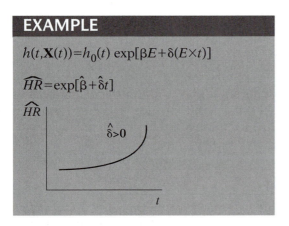

EXAMPLE

$$h(t, \mathbf{X}(t)) = h_0(t) \exp[\beta E + \delta(E \times t)]$$

$$\widehat{HR} = \exp[\hat{\beta} + \hat{\delta} t]$$

We again consider the previous example, with the extended Cox model shown here. For this model, the estimated hazard ratio for the effect of exposure is given by the expression e to the quantity β "hat" plus δ "hat" times t. Thus, depending on whether δ "hat" is positive or negative, the estimated hazard ratio will increase or decrease exponentially as t increases. The graph shown here gives a sketch of how the hazard ratio varies with time if δ "hat" is positive.

Heavyside function:

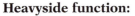
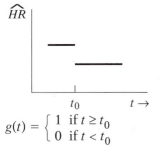

$$g(t) = \begin{cases} 1 & \text{if } t \geq t_0 \\ 0 & \text{if } t < t_0 \end{cases}$$

$$h(t, \mathbf{X}(t)) = h_0(t) \exp[\beta E + \delta E g(t)]$$

We now provide a description of the use of a "heavyside" function. When such a function is used, the hazard ratio formula yields constant hazard ratios for different time intervals, as illustrated in the accompanying graph.

Recall that a heavyside function is of the form $g(t)$, which takes on the value 1 if t is greater than or equal to some specified value of t, called t_0, and takes on the value 0 if t is less than t_0. An extended Cox model which contains a single heavyside function is shown here.

$t \geq t_0$: $g(t) = 1 \Rightarrow E \times g(t) = E$
$h(t,\mathbf{X}) = h_0(t) \exp[(\beta + \delta)E]$
$\widehat{HR} = \exp[\hat{\beta} + \hat{\delta}]$

Note that if $t \geq t_0$, $g(t) = 1$, so the value of $E \times g(t) = E$; the corresponding hazard function is of the form $h_0(t) \times e$ to the quantity $(\beta + \delta)$ times E, and the estimated hazard ratio for the effect of E has the form e to the sum of β "hat" plus δ "hat."

$t < t_0$ $g(t) = 0 \Rightarrow E \times g(t) = 0$
$h(t,\mathbf{X}) = h_0(t) \exp[\beta E]$
$\widehat{HR} = \exp[\hat{\beta}]$

If $t < t_0$, $g(t) = 0$, and the corresponding hazard ratio is simplified to e to the β "hat."

A single heaviside function in the model
$h(t,\mathbf{X}) = h_0(t) \exp[\beta E + \delta(E \times g(t))]$

yields two hazard ratios:
$t \geq t_0$: $\widehat{HR} = \exp(\hat{\beta} + \hat{\delta})$
$t < t_0$: $\widehat{HR} = \exp(\hat{\beta})$

Thus, we have shown that the use of a single heaviside function results in an extended Cox model which gives two hazard ratio values, each value being constant over a fixed time interval.

Alternative model with two heaviside functions:
$h(t,\mathbf{X}) = h_0(t) \exp[\delta_1(E \times g_1(t)) + \delta_2(E \times g_2(t))]$

$g_1(t) = \begin{cases} 1 & \text{if } t \geq t_0 \\ 0 & \text{if } t < t_0 \end{cases}$

$g_2(t) = \begin{cases} 1 & \text{if } t < t_0 \\ 0 & \text{if } t \geq t_0 \end{cases}$

Note: Main effect for E not in model.

There is actually an equivalent way to write this model that uses two heaviside functions in the same model. This alternative model is shown here. The two heavyside functions are called $g_1(t)$ and $g_2(t)$. Each of these functions are in the model as part of a product term with the exposure variable E. Note that this model does not contain a main effect term for exposure.

Two HR's from the alternative model:
$t \geq t_0$: $g_1(t) = 1$, $g_2(t) = 0$
$h(t, \mathbf{X}) = h_0(t) \exp[\delta_1(E \times 1) + \delta_2(E \times 0)]$
$= h_0(t) \exp[\delta_1 E]$
so that $\widehat{HR} = \exp(\hat{\delta}_1)$

For this alternative model, as for the earlier model with only one heaviside function, two different hazard ratios are obtained for different time intervals. To obtain the first hazard ratio, we consider the form that the model takes when $t \geq t_0$. In this case, the value of $g_1(t)$ is 1 and the value of $g_2(t)$ is 0, so the exponential part of the model simplifies to $\delta_1 \times E$; the corresponding formula for the estimated hazard ratio is then e to the δ_1 "hat."

$t < t_0$: $g_1(t) = 0$, $g_2(t) = 1$
$h(t, \mathbf{X}) = h_0(t) \exp[\delta_1(E \times 0) + \delta_2(E \times 1)]$
$= h_0(t) \exp[\delta_2 E]$
so that $\widehat{HR} = \exp(\hat{\delta}_2)$

When $t < t_0$, the value of $g_1(t)$ is 0 and the value of $g_2(t)$ is 1. Then, the exponential part of the model becomes $\delta_2 \times E$, and the corresponding hazard ratio formula is e to the δ_2 "hat."

Alternative model:

$h(t, \mathbf{X}(t)) = h_0(t) \exp [\delta_1(E \times g_1(t)) + \delta_2(E \times g_2(t))]$

Original model:

$h(t, \mathbf{X}(t)) = h_0(t) \exp[\beta E + \delta(E \times g(t))]$

$t \geq t_0: \widehat{HR} = \exp(\hat{\delta}_1) = \exp(\hat{\beta}+\hat{\delta})$

$t < t_0: \widehat{HR} = \exp(\hat{\delta}_2) = \exp(\hat{\beta})$

Thus, using the alternative model, again shown here, we obtain two distinct hazard ratio values. Mathematically, these are the same values as obtained from the original model containing only one heavyside function. In other words, δ_1 "hat" in the alternative model equals β "hat" plus δ "hat" in the original model (containing one heavyside function), and δ_2 "hat" in the alternative model equals β "hat" in the original model.

Heavyside functions:
- two $\widehat{HR}$'s constant within two time intervals
- *extension*: several $\widehat{HR}$'s constant within several time intervals

We have thus seen that heavyside functions can be used to provide estimated hazard ratios that remain constant within each of two separate time intervals of follow-up. We can also extend the use of heavyside functions to provide several distinct hazard ratios that remain constant within several time intervals.

Four time intervals:

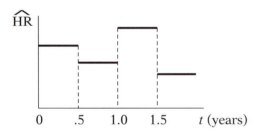

Suppose, for instance, that we wish to separate the data into *four* separate time intervals, and for each interval we wish to obtain a different hazard ratio estimate as illustrated in the graph shown here.

Extended Cox model contains either
- $E, E \times g_1(t), E \times g_2(t), E \times g_3(t)$
  or
- $E \times g_1(t), E \times g_2(t), E \times g_3(t), E \times g_4(t)$

We can obtain four different hazard ratios using an extended Cox model containing *a main effect of exposure and three heavyside functions* in the model as products with exposure. Or, we can use a model containing *no main effect* exposure term, but with product terms involving exposure with *four heavyside functions*.

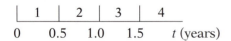

To illustrate the latter model, suppose, as shown on the graph, that the first time interval goes from time 0 to 0.5 of a year; the second time interval goes from 0.5 to 1 year; the third time interval goes from 1 year to a year and a half; and the fourth time interval goes from a year and a half onward.

$$h(t,\mathbf{X}(t)) = h_0(t)\exp[\delta_1, Eg_1,(t)+\delta_2 Eg_2(t)$$
$$+ \delta_3 Eg_3(t) + \delta_4 Eg_4(t)]$$

where

$$g_1(t) = \begin{cases} 1 & \text{if } 0 \le t < 0.5 \text{ year} \\ 0 & \text{if otherwise} \end{cases}$$

$$g_2(t) = \begin{cases} 1 & \text{if } 0.5 \text{ year} \le t < 1.0 \text{ year} \\ 0 & \text{if otherwise} \end{cases}$$

$$g_3(t) = \begin{cases} 1 & \text{if } 1.0 \text{ year} \le t < 1.5 \text{ years} \\ 0 & \text{if otherwise} \end{cases}$$

$$g_4(t) = \begin{cases} 1 & \text{if } t \ge 1.5 \text{ years} \\ 0 & \text{if otherwise} \end{cases}$$

Then, an appropriate extended Cox model containing the four heavyside functions $g_1(t)$, $g_2(t)$, $g_3(t)$, and $g_4(t)$ is shown here. This model assumes that there are four different hazard ratios identified by three cutpoints at half a year, one year, and one and a half years. The formulae for the four hazard ratios are given by separately exponentiating each of the four estimated coefficients, as shown below:

$$4 \; \widehat{HR}\text{'s} \begin{cases} 0 \le t < 0.5: \widehat{HR} = \exp(\hat{\delta}_1) \\ 0.5 \le t < 1.0: \widehat{HR} = \exp(\hat{\delta}_2) \\ 1.0 \le t < 1.5: \widehat{HR} = \exp(\hat{\delta}_3) \\ t \ge 1.5: \widehat{HR} = \exp(\hat{\delta}_4) \end{cases}$$

VII. An Application of the Extended Cox Model to An Epidemiologic Study on the Treatment of Heroin Addiction

EXAMPLE

1991 Australian study (Caplehorn et al.) of heroin addicts
- two methadone treatment clinics
- T = days remaining in treatment (= days until drop out of clinic)
- clinics differ in treatment policies

Dataset name: ADDICTS
Column 1: Subject ID
Column 2: Clinic (1 or 2)
Column 3: Survival status (0 = censored, 1 = departed clinic)
Column 4: Survival time in days
Column 5: Prison Record (0 = none, 1 = any)   covariates
Column 6: Maximum Methadone Dose (mg/day)

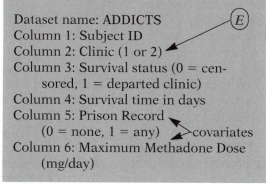

A 1991 Australian study by Caplehorn et al., compared retention in two methadone treatment clinics for heroin addicts. A patient's survival time (T) was determined as the time in days until the patient dropped out of the clinic or was censored at the end of the study clinic. The two clinics differed according to their overall treatment policies.

A listing of some of the variables in the dataset for this study is shown here. The dataset name was called "ADDICTS," and survival analysis programs in the SPIDA package were used in the analysis. Note that the survival time variable is listed in column 4 and the survival status variable, which indicates whether a patient departed from the clinic or was censored, is listed in column 3. The primary exposure variable of interest is the clinic variable, which is coded as 1 or 2. Two other variables of interest are prison record status, listed in column 5 and coded as 0 if none and 1 if any, and maximum methadone dose, in milligrams per day, which is listed in column 6. These latter two variables are considered as covariates.

EXAMPLE (continued)

$$h(t,\mathbf{X}) = h_0(t) \exp[\beta_2(\text{clinic})$$
$$+ \beta_5(\text{prison}) + \beta_6(\text{dose})]$$

Column name	Coeff	StErr	p-value	HR	P(PH)
2 Clinic	−1.009	0.215	0.000	0.365	0.001
5 Prison	1.604	0.329	0.000	1.386	0.333
6 Dose	1.604	0.329	0.000	0.965	0.348

$P(PH)$ for the variables prison and dose are nonsignificant⇒remain in model

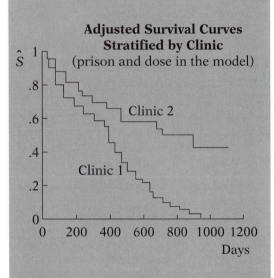

Adjusted Survival Curves Stratified by Clinic
(prison and dose in the model)

Results:
- Curve for clinic 2 consistently lies above curve for clinic 1.
- Curves diverge, with clinic 2 being vastly superior after one year.

Stratifying by **clinic:** cannot obtain hazard ratio for **clinic**

Hazard ratio for **clinic** requires **clinic** in the model.

One of the first models considered in the analysis of the addicts dataset was a Cox PH model containing the three variables, clinic, prison record, and dose. These variables are listed in the addicts dataset as variable numbers, 2, 5, and 6, respectively. A printout of the results for this model is shown here. What stands out from this printout is that the $P(PH)$ value for the clinic variable is zero to three significant places, which indicates that the clinic variable does not satisfy the proportional hazard assumption.

Since the $P(PH)$ values for the other two variables in the model are highly nonsignificant, this suggests that these two variables, namely, prison and dose, can remain in the model.

Further evidence of the PH assumption not being satisfied for the clinic variable can be seen from a graph of adjusted survival curves stratified by clinic, where the prison and dose variables have been kept in the model. Notice that the two curves are much closer together at earlier times, roughly less than one year (i.e., 365 days), but the two curves diverge greatly after one year. This indicates that the hazard ratio for the clinic variable will be much closer to one at early times but quite different from one later on.

The above graph, nevertheless, provides important results regarding the comparison of the two clinics. The curve for clinic 2 consistently lies above the curve for clinic 1, indicating that clinic 2 does better than clinic 1 in retaining its patients in methadone treatment. Further, because the two curves diverge after about a year, it appears that clinic 2 is vastly superior to clinic 1 after one year but only slightly better than clinic 1 prior to one year.

Unfortunately, because the clinic variable has been stratified in the analysis, we cannot use this analysis to obtain a hazard ratio expression for the effect of clinic, adjusted for the effects of prison and dose. We can only obtain such an expression for the hazard ratio if the clinic variable is in the model.

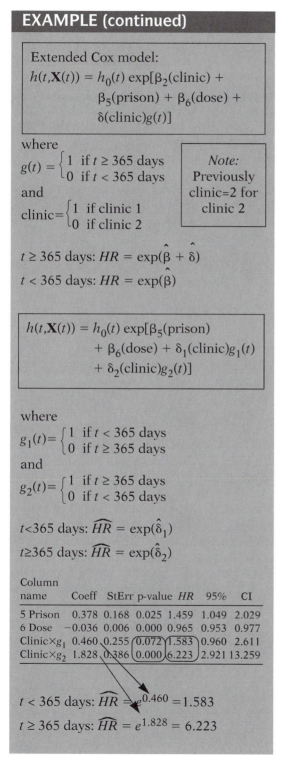

EXAMPLE (continued)

Extended Cox model:
$$h(t, \mathbf{X}(t)) = h_0(t) \exp[\beta_2(\text{clinic}) +$$
$$\beta_5(\text{prison}) + \beta_6(\text{dose}) +$$
$$\delta(\text{clinic})g(t)]$$

where
$$g(t) = \begin{cases} 1 & \text{if } t \geq 365 \text{ days} \\ 0 & \text{if } t < 365 \text{ days} \end{cases}$$

> *Note:*
> Previously
> clinic=2 for
> clinic 2

and
$$\text{clinic} = \begin{cases} 1 & \text{if clinic 1} \\ 0 & \text{if clinic 2} \end{cases}$$

$t \geq 365$ days: $HR = \exp(\hat{\beta} + \hat{\delta})$

$t < 365$ days: $HR = \exp(\hat{\beta})$

$$h(t, \mathbf{X}(t)) = h_0(t) \exp[\beta_5(\text{prison})$$
$$+ \beta_6(\text{dose}) + \delta_1(\text{clinic})g_1(t)$$
$$+ \delta_2(\text{clinic})g_2(t)]$$

where
$$g_1(t) = \begin{cases} 1 & \text{if } t < 365 \text{ days} \\ 0 & \text{if } t \geq 365 \text{ days} \end{cases}$$

and
$$g_2(t) = \begin{cases} 1 & \text{if } t \geq 365 \text{ days} \\ 0 & \text{if } t < 365 \text{ days} \end{cases}$$

$t < 365$ days: $\widehat{HR} = \exp(\hat{\delta}_1)$

$t \geq 365$ days: $\widehat{HR} = \exp(\hat{\delta}_2)$

Column name	Coeff	StErr	p-value	HR	95%	CI
5 Prison	0.378	0.168	0.025	1.459	1.049	2.029
6 Dose	−0.036	0.006	0.000	0.965	0.953	0.977
Clinic×g_1	0.460	0.255	0.072	1.583	0.960	2.611
Clinic×g_2	1.828	0.386	0.000	6.223	2.921	13.259

$t < 365$ days: $\widehat{HR} = e^{0.460} = 1.583$

$t \geq 365$ days: $\widehat{HR} = e^{1.828} = 6.223$

Nevertheless, we can obtain a hazard ratio using an alternative analysis with an extended Cox model that contains a heavyside function, $g(t)$, together with the clinic variable, as shown here. Based on the graphical results shown earlier, a logical choice for the cutpoint of the heavyside function is one year (i.e., 365 days). The corresponding model then provides two hazard ratios: one that is constant above 365 days and the other that is constant below 365 days.

Note that in the extended Cox model here, we have coded the clinc variable as 1 if clinic 1 and 0 if clinic 2, wehereas previously we had coded clinic 2 as 2. the reason for this change in coding, as illustrated by computer output below, is to obtain hazard ratio estimates that are greater than unity.

An equivalent way to write the model is to use two heavyside functions, $g_1(t)$ and $g_2(t)$, as shown here. This latter model contains product terms involving clinic with each heavyside function, and there is no main effect of clinic.

Corresponding to the above model, the effect of clinic is described by two hazard ratios, one for time less than 365 days and the other for greater than 365 days. These hazard ratios are obtained by separately exponentiating the coefficients of each product term, yielding e to the δ_1 "hat" and e to the δ_2 "hat," respectively.

A printout of results using the above model with two heavyside functions is provided here. The results show a borderline nonsignificant hazard ratio ($P = 0.072$) of 1.6 for the effect of clinic when time is less than 365 days in contrast to a highly significant ($P = 0.000$ to three decimal places) hazard ratio of 6.2 when time exceeds 365 days.

Note that the estimated hazard ratio of 1.583 from the printout is computed by exponentiating the estimated coefficient 0.460 of the product term "clinic × g_1" and that the estimated hazard ratio of 6.223 is computed by exponentiating the estimated coefficient 1.828 of the product term "clinic × g_2".

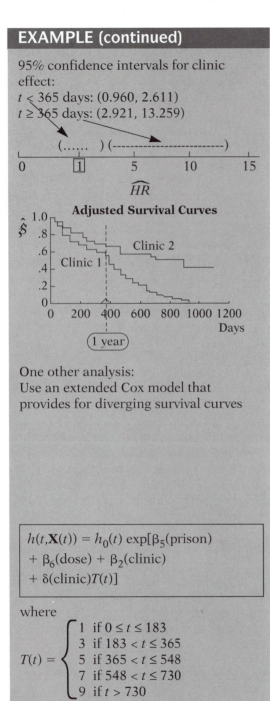

EXAMPLE (continued)

95% confidence intervals for clinic effect:

$t < 365$ days: $(0.960, 2.611)$
$t \geq 365$ days: $(2.921, 13.259)$

Adjusted Survival Curves

One other analysis:
Use an extended Cox model that provides for diverging survival curves

$$h(t, \mathbf{X}(t)) = h_0(t) \exp[\beta_5(\text{prison}) + \beta_6(\text{dose}) + \beta_2(\text{clinic}) + \delta(\text{clinic})T(t)]$$

where

$$T(t) = \begin{cases} 1 & \text{if } 0 \leq t \leq 183 \\ 3 & \text{if } 183 < t \leq 365 \\ 5 & \text{if } 365 < t \leq 548 \\ 7 & \text{if } 548 < t \leq 730 \\ 9 & \text{if } t > 730 \end{cases}$$

Note also that the 95% confidence interval for the clinic effect prior to 365 days—that is, for the product term "clinic $\times g_1(t)$"— is given by the limits 0.960 and 2.611, whereas the corresponding confidence interval after 365 days—that is, for the product term "clinic $\times g_2$"—is given by the limits 2.921 and 13.259. The latter interval is quite wide, showing a lack of precision when t exceeds 365 days; however, when t precedes 365 days, the interval includes the null hazard ratio of 1, indicating a chance effect for this time period.

The results we have just shown support the observations obtained from the graph of adjusted survival curves. That is, these results suggest a large difference in clinic survival times after one year in contrast to a small and probably insignificant difference in clinic survival times prior to one year, with clinic 2 always doing better than clinic 1 at any time.

There is, nevertheless, at least one other approach to the analysis using time-dependent variables that we now describe. This approach considers our earlier graphical observation that the survival curves for each clinic continue to diverge from one another even after one year. In other words, it is reasonable to consider an extended Cox model that allows for such a divergence, rather than a model that assumes the hazard ratios are constant before and after one year.

One way to define an extended Cox model that provides for diverging survival curves is shown here. This model includes, in addition to the clinic variable by itself, a time-dependent variable defined as the product of the clinic variable with a variable we shall call $T(t)$. The variable $T(t)$ is defined to take on the value 1 if t is between 0 and 183 days, 3 if t is between 183 and 365 days, 5 if t is between 365 and 548 days, 7 if t is between 548 and 730 days, and 9 if t exceeds 730 days.

EXAMPLE (continued)

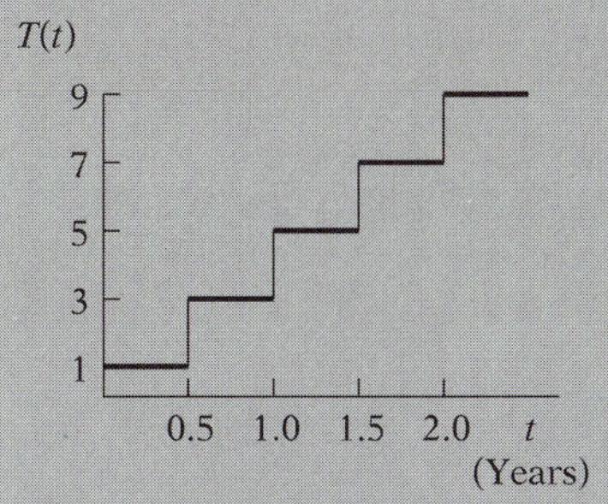

$T(t)$

$$h(t,\mathbf{X}(t)) = h_0(t) \exp[\beta_5(\text{prison})$$
$$+ \beta_6(\text{dose}) + \beta_2(\text{clinic})$$
$$+ \delta(\text{clinic})T(t)]$$

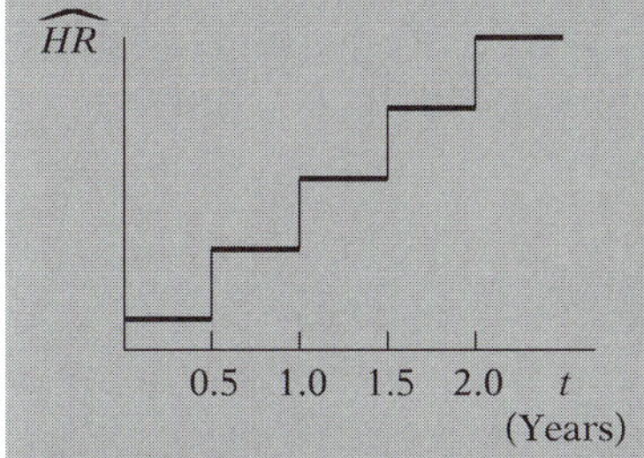

$\widehat{HR}$

$\widehat{HR}$ changes over time.

$0 \le t \le 183; T(t) = 1$:
$$h(t,\mathbf{X}(t)) = h_0(t) \exp[\beta_5(\text{prison})$$
$$+ \beta_6(\text{dose}) + \beta_2(\text{clinic})$$
$$+ \delta(\text{clinic})(1)]$$

So

$$\boxed{\widehat{HR} = \exp(\hat{\beta}_2 + \hat{\delta})}$$

$183 \le t \le 365; T(t) = 3$:
$$h(t,\mathbf{X}(t)) = h_0(t) \exp[\beta_5(\text{prison}) + \beta_6(\text{dose})$$
$$+ \beta_2(\text{clinic}) + \delta(\text{clinic})(3)]$$

$$\boxed{\widehat{HR} = \exp(\hat{\beta}_2 + 3\hat{\delta})}$$

In other words, the value of $T(t)$ changes from 1 to 3 to 5 to 7 to 9 as t changes from less than half a year, to a year, to a year and a half, to two years, and, finally to above two years.

Using the extended Cox model given again here, we can show that the hazard ratio for the effect of clinic increases in increments as we pass through each half year interval up to two years and then remains constant after two years. Notice that the graph shown here is quite similar to the previous graph for the variable $T(t)$, except that here the y-axis gives the estimated hazard ratio, HR "hat," instead of $T(t)$.

To demonstrate how the hazard ratio changes over time for this model, we consider what the model and corresponding estimated hazard ratio expression is during different time intervals.

Starting with the time interval between 0 and 183 days, for which $T(t) = 1$, the exponential part of the model simplifies to terms for the prison and dose variables plus β_2 times the clinic variable plus δ times the clinic variable; the corresponding estimated hazard ratio for the clinic effect is then e to the power β_2 "hat" plus δ "hat."

For the time interval between 183 and 365 days, for which $T(t) = 3$, the exponential part of the model contains the prison, dose and clinic main effect terms as before, plus δ times the clinic variable times 3; the corresponding hazard ratio for the clinic effect is then e to β_2 "hat" plus 3 δ "hat."

EXAMPLE (continued)

$366 \leq t \leq 548$; $T(t) = 5$:

$$\widehat{HR} = \exp(\hat{\beta}_2 + 5\hat{\delta})$$

$549 \leq t \leq 730$; $T(t) = 7$:

$$\widehat{HR} = \exp(\hat{\beta}_2 + 7\hat{\delta})$$

$t \geq 731$; $T(t) = 9$:

$$\widehat{HR} = \exp(\hat{\beta}_2 + 9\hat{\delta})$$

$\hat{\delta} > 0 \Rightarrow \widehat{HR}\uparrow$ as time $\uparrow$

The formulae for the estimated hazard ratios for the other time intervals are shown here. Notice that the formulae change from e to β_2 "hat" plus 5δ "hat" to e to β_2 "hat" plus 7δ "hat" to e to β_2 "hat" plus 9δ "hat."

Thus, if δ "hat" is a positive number, then the estimated hazard ratios will increase in exponential increments as the time intervals change by half-year increments.

Computer results for extended Cox model involving $T(t)$:

Column name	Coeff	StErr	p-value	HR	95%	CI
5 Prison	0.389	0.169	0.021	1.475	1.060	2.054
6 Dose	−0.035	0.006	0.000	0.965	0.953	0.978
2 Clinic	(0.047)	0.355	0.894	1.048	0.523	2.100
Clinic × $T(t)$	(0.282)	0.089	0.001	(1.326)	1.114	1.578

$\widehat{\text{cov}}(\hat{\beta}_2, \hat{\beta}_9) = 0.025$ $-2 \ln L$: 1335.27

$\hat{\beta}_2 = 0.047$, $\hat{\delta} = 0.282$

$e^{\hat{\delta}} = e^{0.282} = 1.326$ is not a hazard ratio.

$\widehat{HR}$ depends on $\hat{\beta}_2$ and $\hat{\delta}$.

We now show results obtained from fitting the extended Cox model we have just been describing. which contains the product term clinic times the time-dependent variable $T(t)$. The covariance estimate shown at the bottom of the table will be used below to compute confidence intervals.

From these results, the estimated coefficient of the clinic variable is β_2 "hat" equals 0.047, and the estimated coefficient δ "hat" obtained for the product term equals 0.282. Note that the value of e to the 0.282 is 1.326, but this value is not an appropriate hazard ratio estimate. In fact, for the model being fit, the hazard ratio depends on the values of both β_2 "hat" and δ "hat."

EXAMPLE (continued)

$$0 \leq t \leq 182: \widehat{HR} = e(\hat{\beta}_2 + \hat{\delta}) = 1.390$$
$$183 \leq t \leq 365: \widehat{HR} = e(\hat{\beta}_2 + 3\hat{\delta}) = 2.442$$
$$366 \leq t \leq 548: \widehat{HR} = e(\hat{\beta}_2 + 5\hat{\delta}) = 4.293$$
$$549 \leq t \leq 730: \widehat{HR} = e(\hat{\beta}_2 + 7\hat{\delta}) = 7.546$$
$$t \geq 731: \widehat{HR} = e(\hat{\beta}_2 + 9\hat{\delta}) = 13.263$$

95% CI formula:

$$\exp\left[\hat{\beta}_2 + T(t) \times \hat{\delta} \pm 1.96\sqrt{\widehat{\mathrm{Var}}\left(\hat{\beta}_2 + T(t) \times \hat{\delta}\right)}\right]$$

$$\mathrm{Var}\left(\hat{\beta}_2 + T(t) \times \hat{\delta}\right) = s^2_{\hat{\beta}_2} + \left[T(t)\right]^2 \times s^2_{\hat{\delta}} + 2T(t)\widehat{\mathrm{cov}}\left(\hat{\beta}_2, \hat{\delta}\right)$$

$$(0.355)^2 \qquad (0.089)^2 \qquad (0.025)$$

Time interval	$\widehat{HR}$	95% CI
$0 \leq t \leq 182$	1.390	(0.600, 3.222)
$183 \leq t \leq 365$	2.442	(0.769, 7.751)
$366 \leq t \leq 548$	4.293	(0.972, 18.954)
$549 \leq t \leq 730$	7.546	(1.220, 46.665)
$t \geq 731$	13.263	(1.525, 115.330)

In particular, the effect of the variable clinic is described by five increasing hazard ratio estimates corresponding to each of the five different time intervals used to define the $T(t)$ function. These five hazard ratio estimates are shown here. These values, which range between 1.390 of the first half-year to 13.263 when t exceeds two years, indicate how the effect of clinic diverges over time for the fitted model.

We can also obtain 95% confidence intervals for each of these hazard ratios using the large sample formula shown here. This formula uses the value of the $T(t)$ function as part of the calculation. The variance expression in the formula is computed using the variances and covariances which can be obtained from the computer results given above. In particular, the variances are $(0.355)^2$ and $(0.089)^2$ for β_2 "hat" and δ "hat," respectively; the covariance value is 0.025.

A table showing the estimated hazard ratios and their corresponding 95% confidence intervals for the clinic effect is given here. Note that all confidence intervals are quite wide.

VIII. An Application of the Extended Cox Model to the Analysis of the Stanford Heart Transplant Data

EXAMPLE

Patients identified as eligible for heart transplant:
T = time until death or censorship
65 patients receive transplants
38 patients do not receive transplants
$n = 138$ patients

Goal: Do patients receiving transplants survive longer than patients not receiving transplants?

We now consider another application of the extended Cox model which involves the use of an internally defined time-dependent variable. In a 1977 report (Crowley and Hu, *J. Amer. Statist. Assoc.*) on the Stanford Heart Transplant Study, patients identified as being eligible for a heart transplant were followed until death or censorship. Sixty-five of these patients received transplants at some point during follow-up, whereas thirty-eight patients did not receive a transplant. There were, thus, a total of $n = 103$ patients. The goal of the study was to assess whether patients receiving transplants survived longer than patients not receiving transplants.

EXAMPLE (continued)

One approach:
Compare two separate groups: 65 transplants vs. 38 nontransplants

Problem:

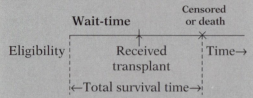

Note: Wait-time contributes to survival time for nontransplants.

Covariates:
Tissue mismatch score ⎱ prognostic only
age at transplant   ⎰ for transplants

Age at eligibility: not considered prognostic for nontransplants

Problems:
• wait-time of transplant recipients
• prognostic factors for transplants only

Alternative approach:
Uses an extended Cox model

Exposure variable:
Heart transplant status at time t, defined as

$$HT(t) = \begin{cases} 0 & \text{if did not receive transplant by time } t, \text{ i.e., if } t < \text{wait-time} \\ 1 & \text{if received transplant prior to time } t, \text{ i.e., if } t \geq \text{wait-time} \end{cases}$$

One approach to the analysis of this data was to separate the dataset into two separate groups, namely, the 65 heart transplant patients and the 38 patients not receiving transplants, and then to compare survival times for these groups.

A problem with this approach, however, is that those patients who received transplants had to wait from the time they were identified as eligible for a transplant until a suitable transplant donor was found. During this "wait-time" period, they were at risk for dying, yet they did not have the transplant. Thus, the wait-time accrued by transplant patients contributes information about the survival of nontransplant patients. Yet, this wait-time information would be ignored if the *total* survival time for each patient were used in the analysis.

Another problem with this approach is that two covariates of interest, namely, *tissue mismatch score* and *age at transplant*, were considered as prognostic indicators of survival only for patients who received transplants. Note that *age at eligibility* was not considered an important prognostic factor for the nontransplant group.

Because of the problems just described, which concern the wait-time of transplants and the effects of prognostic factors attributable to transplants only, an alternative approach to the analysis is recommended. This alternative involves the use of time-dependent variables in an extended Cox model.

The exposure variable of interest in this extended Cox model is heart transplant status at time t, denoted by $HT(t)$. This variable is defined to take on the value 0 at time t if the patient has not received a transplant at this time, that is, if t is less than the wait-time for receiving a transplant. The value of this variable is 1 at time t if the patient has received a transplant prior to or at time t, that is, if t is equal to or greater than the wait-time.

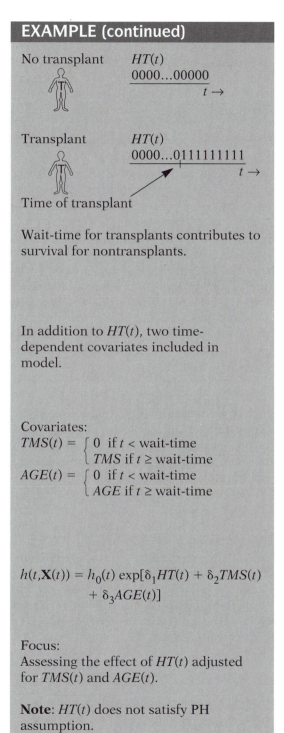

EXAMPLE (continued)

No transplant $HT(t)$

$\dfrac{0000...00000}{t \rightarrow}$

Transplant $HT(t)$

$\dfrac{0000...0111111111}{t \rightarrow}$

Time of transplant

Wait-time for transplants contributes to survival for nontransplants.

In addition to $HT(t)$, two time-dependent covariates included in model.

Covariates:
$$TMS(t) = \begin{cases} 0 & \text{if } t < \text{wait-time} \\ TMS & \text{if } t \geq \text{wait-time} \end{cases}$$
$$AGE(t) = \begin{cases} 0 & \text{if } t < \text{wait-time} \\ AGE & \text{if } t \geq \text{wait-time} \end{cases}$$

$$h(t,\mathbf{X}(t)) = h_0(t) \exp[\delta_1 HT(t) + \delta_2 TMS(t) + \delta_3 AGE(t)]$$

Focus:
Assessing the effect of $HT(t)$ adjusted for $TMS(t)$ and $AGE(t)$.

Note: $HT(t)$ does not satisfy PH assumption.

Thus, for a patient who did not receive a transplant during the study, the value of $HT(t)$ is 0 at all times. For a patient receiving a transplant, the value of $HT(t)$ is 0 at the start of eligibility and continues to be 0 until the time at which the patient receives the transplant; then, the value of $HT(t)$ changes to 1 and remains 1 throughout the remainder of follow-up.

Note that the variable $HT(t)$ has the property that the wait-time for transplant patients contributes to the survival experience of nontransplant patients. In other words, this variable treats a transplant patient as a nontransplant patient prior to receiving the transplant.

In addition to the exposure variable $HT(t)$, two other time-dependent variables are included in our extended Cox model for the transplant data. These variables are covariates to be adjusted for in the assessment of the effect of the $HT(t)$ variable.

These covariates are denoted as $TMS(t)$ and $AGE(t)$ and they are defined as follows: $TMS(t)$ equals 0 if t is less than the wait-time for a transplant but changes to the "tissue mismatch score" (TMS) at the time of the transplant if t is equal to or greater than the wait-time. Similarly, $AGE(t)$ equals 0 if t is less than the wait-time but changes to AGE at time of transplant if t is equal to or greater than the wait-time.

The extended Cox model for the transplant data is shown here. The model contains the three time-dependent variables $HT(t)$, $TMS(t)$ and $AGE(t)$ as described above.

For this model, since $HT(t)$ is the exposure variable of interest, the focus of the analysis concerns assessing the effect of this variable adjusted for the two covariates. Note, however, that because the $HT(t)$ variable is time-dependent by definition, this variable does not satisfy the PH assumption, so that any hazard ratio estimate obtained for this variable is technically time-dependent.

EXAMPLE (continued)

Variable	Coeff	StErr	p-value	e^{coeff}
$HT(t)$	−3.1718	1.1861	0.008	0.0417
$TMS(t)$	0.4442	0.2802	0.112	1.5593
$AGE(t)$	0.0552	0.0226	0.014	1.0567

$$e^{coeff} = e^{-3.1718} = 0.0417 = \frac{1}{23.98}$$

$$\widehat{HR} = \frac{\hat{h}(\text{transplants})}{\hat{h}(\text{nontransplants})} \approx \frac{1}{24}?$$

Not appropriate!

23.98 is inappropriate as a $\widehat{HR}$:
- does not compare two *separate* groups
- exposure variable is *not* time-independent
- wait-time on transplants contributes to survival on nontransplants

Alternative interpretation:
At time t,
$\hat{h}$ ("not yet received transplant")
$\approx 24\,\hat{h}$ ("already received transplant")

More appropriate:

Hazard ratio formula should account for *TMS* and *AGE*.

Transplant?	$HT(t)$	$TMS(t)$	$AGE(t)$
Yes	1	TMS	AGE
No	0	0	0

A summary of computer results for the fit of the above extended Cox model is shown here. These results indicate that the exposure variable $HT(t)$ is significant below the one percent significance level (i.e., the two-sided p-value is 0.008). Thus, transplant status appears to be significantly associated with survival.

To evaluate the strength of the association, note that e to the coefficient of $HT(t)$ equals 0.0417. Since 1 over 0.0417 is 23.98, it appears that there is a 24-fold increase in the hazard of nontransplant patients to transplant patients. The preceding interpretation of the value 0.0417 as a hazard ratio estimate is not appropriate, however, as we shall now discuss further.

First, note that the value of 23.98 inappropriately suggests that the hazard ratio is comparing two separate groups of patients. However, the exposure variable in this analysis is *not* a time-independent variable that distinguishes between two separate groups. In contrast, the exposure variable is time-dependent, and uses the wait-time information on transplants as contributing to the survival experience of non-transplants.

Since the exposure variable is time-dependent, an alternative interpretation of the hazard ratio estimate is that, at any given time t, the hazard for a person *who has not yet received a transplant* (but may receive one later) is approximately 24 times the hazard for a person *who already has received a transplant by that time*.

Actually, we suggest that a more appropriate hazard ratio expression is required to account for a transplant's *TMS* and *AGE* score. Such an expression would compare, at time t, the values of each of the three time-dependent variables in the model. For a person who received a transplant, these values are 1 for $HT(t)$ and *TMS* and *AGE* for the two covariates. For a person who has not received a transplant, the values of all three variables are 0.

EXAMPLE (continued)

i denotes *i*th transplant patient

$\mathbf{X}^*(t) = (HT(t) = 1, TMS(t) = TMS_i, AGE(t) = AGE_i)$
$\mathbf{X}(t) = (HT(t) = 0, TMS(t) = 0, AGE(t) = 0)$

$$\begin{aligned}\widehat{HR}(t) &= \exp[\hat{\delta}_1(1-0) + \hat{\delta}_2(TMS_i - 0) + \\ &\quad \hat{\delta}_3(AGE_i - 0)] \\ &= \exp[\hat{\delta}_1 + \hat{\delta}_2 TMS_i + \hat{\delta}_3 AGE_i] \\ &= \exp[-3.1718 + 0.4442\, TMS_i \\ &\quad + 0.0552\, AGE_i]\end{aligned}$$

$\widehat{HR}(t)$ is time-dependent, i.e., its value at time t depends on TMS_i and AGE_i at time t

TMS range: (0–3.05)
AGE range: (12–64)

Using this approach to compute the hazard ratio, the $\mathbf{X}^*(t)$ vector, which specifies the predictors for a patient i who received a transplant at time t, has the values 1, TMS_i and AGE_i for patient i; the $\mathbf{X}(t)$ vector, which specifies the predictors at time t for a patient who has not received a transplant at time t, has values of 0 for all three predictors.

The hazard ratio formula then reduces to e to the sum of δ_1 "hat" plus δ_2 "hat" times TMS_i plus δ_3 "hat" times AGE_i, where the $\hat{\delta}$ "hat's" are the estimated coefficients of the three time-dependent variables. Substituting the numerical values for these coefficients in the formula gives the exponential expression circled here.

The resulting formula for the hazard ratio is time-dependent in that its value depends on the TMS and AGE values of the ith patient at the time of transplant. That is, different patients can have different values for TMS and AGE at time of transplant. Note that in the dataset, TMS ranged between 0 and 3.05 and AGE ranged between 12 and 64.

We end our discussion of the Stanford Heart Transplant Study at this point. For further insight into the analysis of this dataset, we refer the reader to the 1977 paper by Crowley and Hu (*J. Amer. Statist. Assoc.*).

IX. Summary

Review Cox PH model.

Define time-dependent variable: defined, internal, ancillary.

Extended Cox model:

$$h\big(t, \mathbf{X}(t)\big) = h_0(t) \exp\left[\sum_{i=1}^{p_1} \beta_i X_i + \sum_{j=1}^{p_2} \delta_j X_j(t)\right]$$

$$\widehat{HR}(t) = \exp\left[\sum_{i=1}^{p_1} \hat{\beta}_i\left[X_i^* - X_i\right] + \sum_{j=1}^{p_2} \hat{\delta}_j\left(X_j^*(t) - X_j(t)\right)\right]$$

Function of time

A summary of this presentation on time-dependent variables is now provided. We began by reviewing the main features of the Cox PH model. We then defined a time-dependent variable and illustrated three types of these variables—defined, internal, and ancillary.

Next, we gave the form of the "extended Cox model," shown here again, which allows for time-dependent as well as time-independent variables.

We then described various characteristics of this extended Cox model, including the formula for the hazard ratio. The latter formula is time-dependent so that the PH assumption is not satisfied.

Model for assessing PH assumption:

$$h(t, \mathbf{X}(t)) = h_0(t) \exp\left[\sum_{i=1}^{p} \beta_i X_i + \sum_{i=1}^{p} \delta_i X_i g_i(t)\right]$$

We also showed how to use time-dependent variables to assess the PH assumption for time-independent variables. A general formula for an extended Cox model that simultaneously considers all time-independent variables of interest is shown here.

Examples of $g_i(t)$:
  t, log t, heavyside function

The functions $g_i(t)$ denote functions of time for the ith variable that are to be determined by the investigator. Examples of such functions are $g_i(t) = t$, log t, or a heavyside function.

Heavyside functions:

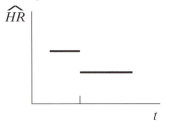

The use of heavyside functions were described and illustrated. Such functions allow for the hazard ratio to be constant within different time intervals.

$h(t, \mathbf{X}(t)) = h_0(t) \exp[\beta E + \delta E g(t)]$

where

$g(t) = \begin{cases} 1 & \text{if } t \geq t_0 \\ 0 & \text{if } t < t_0 \end{cases}$

$h(t, \mathbf{X}(t)) = h_0(t) \exp[\beta_1 E g_1(t) + \beta_2 E g_2(t)]$

where

$g_1(t) = \begin{cases} 1 & \text{if } t \geq t_0 \\ 0 & \text{if } t < t_0 \end{cases}$ $g_2(t) = \begin{cases} 1 & \text{if } t < t_0 \\ 0 & \text{if } t \geq t_0 \end{cases}$

For two time intervals, the model can take either one of two equivalent forms as shown here. The first model contains a main effect of exposure and only one heavyside function. The second model contains two heavyside functions without a main effect of exposure. Both models yield two distinct and equivalent values for the hazard ratio.

EXAMPLE 1

1991 Australian study of heroin addicts
* two methadone maintenance clinics
* *addicts* dataset file
* clnic variable did not satisfy PH assumption

We illustrated the use of time-dependent variables through two examples. The first example considered the comparison of two methadone maintenance clinics for heroin addicts. The dataset file was called *addicts*. In this example, the clinic variable, which was a dichotomous exposure variable, did not satisfy the PH assumption.

EXAMPLE (continued)

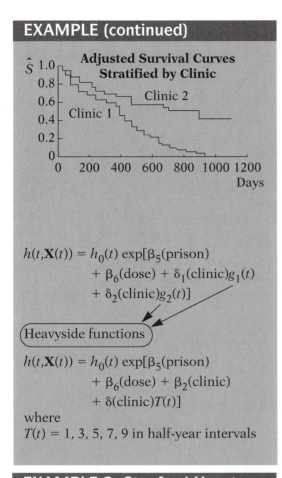

Adjusted Survival Curves Stratified by Clinic

$$h(t,\mathbf{X}(t)) = h_0(t) \exp[\beta_5(\text{prison})$$
$$+ \beta_6(\text{dose}) + \delta_1(\text{clinic})g_1(t)$$
$$+ \delta_2(\text{clinic})g_2(t)]$$

Heavyside functions

$$h(t,\mathbf{X}(t)) = h_0(t) \exp[\beta_5(\text{prison})$$
$$+ \beta_6(\text{dose}) + \beta_2(\text{clinic})$$
$$+ \delta(\text{clinic})T(t)]$$
where
$T(t) = 1, 3, 5, 7, 9$ in half-year intervals

EXAMPLE 2: Stanford Heart Transplant Study

Goals: Do patients receiving transplants survive longer than patients not receiving transplants?

$$h(t,\mathbf{X}(t)) = h_0(t) \exp[\delta_1 HT(t) + \delta_2 TMS(t)$$
$$+ \delta_3 AGE(t)]$$

Exposure variable:

Adjusted survival curves stratified by clinic showed clinic 2 to have consistently higher survival probabilities than clinic 1, with a more pronounced difference in clinics after one year of follow-up. However, this stratification did not allow us to obtain a hazard ratio estimate for clinic. Such an estimate was possible using an extended Cox model containing interaction terms involving clinic with time.

Two extended Cox models were considered. The first used heavyside functions to obtain two distinct hazard ratios, one for the first year of follow-up and the other for greater than one year of follow-up. The model is shown here.

The second extended Cox model used a time-dependent variable that allowed for the two survival curves to diverge over time. This model is shown here.

Both models yielded hazard ratio estimates that agreed reasonably well with the graph of adjusted survival curves stratified by clinic.

The second example considered results obtained in the Stanford Heart Transplant Study. The goal of the study was to assess whether patients receiving transplants survived longer than patients not receiving transplants.

The analysis of these data involved an extended Cox model containing three time-dependent variables. One of these, the exposure variable, and called $HT(t)$, was an indicator of transplant status at time t. The other two variables, $TMS(t)$ and $AGE(t)$, gave tissue mismatch scores and age for transplant patients when time t occurred after receiving a transplant. The value of each of these variables was 0 at times prior to receiving a transplant.

EXAMPLE (continued)

Results: $HT(t)$ highly significant, i.e., transplants have better prognosis than nontransplants.

Hazard ratio estimate problematic:

$$\widehat{HR} = e^{\hat{\delta}_1} = \frac{1}{23.98}$$

More appropriate formula:

$$\widehat{HR} = \exp[-3.1718 + 0.4442\, TMS_i + 0.0552\, AGE_i]$$

The results from fitting the above extended Cox model yielded a highly significant effect of the exposure variable, thus indicating that survival prognosis was better for transplants than for nontransplants.

From these data, we first presented an inappropriate formula for the estimated hazard ratio. This formula used the exponential of the coefficient of the exposure variable, which gave an estimate of 1 over 23.98. A more appropriate formula considered the values of the covariates $TMS(t)$ and $AGE(t)$ at time t. Using the latter, the hazard ratio estimate varied with the tissue mismatch scores and age of each transplant patient.

Chapters

This presentation is now complete. We suggest that the reader review the detailed outline that follows and then answer the practice exercises and test that follow the outline.

1. Introduction to Survival Analysis
2. Kaplan–Meier Curves and the Log–Rank Test
3. The Cox Proportional Hazards Model
4. Evaluating the Proportional Hazards Assumption
5. The Stratified Cox Procedure
6. ✓ Extension of the Cox Proportional Hazards Model for Time-Dependent Variables

This is the final chapter in this text. A listing of the chapters is shown here. For other aspects of survival analysis not covered in the series, we recommend that the reader survey the statistical and epidemiologic published literature on survival analysis.

**Detailed
Outline**

I. **Preview** (page 214)

II. **Review of the Cox PH Model** (pages 214–216)

    A. The formula for the Cox PH model:

$$h(t, \mathbf{X}) = h_0(t) \exp\left[\sum_{i=1}^{p} \beta_i X_i\right]$$

    B. Formula for hazard ratio comparing two individuals:
$\mathbf{X}^* = (x_{11}, x_{12}, \ldots, x_{1k})$ and $\mathbf{X} = (x_{21}, x_{22} \ldots x_{2k})$:

$$\frac{h(t, \mathbf{X}^*)}{h(t, \mathbf{X})} = \exp\left[\sum_{i=1}^{p} \beta_i \left(X_i^* - X_i\right)\right]$$

    C. The meaning of the PH assumption:

- Hazard ratio formula shows that the hazard ratio is independent of time:

$$\frac{h(t, \mathbf{X}^*)}{h(t, \mathbf{X})} = \theta$$

- Hazard ratio for two X's are proportional:
$h(t, \mathbf{X}^*) = \theta \, h(t, \mathbf{X})$

    D. Three methods for checking the PH assumption:

       i. *Graphical:* Compare ln–ln survival curves or observed versus predicted curves

      ii. *Time-dependent covariates:* Use product (i.e., interaction) terms of the form $X \times g(t)$.

     iii. *Goodness-of-fit test:* Use a large sample Z statistic.

    E. Options when the PH assumption is not met:

       i. Use a stratified Cox procedure.

      ii. Use an extended Cox model containing a time-dependent variable of the form $X \times g(t)$.

III. **Definition and Examples of Time-Dependent Variables** (pages 216–219)

    A. Definition: any variable whose values differ over time

    B. Examples of defined, internal, and ancillary time-dependent variables

IV. **The Extended Cox Model for Time-Dependent Variables** (pages 219–221)

    A.

$$h(t, \mathbf{X}(t)) = h_0(t) \exp\left[\sum_{i=1}^{p_1} \beta_i X_i + \sum_{j=1}^{p_2} \delta_j X_j(t)\right]$$

where $\mathbf{X}(t) = (X_1, X_2, \ldots, X_{p_1}, X_1(t), X_2(t), \ldots, X_{p_2}(t))$ denotes the entire collection of predictors at time t, X_i denotes the ith time-independent variable, and $X_j(t)$ denotes the jth time-dependent variable.

B. ML procedure used to estimate regression coefficients.

C. List of computer programs for the extended Cox model.

D. Model assumes that the hazard at time t depends on the value of $X_j(t)$ at the *same* time.

E. Can modify model for lag-time effect.

V. **The Hazard Ratio Formula for the Extended Cox Model** (pages 221–223)

A.
$$HR(t) = \exp\left[\sum_{i=1}^{p_1} \hat{\beta}_i \left[X_i^* - X_i\right] + \sum_{j=1}^{p_2} \hat{\delta}_j \left[X_j^*(t) - X_j(t)\right]\right]$$

B. Because $HR(t)$ is a function of time, the PH assumption is not satisfied.

C. The estimated coefficient of $X_j(t)$ is time-independent, and represents an "overall" effect of $X_j(t)$.

VI. **Assessing Time-Independent Variables That Do Not Satisfy the PH Assumption** (pages 223–229)

A. General formula for assessing PH assumption:
$$h(t, \mathbf{X}(t)) = h_0(t) \exp\left[\sum_{i=1}^{p} \beta_i X_i + \sum_{i=1}^{p} \delta_i X_i g_i(t)\right]$$

B. $g_i(t)$ is a function of time corresponding to X_i

C. Test $H_0: \delta_1 = \delta_2 = \ldots = \delta_p = 0$

D. Heavyside function:
$$g(t) = \begin{cases} 1 & \text{if } t \geq t_0 \\ 0 & \text{if } t < t_0 \end{cases}$$

E. The model with a single heavyside function:
$$h(t, \mathbf{X}(t)) = h_0(t) \exp[\beta E + \delta\, Eg(t)]$$

F. The model with two heavyside functions:
$$h(t, \mathbf{X}(t)) = h_0(t) \exp[\delta_1\, Eg_1(t) + \delta_2\, Eg_2(t)]$$
where
$$g_1(t) = \begin{cases} 1 & \text{if } t \geq t_0 \\ 0 & \text{if } t < t_0 \end{cases} \quad \text{and} \quad g_2(t) = \begin{cases} 1 & \text{if } t < t_0 \\ 0 & \text{if } t \geq t_0 \end{cases}$$

G. The hazard ratios:
$$t \geq t_0: \widehat{HR} = \exp(\hat{\beta} + \hat{\delta}) = \exp(\hat{\delta}_1)$$
$$t < t_0: \widehat{HR} = \exp(\hat{\beta}) = \exp(\hat{\delta}_2)$$

H. Several heavyside functions: examples given with four time-intervals:

- Extended Cox model contains either $\{E, E \times g_1(t), E \times g_2(t), E \times g_3(t)\}$ or $\{E \times g_1(t), E \times g_2(t), E \times g_3(t), E \times g_4(t)\}$
- The model using four product terms and no main effect of E:

$$h(t, \mathbf{X}(t)) = h_0(t) \exp[\delta_1 Eg_1(t) + \delta_2 Eg_2(t) + \delta_3 Eg_3(t) + \delta_4 Eg_4(t)]$$

where

$$g_i(t) = \begin{cases} 1 & \text{if } t \text{ is within interval } i \\ 0 & \text{if otherwise} \end{cases}$$

VII. An Application of the Extended Cox Model to an Epidemiologic Study on the Treatment of Heroin Addiction (pages 229–235)

A. 1991 Australian study of heroin addicts
- two methadone maintenance clinics
- *addicts* dataset file
- clinic variable did not satisfy PH assumption

B. Clinic 2 has consistently higher retention probabilities than clinic 1, with a more pronounced difference in clinics after one year of treatment.

C. Two extended Cox models were considered:
- Use heavyside functions to obtain two distinct hazard ratios, one for less than one year and the other for greater than one year.
- Use a time-dependent variable that allows for the two survival curves to diverge over time.

VIII. An Application of the Extended Cox Model to the Analysis of the Stanford Heart Transplant Data (pages 235–239)

A. The goal of the study was to assess whether patients receiving transplants survived longer than patients not receiving transplants.

B. We described an extended Cox model containing three time-dependent variables:

$$h(t, \mathbf{X}(t)) = h_0(t) \exp[\delta_1 HT(t) + \delta_2 TMS(t) + \delta_3 AGE(t)]$$

C. The exposure variable, called $HT(t)$, was an indicator of transplant status at time t. The other two variables, $TMS(t)$ and $AGE(t)$, gave tissue mismatch scores and age for transplant patients when time t occurred after receiving a transplant.

D. The results yielded a highly significant effect of the exposure variable.

    E. The use of a hazard ratio estimate for this data was problematical.

- An inappropriate formula is the exponential of the coefficient of $HT(t)$, which yields 1/23.98.
- An alternative formula considers the values of the covariates $TMS(t)$ and $AGE(t)$ at time t.

IX. Summary (pages 239–242)

Practice Exercises

The following dataset called "anderson.dat" consists of remission survival times on 42 leukemia patients, half of whom receive a new therapy and the other half of whom get a standard therapy (Freireich et al., *Blood*, 1963). The exposure variable of interest is treatment status ($Rx = 0$ if new treatment, $Rx = 1$ if standard treatment). Two other variables for control are log white blood cell count (i.e., log WBC) and sex. Failure status is defined by the relapse variable (0 if censored, 1 if failure). The dataset is listed as follows:

Subj	Surv	Relapse	Sex	log WBC	Rx
1	35	0	1	1.45	0
2	34	0	1	1.47	0
3	32	0	1	2.2	0
4	32	0	1	2.53	0
5	25	0	1	1.78	0
6	23	1	1	2.57	0
7	22	1	1	2.32	0
8	20	0	1	2.01	0
9	19	0	0	2.05	0
10	17	0	0	2.16	0
11	16	1	1	3.6	0
12	13	1	0	2.88	0
13	11	0	0	2.6	0
14	10	0	0	2.7	0
15	10	1	0	2.96	0
16	9	0	0	2.8	0
17	7	1	0	4.43	0
18	6	0	0	3.2	0
19	6	1	0	2.31	0
20	6	1	1	4.06	0
21	6	1	0	3.28	0
22	23	1	1	1.97	1
23	22	1	0	2.73	1

Subj	Surv	Relapse	Sex	log WBC	Rx
24	17	1	0	2.95	1
25	15	1	0	2.3	1
26	12	1	0	1.5	1
27	12	1	0	3.06	1
28	11	1	0	3.49	1
29	11	1	0	2.12	1
30	8	1	0	3.52	1
31	8	1	0	3.05	1
32	8	1	0	2.32	1
33	8	1	1	3.26	1
34	5	1	1	3.49	1
35	5	1	0	3.97	1
36	4	1	1	4.36	1
37	4	1	1	2.42	1
38	3	1	1	4.01	1
39	2	1	1	4.91	1
40	2	1	1	4.48	1
41	1	1	1	2.8	1
42	1	1	1	5	1

The following printout gives computer results for fitting a Cox PH model containing the three predictives Rx, log WBC, and Sex.

Response: Surv

Column name	Coeff	StErr	p-value	HR	0.95	CI	P(PH)
3 Sex	0.263	0.449	0.558	1.301	0.539	3.139	0.038
4 log WBC	1.594	0.330	0.000	4.922	2.578	9.397	0.828
5 Rx	1.391	0.457	0.002	4.018	1.642	9.834	0.935

n: 42   %Cen: 28.571 $-2 \log L$: 144.218   #iter:6

1. Which of the variables in the model fitted above are time-independent and which are time-dependent?

2. Based on this printout, is the PH assumption satisfied for the model being fit? Explain briefly.

3. Suppose you want to use an extended Cox model to assess the PH assumption for all three variables in the above model. State the general form of an extended Cox model that will allow for this assessment.

4. Suppose you wish to assess the PH assumption for the Sex variable using a heavyside function approach designed to yield a constant hazard ratio for less than 15 weeks of follow-up and a constant hazard ratio for 15 weeks or more of follow-up. State two equivalent alternative extended Cox models that will carry out this approach, one model containing one heavyside function and the other model containing two heavyside functions.

5. The following is a printout of the results obtained by fitting an extended Cox model containing two heavyside functions:

Time-Dependent Cox Regression Analysis
Response: Surv

Column name	Coeff	StErr	p-value	HR	0.95	CI
4 log WBC	1.567	0.333	0.000	4.794	2.498	9.202
5 Rx	1.341	0.466	0.004	3.822	1.533	9.526
0–15 wks	0.358	0.483	0.459	1.430	0.555	3.682
15+ wks	–0.182	0.992	0.855	0.834	0.119	5.831
n:42		%Cen: 28.571		–2 log L: 143.959		#iter:6

Using the above computer results, carry out a test of hypothesis, estimate the hazard ratio, and obtain 95% confidence interval for the treatment effect adjusted for log WBC and the time-dependent Sex variables. What conclusions do you draw about the treatment effect?

6.   We now consider an alternative approach to controlling for Sex using an extended Cox model. We divide the time axis into five time intervals of four weeks duration, and define a single time-dependent covariate that increases linearly with time according to the following formula:

$$
Sex \times Time = \begin{cases}
Sex \times 1 \text{ if } t < 4 \text{ weeks} \\
Sex \times 3 \text{ if } 4 \leq t < 8 \text{ weeks} \\
Sex \times 5 \text{ if } 8 \leq t < 12 \text{ weeks} \\
Sex \times 7 \text{ if } 12 \leq t < 16 \text{ weeks} \\
Sex \times 9 \text{ if } t \geq 16 \text{ weeks}
\end{cases}
$$

For the situation just described, write down the extended Cox model, which contains *Rx*, log WBC, and Sex as main effects plus the time-dependent covariate we have added.

7.   Using the model described in question 6, express the hazard ratio for the effect of Sex adjusted for *Rx* and log WBC for each of the five time intervals used to define the Sex $\times$ Time variable in the model.

8.   The following is a printout of computer results obtained by fitting the model described in question 6.

Time-Dependent Cox Regression Analysis
Response: Surv

Column name	Coeff	StErr	p-value	*HR*	0.95	CI
3 Sex	1.820	1.012	0.072	6.174	0.849	44.896
4 log WBC	1.464	0.336	0.000	4.322	2.236	8.351
5 *Rx*	1.093	0.479	0.022	2.984	1.167	7.626
Sex $\times$ Time	–0.345	0.199	0.083	0.708	0.479	1.046
n:42	%Cen: 28.571		–2 log *L*: 140.831	#iter:6		

Based on the above results, describe the hazard ratio estimate for the treatment effect adjusted for the other variables in the model, and summarize the results of the significance test and interval estimate for this hazard ratio. How do these results compare with the results previously obtained when a heavyside function approach was used? What does this comparison suggest about the drawbacks of using an extended Cox model to adjust for variables not satisfying the PH assumption?

9. The following gives a printout of computer results using a stratified Cox procedure that stratifies on the Sex variable but keeps Rx and log WBC in the model.

Stratified Cox Regression Analysis on Variable: Sex

Response: Surv

Column name	Coeff	StErr	p-value	HR	0.95	CI
4 log WBC	1.390	0.338	0.000	4.016	2.072	7.783
5 Rx	0.931	0.472	0.048	2.537	1.006	6.396
n:42		%Cen: 28.571		$-2 \log L$: 115.119 #iter:6		

Compare the results of the above printout with previously provided results regarding the hazard ratio for the effect of Rx. Is there any way to determine which set of results is more appropriate? Explain.

Test

The following questions consider the analysis of data from a clinical trial concerning gastric carcinoma, in which 90 patients were randomized to either chemotherapy (coded as 2) alone or to a combination of chemotherapy and radiation (coded as 1). See Stablein et al., "Analysis of Survival Data with Nonproportional Hazard Functions," *Controlled Clinical Trials*, vol. 2, pp. 149–159 (1981). A listing of the dataset (called chemo) is given at the end of the presentation.

1. A plot of the log–log Kaplan–Meier curves for each treatment group is shown below. Based on this plot, what would you conclude about the PH assumption regarding the treatment group variable? Explain.

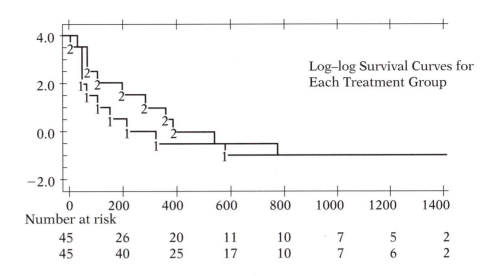

Log–log Survival Curves for
Each Treatment Group

	0	200	400	600	800	1000	1200	1400
Number at risk								
	45	26	20	11	10	7	5	2
	45	40	25	17	10	7	6	2

2. The following is a printout of computer results obtained when fitting
    the PH model containing only the treatment group variable. Based on
    these results, what would you conclude about the PH assumption
    regarding the treatment group variable? Explain.

    Cox Regression Analysis

    Response: Surv (days)

Column name	Coeff	StErr	p-value	HR	0.95	CI	P(PH)
1 Tx	−0.267	0.233	0.253	0.766	0.485	1.21	0
n:90		%Cen: 17.778	−2 log L: 565.488	#iter:4			

3. The following printout shows the results from using a heavyside func-
    tion approach with an extended Cox model to fit these data. The
    model used product terms of the treatment variable (Tx) with each of
    three heavyside functions. The first product term (called Time1)
    involves a heavyside function for the period from 0 to 250 days, the
    second product term (i.e., Time2) involves the period from 250 to 500
    days, and the third product term (i.e., Time3) involves the open-ended
    period from 500 days and beyond.

Time-Dependent Cox Regression Analysis
Response: Surv (days)

Column name	Coeff	StErr	p-value	HR	0.95	CI
Time1	−1.511	0.461	0.001	0.221	0.089	0.545
Time2	0.488	0.450	0.278	1.629	0.675	3.934
Time3	0.365	0.444	0.411	1.441	0.604	3.440
n:90	%Cen: 17.778		−2 log *L*: 551.490 #iter:5			

Write down the hazard function formula for the extended Cox model being used, making sure to explicitly define the heavyside functions involved.

4. Based on the printout, describe the hazard ratios in each of the three time intervals, evaluate each hazard ratio for significance, and draw conclusions about the extent of the treatment effect in each of the three time intervals considered.

5. Inspection of the printout provided in question 3 indicates that the treatment effect in the second and third intervals appears quite similar. Consequently, another analysis was considered that uses only two intervals, from 0 to 250 days versus 250 days and beyond. Write down the hazard function formula for the extended Cox model that considers this situation (i.e., containing two heavyside functions). Also, write down an equivalent alternative hazard function formula which contains the main effect of treatment group plus one heavyside function variable.

6. For the situation described in question 5, the computer results are provided below. Based on these results, describe the hazard ratios for the treatment effect below and above 250 days, summarize the inference results for each hazard ratio, and draw conclusions about the treatment effect within each time interval.

Time-Dependent Cox Regression Analysis
Response: Surv (days)

Column name	Coeff	StErr	p-value	*HR*	0.95	CI
Time1	−1.511	0.461	0.001	0.221	0.089	0.545
Time2	0.427	0.315	0.176	1.532	0.826	2.842

n:90   %Cen: 17.778   −2 log L: 551.528 #iter:5

Answers to Practice Exercises

1. All three variables in the model are time-independent variables.

2. The computer results indicate that the Sex variables do not satisfy the PH assumption because the $P(PH)$ value is 0.038, which is significant at the 0.05 level.

3. $h(t,\mathbf{X}(t)) = h_0(t) \exp[\beta_1(\text{sex}) + \beta_2(\log \text{WBC}) + \beta_3(Rx) + \delta_1(\text{sex})g_1(t)$
$+ \delta_2(\log \text{WBC})g_2(t) + \delta_3(Rx)g_3(t)]$
where the $g_i(t)$ are functions of time.

4. Model 1 (one heavyside function)
$h(t,\mathbf{X}(t)) = h_0(t) \exp[\beta_1(\text{sex}) + \beta_2(\log \text{WBC}) + \beta_3(Rx) + \delta_1(\text{sex})g_1(t)]$
where
$$g_1(t) = \begin{cases} 1 & \text{if } 0 \le t < 15 \text{ weeks} \\ 0 & \text{if } t \ge 15 \text{ weeks} \end{cases}$$

Model 2 (two heavyside functions):
$h(t,\mathbf{X}(t)) = h_0(t) \exp[\beta_2(\log \text{WBC}) + \beta_3(Rx) + \delta_1(\text{sex})g_1(t) + \delta_2(\text{sex})g_2(t)]$
where
$$g_1(t) = \begin{cases} 1 & \text{if } 0 \le t < 15 \text{ weeks} \\ 0 & \text{if } t \ge 15 \text{ weeks} \end{cases}$$
and
$$g_2(t) = \begin{cases} 1 & \text{if } 0 \le t < 15 \text{ weeks} \\ 0 & \text{if } t \ge 15 \text{ weeks} \end{cases}$$

5. The estimated hazard ratio for the effect of Rx is 3.822; this estimate is adjusted for log WBC and for the Sex variable considered as two time-dependent variables involving heavyside functions. The Wald test for significance of Rx has a p-value of 0.004, which is highly significant. The 95% confidence interval for the treatment effect ranges between 1.533 and 9.526, which is quite wide, indicating considerable unreliability of the 3.822 point estimate. Nevertheless, the results indicate a clinically meaningful and significant treatment effect of around 3.8.

6. $h(t, \mathbf{X}(t)) = h_0(t) \exp[\beta_1(\text{sex}) + \beta_2(\log \text{WBC}) + \beta_3(Rx) + \delta_1(\text{sex})g(t)]$,
where

$$g(t) = \begin{cases} 1 & \text{if } t < 4 \text{ weeks} \\ 3 & \text{if } 4 \leq t < 8 \text{ weeks} \\ 5 & \text{if } 8 \leq t < 12 \text{ weeks} \\ 7 & \text{if } 12 \leq t < 16 \text{ weeks} \\ 9 & \text{if } t \geq 16 \text{ weeks} \end{cases}$$

7.   The hazard ratio for the effect of Sex in each time interval, controlling for Rx and log WBC is given as follows:

$t < 4$ weeks	$\widehat{HR} = \exp[\hat{\beta}_1 + \hat{\delta}_1]$
$4 \leq t < 8$ weeks	$\widehat{HR} = \exp[\hat{\beta}_1 + 3\hat{\delta}_1]$
$8 \leq t < 12$ weeks	$\widehat{HR} = \exp[\hat{\beta}_1 + 5\hat{\delta}_1]$
$12 \leq t < 16$ weeks	$\widehat{HR} = \exp[\hat{\beta}_1 + 7\hat{\delta}_1]$
$t \geq 16$ weeks	$\widehat{HR} = \exp[\hat{\beta}_1 + 9\hat{\delta}_1]$

8.   Using the model containing Sex, log WBC, Rx, and Sex $\times$ Time, the estimated hazard ratio for the treatment effect is given by 2.984, with a p-value of 0.022 and a 95% confidence interval ranging between 2.236 and 8.351. The point estimate of 2.984 is quite different from the point estimate of 3.822 for the heavyside function model, although the confidence intervals for both models are wide enough to include both estimates. The discrepancy between point estimates demonstrates that when a time-dependent variable approach is to be used to account for a variable not satisfying the PH assumption, different results may be obtained from different choices of time-dependent variables.

9.   The stratified Cox analysis yields a hazard ratio of 2.537 with a p-value of 0.048 and a 95% CI ranging between 1.006 and 6.396. The point estimate is much closer to the 2.984 for the model containing the Sex $\times$ Time product term than to the 3.822 for the model containing two heavyside functions. One way to choose between models would be to compare goodness-of-fit test statistics for each model; another way is to compare graphs of the adjusted survival curves for each model and determine by eye which set of survival curves fits the data better.

A

Appendix: Computer Programs for Survival Analysis

In this appendix, we provide examples of computer programs for carrying out survival analyses, with particular emphasis on Cox regression procedures. This appendix does not give an exhaustive survey of all computer packages currently available, but rather is intended to provide the reader with a general idea of the similarities and differences among a selected sample of available programs. The packages we consider here are SPIDA, SAS, and BMDP. Of these packages, SPIDA is exclusively for the microcomputer and is therefore not available for a mainframe computer. This author is most familiar with SPIDA (from Macquarie University, Sydney, Australia), so that SPIDA programs for survival analysis are considered exclusively in the text. The packages SAS and BMDP are available for both IBM PC's and mainframes, and are very popular packages throughout the United States.

Below, we provide the syntax and corresponding output from different computer programs applied to the same dataset, the "addicts" dataset, which is listed in Appendix B, is illustrated in Chapter 6 and is the basis for exercises in Chapters 2, 4, and 5. The output that we illustrate includes Kaplan–Meier (KM) and adjusted survival curves, log–log KM and adjusted log–log survival curves, log rank tests and applications of the Cox PH model, the Stratified Cox model, and the extended Cox model (containing time-dependent variables).

The "addicts" Dataset

In a 1991 Australian study by Caplehorn et al., two methadone treatment clinics for heroin addicts were compared to assess patient time remaining under methadone treatment. A patient's survival time (T) was determined as the time in days until the patient dropped out of the clinic or was censored. The two clinics differed according to its live-in policies for patients.

A **listing of the variables** in the dataset is shown below. Note that the survival time variable is listed in column 4 and the survival status variable (which indicates whether a patient departed from the clinic or was censored) is listed in column 3. The primary exposure variable of interest is the clinic variable, which is coded as 1 or 2. Two other variables of interest are prison record status, listed in column 5 and coded as 0 if none and 1 if any, and methadone dose, in milligrams per day, which is listed in column 6. These latter two variables are considered as covariates:

Column 1: Subject ID

Column 2: Clinic (1 or 2)

Column 3: Survival status (0 = censored, 1 = departed clinic)

Column 4: Survival time in days

Column 5: Prison record (0 = none, 1 = any)

Column 6: Maximium methadone dose (mg/day)

SPIDA

The SPIDA package contains four programs for survival analysis:

1. **km:** provides Kaplan–Meier (KM) survival probabilities, log rank statistic, and Peto statistic (alternatively referred to as the Wilcoxon statistic); also, using plotting accessories, provides KM plots and log–log KM plots.

2. **cox:** fits a Cox PH model; also, using plotting accessories, provides adjusted survival and adjusted log–log survival plots.

3. **scox:** fits a stratified Cox model; also, using plotting accessories, provides adjusted stratified survival and log–log survival plots.

4. **tcox:** fits an extended Cox model, where time-dependent variables are defined by specifying different constants for different time intervals; also provides adjusted survival curves.

SPIDA also provides two plotting subroutines, called **splot** and **hsplot,** respectively, which can be used to plot KM survival curves, adjusted survival curves, and corresponding log–log survival curves.

Below we illustrate the use of the above SPIDA programs and subroutines on the addicts dataset. We provide for each illustration of the appropriate command statements and the computer output.

First, we illustrate Kaplan–Meier (KM) probabilities and corresponding KM survival and log–log survival curves for clinics 1 and 2 from the addicts dataset:

des(addicts)

> The **des** command is used to obtain descriptive statistics for the addicts dataset

Column name	Size	Mean	StDev	Min	Max
1 ID	238	134.130	79.292	1	266
2 Clinic	238	1.315	0.466	1	2
3 Status	238	0.630	0.484	0	1
4 Days survival	238	402.571	267.853	2	1076
5 Prison	238	0.466	0.500	0	1
6 Dose	238	60.399	14.450	20	110

```
km (addicts, y=4, s=3, g=2)
```

The **km** command is used to obtain KM probabilities for the two groups in the addicts dataset; also, logrank and Peto statistics are computed

Group	Size	%Cen	LQ	Median	UQ	0.95	Med CI
1	163	25.153	192	428	652	341.000	504
2	75	62.667	280			661.000	

df:1   log rank: 27.893   p-value: 0 Peto: 11.078   p-value:0

```
$sc := km(addicts,y=4,s=3,g=2,sc=1)
splot($sc)
```

Kaplan–Meier (KM) survival curves are plotted using **splot** command. The sc=1 command creates an output file with KM probabilities for each group.

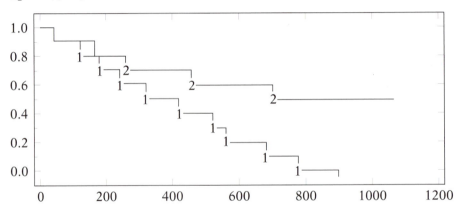

```
splot($sc,loglog=1)
```

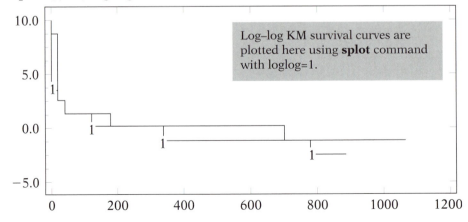

Log–log KM survival curves are plotted here using **splot** command with loglog=1.

We now illustrate the use of the cox and scox procedures to fit Cox PH models to the following data:

```
cox(addicts,y=4,s=3,x=2;5;6)
```

> **cox** procedure is used to fit Cox PH model to addicts dataset with x=2 (clinic) 5 (prison), and 6 (dose) as predictors

Cox Regression Analysis

Response: days survival

Column name	Coeff	StErr	p-value	HR	0.95	CI	P(PH)
2 Clinic	–1.009	0.215	0.000	0.365	0.239	0.556	0.001
5 Prison	0.327	0.167	0.051	1.386	0.999	1.924	0.333
6 Dose	–0.035	0.006	0.000	0.965	0.953	0.977	0.348

n:238   %Cen: 36.975   –2 log *L*: 1346.805   #iter:5

```
$sc := cox(addicts,y=4,s=3,x=2;5;6,sc=((1;2),?,?))
```

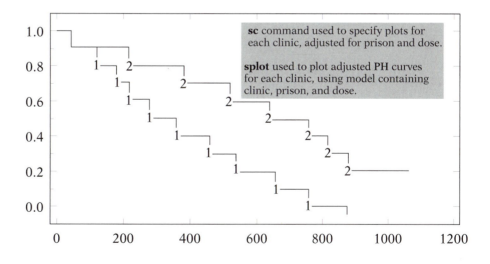

> **sc** command used to specify plots for each clinic, adjusted for prison and dose.
>
> **splot** used to plot adjusted PH curves for each clinic, using model containing clinic, prison, and dose.

```
$sc := scox(addicts,y=4,s=3,strat=2,x=(5,6),sc=?)
```

> **scox** procedure used to stratify on clinic, using prison and dose as predictors in the model.

Stratified Cox Regression Analysis on Variable: clinic

Response: days survival

Column name	Coeff	StErr	p-value	HR	0.95	CI
5 Prison	0.389	0.169	0.021	1.475	1.059	2.054
6 Dose	−0.035	0.006	0.000	0.965	0.953	0.978

n:238   %Cen: 36.975   −2 log *L*: 1195.428   #iter:5

```
splot($sc,h=25)
```

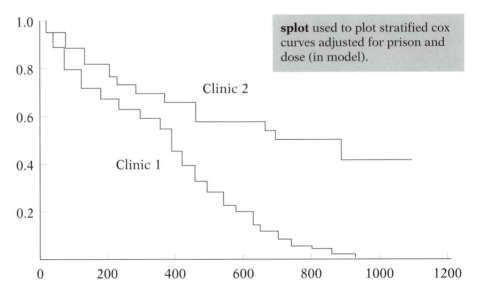

> **splot** used to plot stratified cox curves adjusted for prison and dose (in model).

We now illustrate the use of the tcox procedure to fit extended Cox models to the data, first using a heavyside function approach with two time-dependent variables, and second, using a single time-dependent variable which reflects the continuous diverging appearance of the adjusted survival curves for the two clinics.

> **tcox** procedure used to fit extended cox model using heavyside functions so that hazard ratio for clinic is constant below and a different constant above 365

```
$x := addicts    This statement changes the coding of the clinic variable from (1,2) to (1,0).
$x := $x[;1],2-$x[;2],$x[;3, ,6],0
$tnam := "0-365 days"; "366+ days"
$t := (0,366);(0,366)
tcox($x,y=4,s=3,time=$t,x=(5,6),tcol=((2,7);(7,2)),
tnam=$tnam)
```

Response: days survival

Column name	Coeff	StErr	p-value	HR	0.95	CI
5 Prison	0.378	0.168	0.025	1.459	1.049	2.029
6 Dose	–0.036	0.006	0.000	0.965	0.953	0.977
0–365 days	0.460	0.255	0.072	1.583	0.960	2.611
366+ days	1.828	0.385	0.000	6.223	2.924	13.244

n:238   %Cen: 36.975   –2 log *L*: 1337.149   #iter:5

> **tcox** procedure used to fit extended cox model using a single time-dependent variable defined as the product term **Time1** = **clinic** × **T(t)** where *T(t)* takes on values 1, 3, 5, 7, and 9 so that the hazard ratio for clinic diverges at 183, 366, 549, and 731 days.

```
$x := addicts, (1,3,5,7,9)*(2-addicts[;2])
%name addicts              Changes coding of clinic from (1,2) to (1,0).
tcox($x,y=4,s=3,time=(0,183,366,549,731),x=(2,5,6),tcols=
(7, ,11))
```

Response: days survival

Column name	Coeff	StErr	p-value	HR	0.95	CI
2 Clinic	0.047	0.355	0.894	1.048	0.523	2.100
5 Prison	0.389	0.169	0.021	1.475	1.060	2.054
6 Dose	–0.035	0.006	0.000	0.965	0.953	0.978
Time1	0.282	0.089	0.001	1.326	1.114	1.578

n:238   %Cen: 36.975   –2 log *L*: 1335.272   #iter:6

SAS

The SAS package contains three programs for survival analysis:

1. **LIFETEST:** provides Kaplan–Meier (KM) survival probabilities, log rank statistic, Wilcoxon (i.e., Peto) statistic, KM plots, and log–log KM plots.
2. **PHREG:** fits a Cox PH model, stratified Cox PH model (using **strata** statement to identify variables for stratification), and an extended Cox model (using SAS programming statements to define time-dependent variables). Also, PHREG computes predicted survival probabilities for each study subject failure, computes (using a **baseline** file statement) adjusted survival probabilities for a specified set of predictors, and, using PROC PLOT on an output file, plots adjusted survival and log–log survival probabilities.
3. **LIFEREG:** fits parametric survival models, in particular, Weibull, log normal, log-logistic and gamma distributions; also, using plotting accessories, provides adjusted survival plots.

Both PHREG and LIFEREG procedures can provide regression diagnostic information in terms of residuals; however, no collinearity diagnostics are provided, even though it is possible to create one's own SAS macro for calculating condition indices and variance decomposition proportions from the inverse of the information matrix derived from the likelihood function. Also, PHREG does not provide a P(PH) statistic for testing the PH assumption.

As we have previously done with the SPIDA package, we now illustrate the use of the SAS survival analysis procedures with the **addicts** dataset. First, we provide command statements and printout describing the variables in the dataset:

SAS EXAMPLE

```
/*
! Data file ADDICTS.DAT
!
! Survival times in days of heroin addicts
! from entry to a clinic until departure.
!
! Data provided by John Caplehorn,
! c/- The University of Sydney,
!     Dept of Public Health.
!
! Column 1 = ID of subject
!        2 = clinic (1 or 2)
!        3 = status (0=censored, 1=endpoint)
!        4 = survival time (days)
!        5 = prison record?
!        6 = methadone dose (mg/day)
!
*/
```

LIFETEST PRINTOUT

```
DATA ADDICTS;
   LABEL ID='SUBJECT ID'
         CLINIC='STUDY CLINIC'
         STATUS='CENSORED=0'
         DAYS='SURVIVAL TIME IN DAYS'
         PRISON='PRISON RECORD (Y/N)'
         DOSE='METHADONE DOSE (mg/DAY)';
         INPUT ID CLINIC STATUS DAYS PRISON DOSE;
         CARDS;
    1 1 1   428 0  50
    2 1 1   275 1  55
    3 1 1   262 0  55
    4 1 1   183 0  30
    5 1 1   259 1  65
         •
         •      omitted middle portion of data
         •
  261 1 1    33 1  60
  262 2 1   540 0  80
  263 2 0   551 0  65
  264 1 1    90 0  40
  266 1 1    47 0  45
   ;
RUN;

PROC LIFETEST DATA=ADDICTS METHOD=KM PLOTS=(S,LLS);
   TIME DAYS*STATUS(0);
   STRATA CLINIC;
RUN;
```

PROC LIFETEST computes Kaplan–Meier estimates and plots, including log–log plots. Also computes log–rank test statistic.

We now illustrate SAS's PROC LIFETEST by producing Kaplan–Meier survival probabilities and corresponding survival and log–log plots (using PROC PLOT):

LIFETEST PRINTOUT

Product-Limit Survival Estimates
Clinic = 1

Days	Survival	Failure	Survival standard error	Number failed	Number left
0.00	1.0000	0	0	0	163
2.00*	•	•	•	0	162
7.00	0.9938	0.00617	0.00615	1	161
17.00	0.9877	0.0123	0.00868	2	160
19.00	0.9815	0.0185	0.0106	3	159
•					•
•		Omitted middle portion of data			•
•					•
840.00*	•	•	•	119	4
857.00	0.0543	0.9457	0.0262	120	3
892.00	0.0362	0.9638	0.0229	121	2
899.00	0.0181	0.9819	0.0172	122	1
905.00*	•	•	•	122	0

*Censored observation.

Quantiles:	75%	652.00	Mean:	431.47
	50%	428.00	Standard error:	22.51
	25%	192.00		

NOTE: The last observation was censored, so the estimate of the mean is biased.

Product-Limit Survival Estimates
Clinic = 2

Days	Survival	Failure	Survival standard error	Number failed	Number left
0.00	1.0000	0	0	0	75
2.00*	•	•	•	0	74

LIFETEST PRINTOUT

Days	Survival	Failure	Survival standard error	Number failed	Number left
13.00	0.9865	0.0135	0.0134	1	73
26.00	0.9730	0.0270	0.0189	2	72
35.00	0.9595	0.0405	0.0229	3	71
•					•
•		Omitted middle portion of data			•
•					•
932.00*	•	•	•	28	5
944.00*	•	•	•	28	4
969.00*	•	•	•	28	3
1021.00*	•	•	•	28	2
1052.00*	•	•	•	28	1
1076.00*	•	•	•	28	0

*Censored observation.

Quantiles: 75%   •   Mean: 629.82
            50%   •   Standard Error: 39.34
            25%   280.00

NOTE: The last observation was censored so the estimate of the mean is biased.

Summary of the Number of Censored and Uncensored Values

CLINIC	Total	Failed	Censored	%Censored
1	163	122	41	25.1534
2	75	28	47	62.6667
Total	238	150	88	36.974

LIFETEST PRINTOUT

SURVIVAL FUNCTION ESTIMATES

Kaplan–Meier Curves

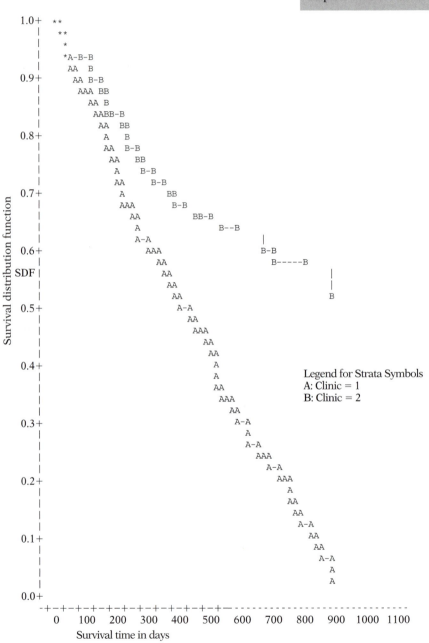

Legend for Strata Symbols
A: Clinic = 1
B: Clinic = 2

LIFETEST PRINTOUT

LOG(–LOG(SURVIVAL FUNCTION)) ESTIMATES

Log–Log Kaplan–Meier survival curves.

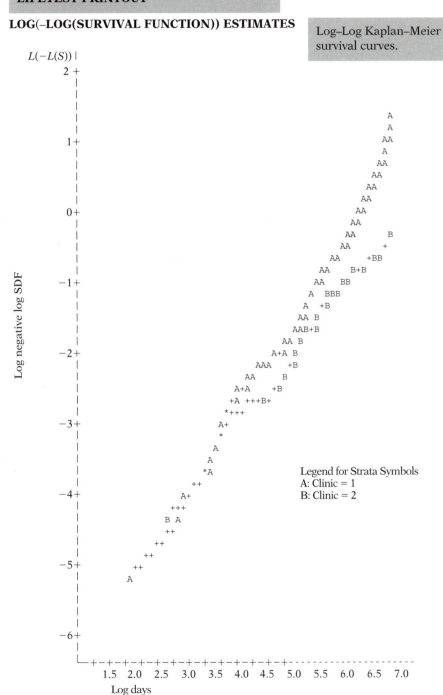

Legend for Strata Symbols
A: Clinic = 1
B: Clinic = 2

Log days

LIFETEST PRINTOUT

Testing Homogeneity of Survival Curves over Strata

Rank statistics

CLINIC	Log–rank	Wilcoxon
1	31.09184	2929
2	–31.0918	–2929

Covariance Matrix for the Log–Rank Statistics

CLINIC	1	2
1	34.6579	–34.6579
2	–34.6579	34.6579

Covariance Matrix for the Wilcoxon Statistics

CLINIC	1	2
1	737868	–737868
2	–737868	737868

Test of Equality over Strata

Test	Chi-Square	DF	PR > Chi-Square
Log–rank	27.8927	1	0.0001
Wilcoxon	11.6268	1	0.0007
–2 log *(LR)*	26.0236	1	0.0001

```
PROC MEANS DATA=ADDICTS NOPRINT;
   VAR PRISON DOSE;
   OUTPUT OUT=RISK MEAN=PRISON DOSE;
RUN;

DATA INRISK;
SET RISK;
DO I=1 TO 2;
CLINIC=I;
OUTPUT;
END;
RUN;
```

PROC MEANS is used to calculate the **overall** means for the prison and dose variables and the "OUTPUT" statement sets up an output file called "RISK" to be used by PROC PHREG for plotting adjusted survival and log–log survival curves.

The dataset "INRISK" is created from the dataset "RISK" to contain two lines of data, one for each clinic, with the overall means for prison and dose on each line.

PROC PRINT provides output for dataset "INRISK"

```
PROC PRINT DATA=INRISK;
   VAR CLINIC PRISON DOSE;
RUN;
```

PRINTOUT OF "INRISK"

OBS	CLINIC	PRISON	DOSE
1	1	0.46639	60.3992
2	2	0.46639	60.3992

We now apply **PROC PHREG** to the addicts dataset to fit Cox PH, stratified Cox, and extended Cox models as described below:

Fit Cox PH model with predictors CLINIC, PRISON, and DOSE.

```
PROC PHREG DATA=ADDICTS;
   MODEL DAYS*STATUS(0)=CLINIC PRISON DOSE / RL;
   ID ID;
   BASELINE COVARIATES=INRISK OUT=MODEL1 SURVIVAL=S1 / NOMEAN;
RUN;
```

Plot adjusted survival curves separately for each clinic.

```
PROC PLOT DATA=MODEL1;
   TITLE2 'PLOT OF SURVIVAL FUNCTION VS. TIME';
   TITLE3 'ADJUSTED FOR CLINIC, DOSE, AND PRISON';
   PLOT S1*DAYS=CLINIC;
RUN;
```

PHREG PRINTOUT

The PHREG Procedure

Dataset: WORK.ADDICTS
Dependent Variable: DAYS   SURVIVAL TIME IN DAYS
Censoring Variable: STATUS   CENSORED = 0
Censoring Value(s): 0
Ties Handling: BRESLOW

Summary of the Number of
Event and Censored Values

Total	Event	Censored	Percent censored
238	150	88	36.97

PHREG PRINTOUT

Testing Global Null Hypothesis: BETA = 0

Criterion	Without covariates	With covariates	Model Chi-Square
–2 log L	1411.324	1346.805	64.519 with 3 DF (p=0.0001)
Score	—	—	56.273 with 3 DF (p=0.0001)
Wald	—	—	54.094 with 3 DF (p=0.0001)

Analysis of Maximum Likelihood Estimates

Variable	DF	Parameter estimate	Standard error	Wald Chi-Square	Pr > Chi-Square
CLINIC	1	–1.008870	0.21487	22.04524	0.0001
PRISON	1	0.326511	0.16722	3.81253	0.0509
DOSE	1	–0.035396	0.00638	30.78505	0.0001

Analysis of Maximum Likelihood Estimates

Conditional Risk Ratio and 95% Confidence Limits

Variable	Risk ratio	Lower	Upper	Label
CLINIC	0.365	0.239	0.556	Study clinic
PRISON	1.386	0.999	1.924	Prison record (Y/N)
DOSE	0.965	0.953	0.977	Methadone dose (mg/day)

PLOT OF SURVIVAL FUNCTION VS. TIME ADJUSTED FOR CLINIC, DOSE, AND PRISON

Plot of S1*DAYS. Symbol is value of CLINIC.

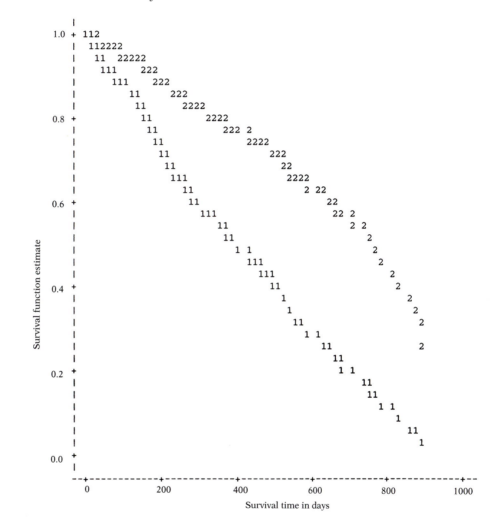

```
PROC PHREG DATA=ADDICTS;
   MODEL DAYS*STATUS(0)=PRISON DOSE / RL;
   STRATA CLINIC;
   ID ID;
   BASELINE COVARIATES=INRISK OUT=MODEL2 SURVIVAL=S2
   LOGLOGS=LLS / NOMEAN;
RUN;
```

> Fit Cox PH model with predicators Prison and Dose, stratified by Clinic.

PHREG PRINTOUT

The PHREG Procedure

Dataset: WORK.ADDICTS
Dependent Variable: DAYS   SURVIVAL TIME IN DAYS
Censoring Variable: STATUS CENSORED = 0
Censoring Value(s): 0
Ties Handling: BRESLOW

Summary of the Number of Event and Censored Values

Stratum	CLINIC	Total	Event	Censored	Percent censored
1	1	163	122	41	25.15
2	2	75	28	47	62.67
Total		238	150	88	36.97

Testing Global Null Hypothesis: BETA=0

Criterion	Without covariates	With covariates	Model chi-square
$-2 \log L$	1229.367	1195.428	33.939 with 2 DF (p = 0.0001)
Score	—	—	33.363 with 2 DF (p = 0.0001)
Wald	—	—	32.690 with 2 DF (p = 0.0001)

Analysis of Maximum Likelihood Estimates

Variable	DF	Parameter estimate	Standard error	Wald chi-square	Pr > chi-square
PRISON	1	0.388788	0.16892	5.29770	0.0214
DOSE	1	–0.035145	0.00647	29.55175	0.0001

Conditional Risk Ratio and 95% Confidence Limits

Variable	Risk ratio	Lower	Upper	Label
PRISON	1.475	1.059	2.054	Prison record (Y/N)
DOSE	0.965	0.953	0.978	Methadone dose (mg/day)

```
DATA MODEL2;
   SET MODEL2;
   LOG_T=LOG(DAYS);
   LABEL LOG_T='LOG OF TIME (DAYS)';
RUN;

PROC PLOT DATA=MODEL2;
   TITLE2 'PLOTS OF SURVIVAL FUNCTION AND LOG(-LOG(S)) VS.
   TIME';
   TITLE3 'ADJUSTED FOR DOSE AND PRISON';
   TITLE4 'STRATIFIED BY CLINIC';
   PLOT S2*DAYS=CLINIC LLS*LOG_T=CLINIC;
RUN;
```

> Plot-adjusted survival and log–log survival curves for PH model with predictors PRISON and DOSE, stratified by CLINIC.

PHREG PRINTOUT

PLOT OF SURVIVAL FUNCTION VS. TIME ADJUSTED FOR DOSE AND PRISON STRATIFIED BY CLINIC

Plot of S2*DAYS. Symbol is value of CLINIC.

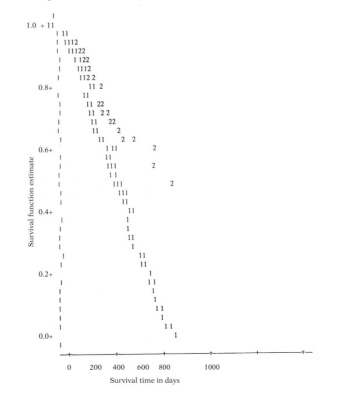

PLOT OF LOG(–LOG(S)) VS. TIME, ADJUSTED FOR DOSE AND PRISON STRATIFIED BY CLINIC.

Plot of LLS*LOG_T. Symbol is value of CLINIC.

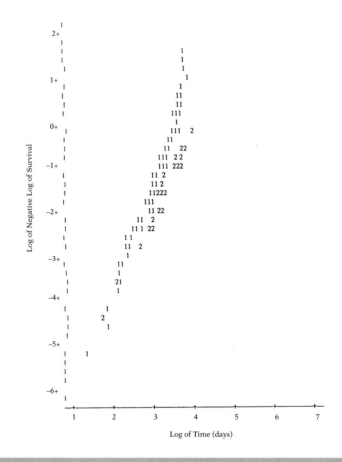

Fit extended Cox model with predictors **PRISON**, **DOSE**, **CLINICT1**, and **CLINICT2**, where latter two variables are time-dependent and involve the product of **CLINIC** variable with heavyside functions defined by 365-day cutoff.

```
PROC PHREG DATA=ADDICTS;
   TITLE2 ' ';
   TITLE3 ' ';
   TITLE4 ' ';
   MODEL DAYS*STATUS(0)=PRISON DOSE CLINICT1 CLINICT2 / RL;
   CLINICT1=0;
   IF DAYS < 365 THEN CLINICT1=CLINIC;
   CLINICT2=0;
   IF DAYS >= 365 THEN CLINICT2=CLINIC;
RUN;
```

PHREG PRINTOUT

The PHREG Procedure

Dataset: WORK.ADDICTS
Dependent Variable: DAYS   SURVIVAL TIME IN DAYS
Censoring Variable: STATUS   CENSORED = 0
Censoring Value(s): 0
Ties Handling: BRESLOW

Summary of the Number of Event and Censored Values

Total	Event	Censored	Percent censored
238	150	88	36.97

Testing Global Null Hypothesis: BETA=0

Criterion	Without covariates	With covariates	Model chi-square
$-2 \log L$	1411.324	1337.149	74.175 with 4 DF (p = 0.0001)
Score	•	•	64.137 with 4 DF (p = 0.0001)
Wald	•	•	57.444 with 4 DF (p = 0.0001)

Analysis of Maximum Likelihood Estimates*

Variable	DF	Parameter estimate	Standard error	Wald chi-square	Pr > chi-square
PRISON	1	0.377704	0.16840	5.03045	0.0249
DOSE	1	−0.035512	0.00644	30.45033	0.0001
CLINICT1	1	−0.459563	0.25529	3.24055	0.0718
CLINICT2	1	−1.828228	0.38595	22.43922	0.0001

* Coding used for clinic is 1=clinic1, 2=clinic2

Conditional Risk Ratio and 95% Confidence Limits

Variable	Risk ratio	Lower	Upper	Label
PRISON	1.459	1.049	2.029	PRISON RECORD (Y/N)
DOSE	0.965	0.953	0.977	METHADONE DOSE (mg/day)
CLINICT1	0.632	0.383	1.042	
CLINICT2	0.161	0.075	0.342	

```
PROC PHREG DATA=ADDICTS;
   MODEL DAYS*STATUS(0)=CLINIC PRISON DOSE CLINIC_T / RL
   COVB;
   IF 0<=DAYS<=183 THEN T=1;
   IF 183<DAYS<=365 THEN T=3;
   IF 365<DAYS<=548 THEN T=5;
   IF 548<DAYS<=730 THEN T=7;
   IF DAYS>730 THEN T=9;
   CLINIC_T=CLINIC*T;
RUN;
```

Fit extended Cox model with predictors CLINIC, PRISON, DOSE, and a time-dependent CLINIC_T variable defined to allow diverging survival curves over time.

The PHREG Procedure

Datset: WORK.ADDICTS
Dependent Variable: DAYS   SURVIVAL TIME IN DAYS
Censoring Variable: STATUS   CENSORED=0
Censoring Value(s): 0
Ties Handling: BRESLOW

Summary of the Number of Event and Censored Values

Total	Event	Censored	Percent censored
238	150	88	36.97

Testing Global Null Hypothesis: BETA=0

Criterion	Without covariates	With covariates	Model chi-square
–2 log L	1411.324	1335.518	75.806 with 4 DF (p = 0.0001)
Score	•	•	66.449 with 4 DF (p = 0.0001)
Wald	•	•	57.647 with 4 DF (p = 0.0001)

Analysis of Maximum Likelihood Estimates

Variable	DF	Parameter estimate	Standard error	Wald chi-square	Pr > chi-square
CLINIC	1	0.028900	0.35290	0.00671	0.9347
PRISON	1	0.388220	0.16880	5.28969	0.0215
DOSE	1	–0.035283	0.00644	30.00208	0.0001
CLINIC_T	1	–0.278001	0.08827	9.91870	0.0016

| PHREG PRINTOUT | **Conditional Risk Ratio and 95% Confidence Limits** |

Conditional Risk Ratio and 95% Confidence Limits

Variable	Risk ratio	Lower	Upper	Label
CLINIC	1.029	0.515	2.056	STUDY CLINIC
PRISON	1.474	1.059	2.052	PRISON RECORD (Y/N)
DOSE	0.965	0.953	0.978	METHADONE DOSE (mg/DAY)
CLINIC_T	0.757	0.637	0.900	

BMDP

The BMDP package contains two programs for survival analysis;

1. **1L:** provides Kaplan–Meier (KM) survival probabilities, log–rank statistic (called in the program the generalized Savage Mantel-Cox test), generalized Wilcoxon (i.e., Peto) test, KM plots, and log–log KM plots.
2. **2L:** fits the Cox PH model, stratified Cox PH model (using a **stratification** statement in the **/regression** paragraph to identify variables for stratification), and an extended Cox model (using a **function** statement to define time-dependent variables). Also computes and plots adjusted survival and log–log survival probabilities for a specified set of predictors.

As with SAS's PROC PHREG, the 2L program also provides regression diagnostic information in terms of residuals; however, no collinearity diagnostics are provided, even though it is possible to create one's own BMDP macro for calculating condition indices and variance decomposition proportions from the inverse of the information matrix derived from the likelihood function. Also, the 2L program *does not* provide a GOF statistic for testing the PH assumption.

We now illustrate the use of the BMDP survival analysis procedures with the addicts dataset. First, we use **1L** to provide command statements and printout for obtaining Kaplan–Meier survival probabilities corresponding survival curves:

BMDP EXAMPLE

```
PROGRAM INSTRUCTIONS
/INPUT     UNIT IS 11.
           VARIABLES = 6.
           FORMAT = FREE.
/VARIABLE  NAMES = ID, CLINIC, STATUS, DAYS, PRISON, DOSE.
/FORM      TIME = DAYS.
           UNIT = DAYS.
           STATUS = STATUS.
```

```
                                     RESPONSE = 1.
                        /GROUP     CODES(CLINIC) = 1, 2.
                                   NAMES(CLINIC) = CLINIC_1, CLINIC_2.
                        /ESTIMATE  METHOD = PRODUCT.
                                   PLOTS = SURV, LOG.
                                   BROOK = 95.
                                   GROUPING = CLINIC.
                                   STATISTICS = ALL.
                                   EXPECTED.
                        /END
```

These commands produce tables of KM survival probabilities, log–rank and Peto test statistics, and survival and log–log survival curves for each clinic.

1L PRINTOUT

TIME VARIABLE IS DAYS

KM probabilities for Clinic 1.

PRODUCT-LIMIT SURVIVAL ANALYSIS   GROUPING VARIABLE IS CLINIC   LEVEL IS CLINIC_1

CASE LABEL	CASE NUMBER	TIME DAYS	STATUS	CUMULATIVE SURVIVAL	STANDARD ERROR	CUM DEAD	CUM LOST	REMAIN AT RISK
	217	2.00	CENSORED			0	0	162
	175	7.00	DEAD	0.9938	0.0062	1	0	161
	164	17.00	DEAD	0.9877	0.0087	2	0	160
	220	19.00	DEAD	0.9815	0.0106	3	0	159
	193	28.00	CENSORED			3	0	158
	203	28.00	CENSORED			3	0	157
	•							•
	•		Omitted middle portion of data					•
	•							•
	55	857.00	DEAD	0.0543	0.0262	120	0	3
	9	892.00	DEAD	0.0362	0.0229	121	0	2
	54	899.00	DEAD	0.0181	0.0172	122	0	1
	70	905.00	CENSORED			122	0	0

MEAN SURVIVAL TIME =   431.57   LIMITED TO   905.00   S.E. =   22.526

QUANTILE	ESTIMATE	ASYMPTOTIC STANDARD ERROR
75TH	192.00	15.79
MEDIAN (50TH)	428.00	48.59
25TH	652.00	54.25

BROOKMEYER-CROWLEY 95% CONFIDENCE INTERVAL FOR MEDIAN SURVIVAL TIME
(341.00, 504.00)

*** NOTE   *** BROOKMEYER-CROWLEY CONFIDENCE INTERVAL ASSUMES NO TIES

1L PRINTOUT

PRODUCT-LIMIT SURVIVAL ANALYSIS   GROUPING VARIABLE IS CLINIC   LEVEL IS CLINIC_2

TIME VARIABLE IS DAYS

KM probabilities for Clinic 2.

CASE LABEL	CASE NUMBER	TIME DAYS	STATUS	CUMULATIVE SURVIVAL	STANDARD ERROR	CUM DEAD	CUM LOST	REMAIN AT RISK
	143	2.00	CENSORED			0	0	74
	123	13.00	DEAD	0.9865	0.0134	1	0	73
	116	26.00	DEAD	0.9730	0.0189	2	0	72
	106	35.00	DEAD	0.9595	0.0229	3	0	71
	210	41.00	DEAD	0.9459	0.0263	4	0	70
	104	53.00	CENSORED			4	0	69
	•							•
	•		Omitted middle portion of data					•
	•							•
	125	969.00	CENSORED			28	0	3
	153	1021.00	CENSORED			28	0	2
	126	1052.00	CENSORED			28	0	1
	142	1076.00	CENSORED			28	0	0

MEAN SURVIVAL TIME = 732.20 LIMITED TO 1076.00 S.E. = 51.438

QUANTILE	ESTIMATE	STANDARD ERROR
75TH	280.00	69.41

LOWER ONE-SIDED BROOKMEYER-CROWLEY 95% CONFIDENCE LIMIT FOR MEDIAN SURVIVAL TIME = 661.00

** NOTE   *** BROOKMEYER-CROWLEY CONFIDENCE INTERVAL ASSUMES NO TIES AMONG OBSERVED RESPONSE TIMES. AT LEAST ONE SUCH TIE OCCURRED.

SUMMARY TABLE

	TOTAL	DEAD	CENSORED	PROPORTION CENSORED
CLINIC_1	163	122	41	0.2515
CLINIC_2	75	28	47	0.6267
TOTALS	238	150	88	

```
                SUMS FOR OBSERVED AND EXPECTED RESPONSES (MANTEL-COX TEST)

                          OBSERVED    EXPECTED    (OBS/EXP)
               CLINIC_1    122.0       90.91       1.34
               CLINIC_2     28.0       59.09       0.47
```

The "log–rank" statistic is called the generalized Savage (Mantel-Cox) statistic in BMDP and the "Peto" statistic is called the Generalized Wilcoxon (Breslow) statistic in BMDP

```
                              TEST STATISTICS

                                            STATISTIC  D.F.  P-VALUE
               GENERALIZED SAVAGE (MANTEL-COX)          27.895   1   0.0000
               TARONE-WARE                              17.597   1   0.0000
               GENERALIZED WILCOXON (BRESLOW)           11.627   1   0.0007
               GENERALIZED WILCOXON (PETO-PRENTICE) 15.652   1   0.0001
```

```
                        PATTERN OF CENSORED DATA

CLINIC_1   ** * ******   * **  * *** ******        ****  *
CLINIC_2   *  **  *    *     * * *  * * ****** * * ***   *   **  * **

          .+....+....+....+....+....+....+....+....+....+....+....+....+.
             100.      300.      500.      700.      900.     1100
          0.00      200.      400.      600.      800.      1000      1200

                     PATTERN OF TRUE RESPONSE TIMES

CLINIC_1   ***********************************  ****  ***  *
CLINIC_2    ** ****** ****  * **   **    *        * *        *

          .+....+....+....+....+....+....+....+....+....+....+....+....+.
             100.      300.      500.      700.      900.     1100
          0.00      200.      400.      600.      800.      1000      1200
```

1L PRINTOUT

CUMULATIVE PROPORTION
SURVIVING GROUP VAR: CLINIC

KM survival curves for Clinics 1 and 2.

A is CLINIC_1   B is CLINIC_2

```
        .+....+....+....+....+....+....+....+....+....+....+....+....+.
  1.0  +B.                                                            +
    -   B.                                                            -
    -    B..                                                          -
    -    AABB.                                                        -
    -     AA.BB                                                       -
    -       AAB.                                                      -
    -       AABB.                                                     -
    -       AA BB.                                                    -
 0.80  +      AA   B.                                                 +
    -          A    .                                                 -
    -          AA   B-
    -           A.  B.B..                                             -
    -            A        B.                                          -
    -           AA.        B...B                                      -
    -            A          B....                                     -
    -           AAA              B......                              -
 0.60  +          AA.                B..                              +
    -              A.                 B.........                      -
    -              A.                         .                       -
    -               AA                          B..........          -
    -               AA.                                               -
    -                AA                                               -
    -                AA.                                              -
    -                 AA                                              -
 0.40  +                A                                             +
    -                  A.                                             -
    -                   A.                                            -
    -                    A.                                           -
    -                    AA.                                          -
    -                     A.                                          -
    -                      AA                                         -
    -                       AA                                        -
 0.80  +                       A.AA                                   +
    -                            AA                                   -
    -                            AA                                   -
    -                             A..                                 -
    -                               A.                                -
    -                                A.                               -
    -                                 A.                              -
    -                                  A                              -
  0.0  +                                                              +
        .+....+....+....+....+....+....+....+....+....+....+....+....+.
          100.      300.      500.      700.      900.      1100
      0.00      200.      400.      600.      800.      1000      1200
```

DAYS

| 1L PRINTOUT | LOG OF CUMULATIVE PROPORTION SURVIVING GROUP VAR: CLINIC | log–log KM curves for Clinics 1 and 2. |

A is CLINIC_1   B is CLINIC_2

```
       .+....+....+....+....+....+....+....+....+....+....+....+....+.
       -                                                            -
       -                                                            -
 1.0 +                                                              +
 0.9 +BBB.                                                          +
 0.8 +  B.BBBBB.                                                    +
     -      AAABBBB.                                                -
 0.7 +         AA. BB.B..                                          +
 0.6 +          AAA     BB...B....                                 +
     -           AAAAA        B.....B..                            -
 0.5 +            AAA.             B.........                      +
     -              AAA.                   B..........            -
 0.4 +               AAA                                          +
     -                AA                                          -
     -                AA                                          -
 0.3 +                AA                                          +
     -                AAA.                                        -
     -                  A.                                        -
     -                 AA                                         -
 0.2 +                 AA                                         +
     -                 A.A.                                       -
     -                  A.                                        -
     -                  A.                                        -
     -                  A                                         -
     -                  A                                         -
     -                  A..                                       -
 0.1 +                    .                                       +
     -                  A.                                        -
     -                  A                                         -
     -                   .                                        -
     -                  A.                                        -
     -                   .                                        -
     -                   .                                        -
     -                  A..                                       -
     -                   .                                        -
     -                   .                                        -
     -                   .                                        -
     -                  A                                         -
     -                  A                                         -
     -                                                            -
     -                                                            -
 0.  +                                                            +
       .+....+....+....+....+....+....+....+....+....+....+....+....+.
         100.     300.     500.     700.     900.     1100
       0.00    200.     400.     600.     800.     1000     1200
```

DAYS

PROGRAM INSTRUCTIONS

/INPUT	UNIT IS 11.
	VARIABLES = 6.
	FORMAT = FREE.

> These commands use Procedure **2L** to fit Cox PH model with predictors CLINIC, PRISON, and DOSE.

/VARIABLE   NAMES = ID, CLINIC, STATUS, DAYS, PRISON, DOSE.

/FORM	TIME = DAYS
	UNIT = DAYS
	STATUS = STATUS
	RESPONSE = 1.

> Also, adjusted survival curves are plotted for each clinic.

| /GROUP | CODES(CLINIC) = 1, 2. |
| | NAMES(CLINIC) = CLINIC_1, CLINIC_2. |

/REGRESS   COVARIATES=CLINIC, DOSE, PRISON.

/PLOT	TYPE = SURV
	PATTERN = 1, 58.957, 0.46.
	PATTERN = 2, 63.533, 0.48.

/END

2L PRINTOUT

COX PROPORTIONAL HAZARDS MODEL
―――――――――――――――――
RISK TYPE IS LOGLIN

INDEPENDENT VARIABLES
     2 CLINIC   6 DOSE   5 PRISON

   LOG LIKELIHOOD =   −673.4024
GLOBAL CHI-SQUARE =   56.27 D.F.= 3 P-VALUE =0.0000
NORM OF THE SCORE VECTOR= 0.159E−01

VARIABLE	COEFFICIENT	STANDARD ERROR	COEFF./ S.E.	EXP (COEFF.)
2 CLINIC	−1.0088	0.2149	−4.6949	0.3657
6 DOSE	−0.0354	0.0064	−5.5484	0.9652
5 PRISON	0.3265	0.1672	1.9525	1.3861

Estimated Survivor Function

Adjusted survival curves plotted for each clinic for PH model containing CLINIC, PRISON and DOSE variables

```
      .+.....+.....+.....+.....+.....+.....+.....+.....+.....+.....+.
 1.0  +*B                                                          +
    - ABB                                                          -
    - AA BBBB                                                      -
    -  A     BB                                                    -
    -   A      BB                                                  -
0.90  +    AA      B                                               +
    -      A       BBB                                             -
    -       A        B                                            -
    -       AA        BBB                                         -
    -        AA          BBB                                      -
0.80  +        A            B                                      +
    -          A            BBBB                                  -
    -          A               BB                                 -
    -         AA                 BB                               -
    -          AA                  B                              -
0.70  +         A                   BB                             -
    -           AA                   BB                           -
    -            A                     BB                         -
    -             A                     BB                        -
    -             AA                      B                       -
0.60  +            AA                       BB                     +
    -              AA                       BB                    -
    -               AA                        B                  -
    -                A                         BB                -
    -                A                          BB               -
0.50  +                A                          B               +
    -                 A                           B              -
    -                 AAA                          B            -
    -                  A                            B           -
    -                  AA                            B          -
0.40  +                   AA                          BB          +
    -                     A                            BB        -
    -                     A                                      -
    -                     A                                      -
    -                     AA                                     -
0.30  +                      AAA                                  +
    -                        A                                   -
    -                        AA                                  -
    -                         AA                                 -
    -                          A                                 -
0.20  +                          AA                              +
    -                            AA                              -
    -                             A                              -
    -                             AA                             -
    -                              AA                            -
0.10  +                               AA                          +
    -                                A                            -
    -                                AAA                          -
    -                                  A                          -
    -                                                            -
 0.0  +    .+.....+.....+.....+.....+.....+.....+.....+.....+.....+.
         100.       300.       500.       700.       900.
      0.00       200.      400.      600.      800.      1000
```

DAYS

These commands fit a Cox PH model with predictors **PRISON** and **DOSE**, stratified by **CLINIC**. Adjusted (for **CLINIC**) survival and log–log survival curves are also plotted.

```
/REGRESS      COVARIATES=DOSE, PRISON.
              STRATA = CLINIC.
/PLOT         TYPE = SURV, LOG.
              PATTERN = 60.399, 0.466.
/END
```

2L PRINTOUT

```
              COX PROPORTIONAL HAZARDS MODEL
              ─────────────────────────────
              RISK TYPE IS LOGLIN


   INDEPENDENT VARIABLES
        6 DOSE          5 PRISON


     LOG LIKELIHOOD =   −597.7140
   GLOBAL CHI-SQUARE =     33.36  D.F.=  2   P-VALUE =0.0000
   NORM OF THE SCORE VECTOR=  0.221E-06


                              STANDARD   COEFF./       EXP
   VARIABLE    COEFFICIENT     ERROR       S.E.      (COEFF.)
   6 DOSE        −0.0351       0.0065     −5.4362      0.9655
   5 PRISON       0.3888       0.1689      2.3017      1.4752



   PLOT DIRECTORY
                CONVERSION          6            5
   PATTERN      FACTOR **          DOSE        PRISON
      1           1.000           60.399        .466
```

```
** USE THE CONVERSION FACTOR AS AN EXPONENT TO CONVERT
THE ESTIMATE FOR THE BASELINE SURVIVOR FUNCTION TO THE
SURVIVOR FUNCTION FOR A PARTICULAR COVARIATE PATTERN. THE
PROPORTIONAL HAZARDS BASELINE SURVIVOR FUNCTION IS
PRINTED WHEN YOU REQUEST THE SURVIVAL OPTION IN THE PRINT
PARAGRAPH.
```

2L PRINTOUT	Adjusted survival curves by CLINIC for stratified Cox model containing PRISON and DOSE, stratified by CLINIC.

Estimated Survivor Function

```
       .+.....+.....+.....+.....+.....+.....+.....+.....+.....+.....+.
  1.0  +*                                                            +
   -  *                                                              -
   - A*                                                              -
   - A*BB                                                            -
   -   A BB                                                          -
  0.90 +    A  B                                                     +
   -        AABB                                                     -
   -        AABB                                                     -
   -        AA B                                                     -
   -         A BB                                                    -
  0.80 +        A  B                                                 +
   -         AA  BB                                                  -
   -          A  B                                                   -
   -          A  BB                                                  -
   -          AA  BB                                                 -
  0.70 +          A    BBB                                           +
   -             AA      BBB                                         -
   -             AA        BB                                        -
   -             A          BBB                                      -
   -            AAA           BBBBB                                  -
  0.60 +            A             BBBB                               +
   -               AA               BB                              -
   -               A                 BB                             -
   -               AA                 BBB                           -
   -               AAA                   BBB                         -
  0.50 +               A                      BBB                   +
   -                   A                                            -
   -                  AA                                            -
   -                  AA                                            -
   -                   A                                            -
  0.40 +                   A                                        +
   -                       A                                        -
   -                       A                                        -
   -                       A                                        -
   -                        A                                       -
  0.30 +                      AAA                                   +
   -                        A                                       -
   -                        A                                       -
   -                       AA                                       -
   -                        A                                       -
  0.20 +                      AAA                                   +
   -                         AA                                     -
   -                          A                                     -
   -                         AA                                     -
   -                          A                                     -
  0.10 +                          AA                                +
   -                             A                                  -
   -                             A                                  -
   -                            AAA                                 -
   -                              A                                 -
  0.0  +                                                            +
       .+.....+.....+.....+.....+.....+.....+.....+.....+.....+.....+.
          100.       300.       500.       700.       900.
       0.00      200.       400.       600.       800.       1000
                                                          DAYS
```

2L PRINTOUT	Adjusted log–log survival curves by CLINIC for stratified Cox model containing PRISON and DOSE, stratified by CLINIC.

Log Minus Log Survivor Function

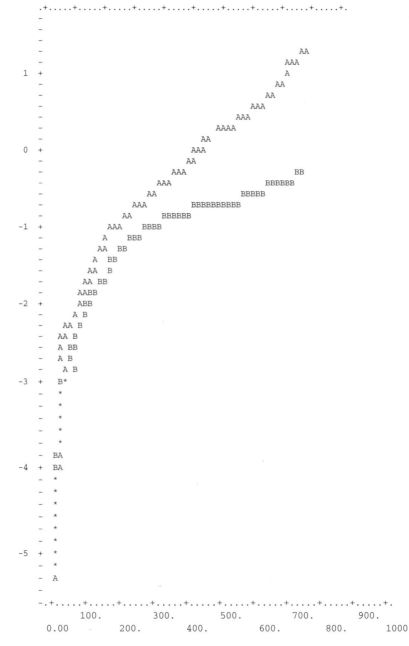

DAYS

> Fit extended Cox model with predictors **PRISON, DOSE, CLINICT1**, and **CLIN-ICT2**, where latter two variables are time-dependent and defined by the **FUNC-TION** statement as separate products of the **CLINIC** variable with heavyside functions defined by 365-day cutoff.

PROGRAM INSTRUCTIONS

```
/REGRESS     COVARIATES=DOSE, PRISON.
             ADD = CLINICT1, CLINICT2.
             AUXILIARY = CLINIC, DAYS.

/FUNCTION    CLINICT1 = 0.
             CLINICT2 = 0.
             IF (DAYS < 365) THEN CLINICT1=CLINIC.
             IF (DAYS >= 365) THEN CLINICT2=CLINIC.

             /END
```

2L PRINTOUT

COX PROPORTIONAL HAZARDS MODEL
───────────────────────────────
RISK TYPE IS LOGLIN

INDEPENDENT VARIABLES
     6 DOSE   5 PRISON   7 CLINICT1   8 CLINICT2

```
   LOG LIKELIHOOD =   -668.5774
GLOBAL CHI-SQUARE =    64.14  D.F.=  4  P-VALUE =0.0000
NORM OF THE SCORE VECTOR=  0.1433E-04
```

VARIABLE	COEFFICIENT	STANDARD ERROR	COEFF./ S.E.	EXP (COEFF.)
6 DOSE	−0.0355	0.0064	−5.5182	0.9651
5 PRISON	0.3777	0.1684	2.2429	1.4589
7 CLINICT1	−0.4596	0.2553	−1.8002	0.6316
8 CLINICT2	−1.8282	0.3859	−4.7370	0.1607

Fit extended Cox model with predictors CLINIC, PRISON, DOSE, and a time-dependent CLINIC_T variable defined by the **FUNCTION** statement to allow diverging survival curves over time.

```
PROGRAM INSTRUCTIONS

/REGRESS       COVARIATES=CLINIC, PRISON, DOSE.
               ADD = CLINIC_T.

/FUNCTION      IF (TIME >= 0 AND TIME <= 183) THEN
               CLINIC_T=CLINIC.
               IF (TIME >183 AND TIME <= 365) THEN
               CLINIC_T=CLINIC*3.
               IF (TIME >365 AND TIME <= 548) THEN
               CLINIC_T=CLINIC*5.
               IF (TIME >548 AND TIME <= 730) THEN
               CLINIC_T=CLINIC*7.
               IF (TIME >730) THEN CLINIC_T=CLINIC*9.
/END
```

2L PRINTOUT

```
         COX PROPORTIONAL HAZARDS MODEL
         ──────────────────────
         RISK TYPE IS LOGLIN

INDEPENDENT VARIABLES
      2 CLINIC      5 PRISON        6 DOSE        7 CLINIC_T

   LOG LIKELIHOOD =  -667.7591
GLOBAL CHI-SQUARE =     66.45  D.F.=  4  P-VALUE =0.0000
NORM OF THE SCORE VECTOR=  0.677E-04
```

VARIABLE	COEFFICIENT	STANDARD ERROR	COEFF./ S.E.	EXP (COEFF.)
2 CLINIC	0.0289	0.3529	0.0819	1.0293
5 PRISON	0.3882	0.1688	2.2999	1.4744
6 DOSE	−0.0353	0.0064	−5.4774	0.9653
7 CLINIC_T	−0.2780	0.0883	−3.1494	0.7573

Note: The Clinic variable is coded as 1=clinic1, 2=clinic2, and is *not* recoded to a (1,0) variable for this analysis.

B
Appendix: Datasets

In this appendix, we provide listings of datasets that are illustrated in the textbook using examples of computer output either as part of a chapter's main presentation or as part of the practice exercises or test. A table of contents for this appendix is given as follows:

ADDICTS.DAT

Survival times in days of heroin addicts from entry to a clinic until departure. Data provided by John Caplehorn (The University of Sydney, Department of Public Health).

Column 1 = ID of subject
2 = Clinic (1 or 2)
3 = status (0=censored, 1=endpoint)
4 = survival time (days)
5 = prison record?
6 = methadone dose (mg/day)

/nr = 238
/field = (n4,2n2,n5,n2,n4)

1	2	3	4	5	6	1	2	3	4	5	6	1	2	3	4	5	6
1	1	1	428	0	50	31	1	0	602	0	60	62	1	1	452	0	60
2	1	1	275	1	55	32	1	1	652	0	80	63	1	1	760	0	60
3	1	1	262	0	55	33	1	1	293	0	65	64	1	1	496	0	65
4	1	1	183	0	30	34	1	0	564	0	60	65	1	1	258	1	40
5	1	1	259	1	65	36	1	1	394	1	55	66	1	1	181	1	60
6	1	1	714	0	55	37	1	1	755	1	65	67	1	1	386	0	60
7	1	1	438	1	65	38	1	1	591	0	55	68	1	0	439	0	80
8	1	0	796	1	60	39	1	0	787	0	80	69	1	0	563	0	75
9	1	1	892	0	50	40	1	1	739	0	60	70	1	1	337	0	65
10	1	1	393	1	65	41	1	1	550	1	60	71	1	0	613	1	60
11	1	0	161	1	80	42	1	1	837	0	60	72	1	1	192	1	80
12	1	1	836	1	60	43	1	1	612	0	65	73	1	0	405	0	80
13	1	1	523	0	55	44	1	0	581	0	70	74	1	1	667	0	50
14	1	1	612	0	70	45	1	1	523	0	60	75	1	0	905	0	80
15	1	1	212	1	60	46	1	1	504	1	60	76	1	1	247	0	70
16	1	1	399	1	60	48	1	1	785	1	80	77	1	1	821	0	80
17	1	1	771	1	75	49	1	1	774	1	65	78	1	1	821	1	75
18	1	1	514	1	80	50	1	1	560	0	65	79	1	0	517	0	45
19	1	1	512	0	80	51	1	1	160	0	35	80	1	0	346	1	60
21	1	1	624	1	80	52	1	1	482	0	30	81	1	1	294	0	65
22	1	1	209	1	60	53	1	1	518	0	65	82	1	1	244	1	60
23	1	1	341	1	60	54	1	1	683	0	50	83	1	1	95	1	60
24	1	1	299	0	55	55	1	1	147	0	65	84	1	1	376	1	55
25	1	0	826	0	80	57	1	1	563	1	70	85	1	1	212	0	40
26	1	1	262	1	65	58	1	1	646	1	60	86	1	1	96	0	70
27	1	0	566	1	45	59	1	1	899	0	60	87	1	1	532	0	80
28	1	1	368	1	55	60	1	1	857	0	60	88	1	1	522	1	70
30	1	1	302	1	50	61	1	1	180	1	70	89	1	1	679	0	35

1	2	3	4	5	6	1	2	3	4	5	6	1	2	3	4	5	6
90	1	0	408	0	50	134	2	1	232	1	70	184	2	0	222	0	40
91	1	0	840	0	80	135	2	1	13	1	60	186	2	0	683	0	100
92	1	0	148	1	65	137	2	0	563	0	70	187	2	0	496	0	40
93	1	1	168	0	65	138	2	0	969	0	80	188	2	1	389	0	55
94	1	1	489	0	80	143	2	0	1052	0	80	189	1	1	126	1	75
95	1	0	541	0	80	144	2	0	944	1	80	190	1	1	17	1	40
96	1	1	205	0	50	145	2	0	881	0	80	192	1	1	350	0	60
97	1	0	475	1	75	146	2	1	190	1	50	193	2	0	531	1	65
98	1	1	237	0	45	148	2	1	79	0	40	194	1	0	317	1	50
99	1	1	517	0	70	149	2	0	884	1	50	195	1	0	461	1	75
100	1	1	749	0	70	150	2	1	170	0	40	196	1	1	37	0	60
101	1	1	150	1	80	153	2	1	286	0	45	197	1	1	167	1	55
102	1	1	465	0	65	156	2	0	358	0	60	198	1	1	358	0	45
103	2	1	708	1	60	158	2	0	326	1	60	199	1	1	49	0	60
104	2	0	713	0	50	159	2	0	769	1	40	200	1	1	457	1	40
105	2	0	146	0	50	160	2	1	161	0	40	201	1	1	127	0	20
106	2	1	450	0	55	161	2	0	564	1	80	202	1	1	7	1	40
109	2	0	555	0	80	162	2	1	268	1	70	203	1	1	29	1	60
110	2	1	460	0	50	163	2	0	611	1	40	204	1	1	62	0	40
111	2	0	53	1	60	164	2	1	322	0	55	205	1	0	150	1	60
113	2	1	122	1	60	165	2	0	1076	1	80	206	1	1	223	1	40
114	2	1	35	1	40	166	2	0	2	1	40	207	1	0	129	1	40
118	2	0	532	0	70	168	2	0	788	0	70	208	1	0	204	1	65
119	2	0	684	0	65	169	2	0	575	0	80	209	1	1	129	1	50
120	2	0	769	1	70	170	2	1	109	1	70	210	1	1	581	0	65
121	2	0	591	0	70	171	2	0	730	1	80	211	1	1	176	0	55
122	2	0	769	1	40	172	2	0	790	0	90	212	1	1	30	0	60
123	2	0	609	1	100	173	2	0	456	1	70	213	1	1	41	0	60
124	2	0	932	1	80	175	2	1	231	1	60	214	1	0	543	0	40
125	2	0	932	1	80	176	2	1	143	1	70	215	1	0	210	1	50
126	2	0	587	0	110	177	2	0	86	1	40	216	1	1	193	1	70
127	2	1	26	0	40	178	2	0	1021	0	80	217	1	1	44	0	55
128	2	0	72	1	40	179	2	0	684	1	80	218	1	1	367	0	45
129	2	0	641	0	70	180	2	1	878	1	60	219	1	1	348	1	60
131	2	0	367	0	70	181	2	1	216	0	100	220	1	0	28	0	50
132	2	0	633	0	70	182	2	0	808	0	60	221	1	0	337	0	40
133	2	1	661	0	40	183	2	1	268	1	40	222	1	0	175	1	60

1	2	3	4	5	6	1	2	3	4	5	6	1	2	3	4	5	6
223	2	1	149	1	80	238	2	0	531	1	45	252	1	1	180	1	60
224	1	1	546	1	50	239	1	0	98	0	40	253	1	1	314	0	70
225	1	1	84	0	45	240	1	1	145	1	55	254	1	0	480	0	50
226	1	0	283	1	80	241	1	1	50	0	50	255	1	0	325	1	60
227	1	1	533	0	55	242	1	0	53	0	50	256	2	1	280	0	90
228	1	1	207	1	50	243	1	0	103	1	50	257	1	1	204	0	50
229	1	1	216	0	50	244	1	0	2	1	60	258	2	1	366	0	55
230	1	0	28	0	50	245	1	1	157	1	60	259	2	0	531	1	50
231	1	1	67	1	50	246	1	1	75	1	55	260	1	1	59	1	45
232	1	0	62	1	60	247	1	1	19	1	40	261	1	1	33	1	60
233	1	0	111	0	55	248	1	1	35	0	60	262	2	1	540	0	80
234	1	1	257	1	60	249	2	0	394	1	80	263	2	0	551	0	65
235	1	1	136	1	55	250	1	1	117	0	40	264	1	1	90	0	40
236	1	0	342	0	60	251	1	1	175	1	60	266	1	1	47	0	45
237	2	1	41	0	40												

ANDERSON.DAT Survival times in weeks (in remission) of 42 leukemia patients in clinical trial to compare treatment with placebo. Data from Freireich et al., "The effect of 6-mercaptopurine on the duration of steroid-induced remissions in acute leukemia," *Blood* **21,** 699–716, 1963.

Column 1 = survival time (weeks)
        2 = status (0 = censored, 1 = relapse)
        3 = sex (1 = male, 0 = female)
        4 = log WBC
        5 = *Rx* (1 = placebo, 0 = treatment)
/nr = 42
/field = (n3,2n2,n5,n2)

1	2	3	4	5	1	2	3	4	5	1	2	3	4	5
35	0	1	1.45	0	9	0	0	2.80	0	8	1	0	3.52	1
34	0	1	1.47	0	7	1	0	4.43	0	8	1	0	3.05	1
32	0	1	2.20	0	6	0	0	3.20	0	8	1	0	2.32	1
32	0	1	2.53	0	6	1	0	2.31	0	8	1	1	3.26	1
25	0	1	1.78	0	6	1	1	4.06	0	5	1	1	3.49	1
23	1	1	2.57	0	6	1	0	3.28	0	5	1	0	3.97	1
22	1	1	2.32	0	23	1	1	1.97	1	4	1	1	4.36	1
20	0	1	2.01	0	22	1	0	2.73	1	4	1	1	2.42	1
19	0	0	2.05	0	17	1	0	2.95	1	3	1	1	4.01	1
17	0	0	2.16	0	15	1	0	2.30	1	2	1	1	4.91	1
16	1	1	3.60	0	12	1	0	1.50	1	2	1	1	4.48	1
13	1	0	2.88	0	12	1	0	3.06	1	1	1	1	2.80	1
11	0	0	2.60	0	11	1	0	3.49	1	1	1	1	5.00	1
10	0	0	2.70	0	11	1	0	2.12	1					
10	1	0	2.96	0										

CHEMO.DAT

Survival times in days from a clinical trial on gastric carcinoma, involving 90 patients randomized to either chemotherapy alone or to a combination of chemotherapy and radiation. Data from Stablein et al., "The analysis of survival data with nonproportional hazard functions," *Controlled Clinical Trials* **2**, 149–159, 1981.

Column 1 = Rx (1 = chemotherapy, 2 = chemotherapy and radiation)
    2 = status (0 = censored, 1 = died)
    3 = survival time (days)
/nr = 3
/field = (s1,c15)

1	2	3	1	2	3	1	2	3	1	2	3	1	2	3
1	1	17	1	1	197	1	0	882	2	1	301	2	1	535
1	1	42	1	1	208	1	0	892	2	1	342	2	1	562
1	1	44	1	1	234	1	0	1031	2	1	354	2	1	675
1	1	48	1	1	235	1	0	1033	2	1	356	2	1	676
1	1	60	1	1	254	1	0	1306	2	1	358	2	1	748
1	1	72	1	1	307	1	0	1335	2	1	380	2	1	748
1	1	74	1	1	315	1	1	1366	2	0	381	2	1	778
1	1	95	1	1	401	1	0	1452	2	1	383	2	1	786
1	1	103	1	1	445	1	0	1472	2	1	383	2	1	797
1	1	108	1	1	464	2	1	1	2	1	388	2	0	945
1	1	122	1	1	484	2	1	63	2	1	394	2	1	955
1	1	144	1	1	528	2	1	105	2	1	408	2	1	968
1	1	167	1	1	542	2	1	129	2	1	460	2	0	1180
1	1	170	1	1	567	2	1	182	2	1	489	2	1	1245
1	1	183	1	1	577	2	1	216	2	1	499	2	1	1271
1	1	185	1	1	580	2	1	250	2	1	524	2	0	1277
1	1	193	1	1	795	2	1	262	2	0	529	2	0	1397
1	1	195	1	1	855	2	1	301	2	1	535	2	0	1512
1	1	197	1	0	882	2	1	301	2	1	562	2	0	1519

STANF.DAT   Survival times in days for 249 patients in Stanford Heart Transplant Trial. Data from Kalbfleisch, J., and Prentice, R., *The Statistical Analysis of Failure Time Data,* John Wiley and Sons, New York, 1980.

Column 1 = pretransplant survival time
        2 = status at first endpoint (0 = alive, 1 = dead)
        3 = posttransplant survival time
        4 = status at second endpoint (Feb 1980)
        5 = age at transplant
        6 = tissue mismatch score
/field = (n3,n2,s1,n4,n2,n3,s1,n4)

1	2	3	4	5	6	1	2	3	4	5	6
49	1	—	—	—	—	70	0	1	1	54	0.47
5	1	—	—	—	—	34	1	—	—	—	—
0	0	15	1	54	1.11	15	0	836	1	44	1.58
35	0	3	1	40	1.66	15	1	—	—	—	—
17	1	—	—	—	—	16	0	60	1	64	0.69
2	1	—	—	—	—	50	0	1996	1	49	0.91
50	0	623	1	51	1.32	22	0	3694	0	40	0.38
39	1	—	—	—	—	11	1	—	—	—	—
84	1	—	—	—	—	45	0	54	1	49	2.09
11	0	46	1	42	0.61	18	0	47	1	62	0.87
25	0	126	1	48	0.36	4	0	0	1	41	0.87
7	1	—	—	—	—	1	0	51	1	50	—
16	0	64	1	54	1.89	40	0	2878	1	49	0.75
36	0	1350	1	54	0.87	57	0	3410	1	45	0.98
0	1	—	—	—	—	2	1	—	—	—	—
27	0	279	1	49	1.12	1	1	—	—	—	—
35	1	—	—	—	—	39	1	—	—	—	—
19	0	23	1	56	2.05	0	0	44	1	36	0.00
36	1	—	—	—	—	1	0	994	1	48	0.81
17	0	10	1	56	2.76	20	0	51	1	47	1.38
7	0	1024	1	43	1.13	8	1	—	—	—	—
11	0	39	1	42	1.38	35	0	1478	1	36	1.35
2	0	730	1	58	0.96	82	0	897	1	46	—
82	0	136	1	52	1.62	31	0	254	1	48	1.08
24	0	1961	1	33	1.06	101	1	—	—	—	—
112	0	—	—	—	—	40	0	148	1	47	—
262	1	—	—	—	—	2	1	—	—	—	—

— denotes missing data

1	2	3	4	5	6	1	2	3	4	5	6
9	0	51	1	52	1.51	309	0	146	1	45	0.16
66	0	3021	0	38	0.98	27	0	431	1	47	0.33
148	1	—	—	—	—	4	0	161	1	43	1.20
20	0	323	1	48	1.82	1	0	14	1	40	—
77	0	2984	0	32	0.19	12	0	2313	0	26	0.46
2	0	66	1	49	0.66	20	0	1634	1	23	1.78
1	1	—	—	—	—	95	0	48	1	28	0.77
57	0	—	—	—	—	20	1	—	—	—	—
26	0	2723	0	32	1.93	37	0	2127	1	35	0.67
32	0	550	1	48	0.12	56	0	263	1	49	0.48
11	0	66	1	51	1.12	50	0	2106	0	40	0.86
31	1	—	—	—	—	70	1	—	—	—	—
56	0	227	1	19	1.02	1	0	293	1	43	0.70
2	0	65	1	45	1.68	5	0	2025	0	30	1.44
9	0	2805	0	48	1.20	29	0	2000	0	45	1.46
4	0	25	1	53	1.68	1	0	2006	0	15	1.26
30	0	2734	0	47	0.97	1	0	1995	0	47	1.65
3	0	631	1	26	1.46	10	0	1945	0	38	1.28
26	0	63	1	56	2.16	6	0	65	1	55	0.69
4	0	12	1	29	0.61	2	0	731	1	38	0.42
1	1	—	—	—	—	40	0	1866	0	49	0.51
45	0	2474	1	52	1.70	18	0	538	1	49	2.76
20	1	—	—	—	—	0	0	1846	0	44	0.83
209	0	547	1	49	0.81	26	0	68	1	35	0.85
66	0	29	1	53	1.08	19	0	1778	0	27	0.70
25	0	1384	1	46	1.41	68	0	928	1	50	1.12
5	0	544	1	52	1.94	55	1	—	—	—	—
31	0	48	1	53	3.05	11	0	1722	0	40	0.95
36	0	297	1	42	0.60	1	0	1718	0	39	1.77
4	1	—	—	—	—	30	0	22	1	27	1.64
7	0	1318	1	48	1.44	29	0	7	1	28	1.00
59	0	50	1	46	2.25	25	0	40	1	42	1.59
30	0	1352	1	54	0.68	47	0	1612	0	51	1.25
138	0	68	1	51	1.33	46	0	25	1	52	0.53
159	0	26	1	52	0.82	1	0	1638	0	48	0.43
340	1	—	—	—	—	59	0	1547	0	50	0.18

— denotes missing data

1	2	3	4	5	6	1	2	3	4	5	6
15	0	1534	1	44	1.71	13	1	—	—	—	—
70	1	—	—	—	—	53	1	—	—	—	—
32	0	1271	1	32	1.05	36	0	993	0	30	0.95
63	0	—	—	—	—	59	0	950	0	46	—
11	0	44	1	46	1.71	45	0	121	1	45	—
52	0	1232	1	18	0.70	4	0	729	1	49	1.10
4	0	1247	1	41	0.43	35	0	202	1	48	1.24
10	0	191	1	42	1.74	48	0	841	0	48	0.86
42	0	1393	0	46	0.95	20	0	1	1	21	0.47
1	1	—	—	—	—	88	0	752	1	43	1.50
35	0	1202	1	38	—	0	0	834	0	49	—
51	0	274	1	31	0.58	1	0	265	1	49	1.22
34	0	1373	0	41	1.38	121	0	132	1	46	1.09
3	1	—	—	—	—	76	0	738	0	41	0.53
7	0	1378	0	41	1.65	26	0	86	1	12	1.26
6	0	31	1	33	0.36	10	0	328	1	34	1.02
14	1	—	—	—	—	2	0	793	0	19	1.98
46	0	381	1	45	0.98	10	0	781	0	20	1.12
16	0	1341	0	50	1.13	86	0	663	0	36	0.47
70	0	1262	0	34	1.68	33	1	—	—	—	—
3	0	42	1	19	0.63	35	0	—	—	—	—
27	0	1261	0	47	0.82	30	0	221	1	35	1.04
17	0	47	1	36	0.16	75	0	90	1	38	1.00
11	0	1264	0	52	0.64	9	0	660	0	42	0.75
82	0	48	1	51	0.99	79	1	—	—	—	—
202	0	30	1	34	0.84	106	0	36	1	45	0.20
86	0	1150	1	32	2.25	36	1	—	—	—	—
70	0	626	1	53	1.74	12	—	618	0	50	0.82
38	0	1193	0	24	1.15	9	1	—	—	—	—
71	0	45	1	48	0.65	29	1	—	—	—	—
43	1	—	—	—	—	14	0	619	0	47	0.90
63	0	1107	0	18	0.25	17	1	—	—	—	—
129	0	1040	1	43	0.50	5	0	576	0	53	2.25
69	1	—	—	—	—	26	0	548	0	30	0.47
12	0	1116	0	14	0.54	1	0	563	0	41	—
25	0	1102	0	39	1.35	12	0	549	0	40	2.53
39	0	195	1	39	0.73	32	0	169	1	51	1.89

— denotes missing data

1	2	3	4	5	6	1	2	3	4	5	6
33	0	122	1	51	1.33	89	0	22	1	45	—
19	0	534	0	20	—	223	0	—	—	—	—
8	0	541	0	47	0.43	59	0	231	1	52	—
16	1	—	—	—	—	65	0	188	1	52	—
18	1	—	—	—	—	82	0	149	0	21	—
62	0	464	0	38	2.07	27	0	176	0	29	1.72
2	1	—	—	—	—	192	0	—	—	—	—
82	0	10	1	13	1.49	67	0	119	0	20	—
1	1	—	—	—	—	18	1	—	—	—	—
70	0	136	1	55	—	176	0	—	—	—	—
167	0	322	0	36	1.73	9	0	138	1	41	—
52	0	5	1	20	—	11	1	—	—	—	—
15	0	382	1	36	—	146	0	—	—	—	—
9	0	468	0	24	1.39	125	0	—	—	—	—
63	0	406	0	39	1.18	15	0	107	0	46	—
15	1	—	—	—	—	23	0	98	0	19	—
2	0	391	0	27	1.17	31	1	—	—	—	—
13	1	—	—	—	—	30	0	89	0	27	—
11	0	374	0	47	—	22	0	56	0	27	—
92	0	292	1	43	1.40	24	1	—	—	—	—
17	0	50	1	50	0.50	10	0	60	0	13	—
36	0	139	1	51	0.96	25	0	2	0	39	—
117	0	145	1	50	0.96	14	0	—	—	—	—
51	0	278	1	41	0.98	12	0	1	0	27	—
18	1	—	—	—	—						

— denotes missing data

VETS.DAT

Survival data for 137 patients from Veteran's Administration Lung Cancer Trial. Data from Kalbfleisch, J., and Prentice, R., *The Statistical Analysis of Failure Time Data*, John Wiley and Sons, New York, 1980.

Column 1 = treatment (1 = standard, 2 = test)
      2 = cell type 1 (1 = large, 0 = other)
      3 = cell type 2 (1 = adeno, 0 = other)
      4 = cell type 3 (1 = small, 0 = other)
      5 = cell type 4 (1 = squamous, 0 = other)
      6 = survival time (days)
      7 = performance status (0 = worst, . . . , 100 = best)
      8 = disease duration (months)
      9 = age (years)
    10 = prior therapy (0 = none, 10 = some)
    11 = status (0 = censored, 1 = Died)
/field = (n2, 4n1, N4, 4N3, N2)

1	2	3	4	5	6	7	8	9	10	11
1	0	0	0	1	72	60	7	69	0	1
1	0	0	0	1	411	70	5	64	10	1
1	0	0	0	1	228	60	3	38	0	1
1	0	0	0	1	126	60	9	63	10	1
1	0	0	0	1	118	70	11	65	10	1
1	0	0	0	1	10	20	5	49	0	1
1	0	0	0	1	82	40	10	69	10	1
1	0	0	0	1	110	80	29	68	0	1
1	0	0	0	1	314	50	18	43	0	1
1	0	0	0	1	100	70	6	70	0	0
1	0	0	0	1	42	60	4	81	0	1
1	0	0	0	1	8	40	58	63	10	1
1	0	0	0	1	144	30	4	63	0	1
1	0	0	0	1	25	80	9	52	10	0
1	0	0	0	1	11	70	11	48	10	1
1	0	0	1	0	30	60	3	61	0	1
1	0	0	1	0	384	60	9	42	0	1
1	0	0	1	0	4	40	2	35	0	1
1	0	0	1	0	54	80	4	63	10	1
1	0	0	1	0	13	60	4	56	0	1
1	0	0	1	0	123	40	3	55	0	0
1	0	0	1	0	97	60	5	67	0	0
1	0	0	1	0	153	60	14	63	10	1

1	2	3	4	5	6	7	8	9	10	11
1	0	0	1	0	59	30	2	65	0	1
1	0	0	1	0	117	80	3	46	0	1
1	0	0	1	0	16	30	4	53	10	1
1	0	0	1	0	151	50	12	69	0	1
1	0	0	1	0	22	60	4	68	0	1
1	0	0	1	0	56	80	12	43	10	1
1	0	0	1	0	21	40	2	55	10	1
1	0	0	1	0	18	20	15	42	0	1
1	0	0	1	0	139	80	2	64	0	1
1	0	0	1	0	20	30	5	65	0	1
1	0	0	1	0	31	75	3	65	0	1
1	0	0	1	0	52	70	2	55	0	1
1	0	0	1	0	287	60	25	66	10	1
1	0	0	1	0	18	30	4	60	0	1
1	0	0	1	0	51	60	1	67	0	1
1	0	0	1	0	122	80	28	53	0	1
1	0	0	1	0	27	60	8	62	0	1
1	0	0	1	0	54	70	1	67	0	1
1	0	0	1	0	7	50	7	72	0	1
1	0	0	1	0	63	50	11	48	0	1
1	0	0	1	0	392	40	4	68	0	1
1	0	0	1	0	10	40	23	67	10	1
1	0	1	0	0	8	20	19	61	10	1
1	0	1	0	0	92	70	10	60	0	1
1	0	1	0	0	35	40	6	62	0	1
1	0	1	0	0	117	80	2	38	0	1
1	0	1	0	0	132	80	5	50	0	1
1	0	1	0	0	12	50	4	63	10	1
1	0	1	0	0	162	80	5	64	0	1
1	0	1	0	0	3	30	3	43	0	1
1	0	1	0	0	95	80	4	34	0	1
1	1	0	0	0	177	50	16	66	10	1
1	1	0	0	0	162	80	5	62	0	1
1	1	0	0	0	216	50	15	52	0	1
1	1	0	0	0	553	70	2	47	0	1
1	1	0	0	0	278	60	12	63	0	1
1	1	0	0	0	12	40	12	68	10	1
1	1	0	0	0	260	80	5	45	0	1

1	2	3	4	5	6	7	8	9	10	11
1	1	0	0	0	200	80	12	41	10	1
1	1	0	0	0	156	70	2	66	0	1
1	1	0	0	0	182	90	2	62	0	0
1	1	0	0	0	143	90	8	60	0	1
1	1	0	0	0	105	80	11	66	0	1
1	1	0	0	0	103	80	5	38	0	1
1	1	0	0	0	250	70	8	53	10	1
1	1	0	0	0	100	60	13	37	10	1
2	0	0	0	1	999	90	12	54	10	1
2	0	0	0	1	112	80	6	60	0	1
2	0	0	0	1	87	80	3	48	0	0
2	0	0	0	1	231	50	8	52	10	0
2	0	0	0	1	242	50	1	70	0	1
2	0	0	0	1	991	70	7	50	10	1
2	0	0	0	1	111	70	3	62	0	1
2	0	0	0	1	1	20	21	65	10	1
2	0	0	0	1	587	60	3	58	0	1
2	0	0	0	1	389	90	2	62	0	1
2	0	0	0	1	33	30	6	64	0	1
2	0	0	0	1	25	20	36	63	0	1
2	0	0	0	1	357	70	13	58	0	1
2	0	0	0	1	467	90	2	64	0	1
2	0	0	0	1	201	80	28	52	10	1
2	0	0	0	1	1	50	7	35	0	1
2	0	0	0	1	30	70	11	63	0	1
2	0	0	0	1	44	60	13	70	10	1
2	0	0	0	1	283	90	2	51	0	1
2	0	0	0	1	15	50	13	40	10	1
2	0	0	1	0	25	30	2	69	0	1
2	0	0	1	0	103	70	22	36	10	0
2	0	0	1	0	21	20	4	71	0	1
2	0	0	1	0	13	30	2	62	0	1
2	0	0	1	0	87	60	2	60	0	1
2	0	0	1	0	2	40	36	44	10	1
2	0	0	1	0	20	30	9	54	10	1
2	0	0	1	0	7	20	11	66	0	1
2	0	0	1	0	24	60	8	49	0	1
2	0	0	1	0	99	70	3	72	0	1

1	2	3	4	5	6	7	8	9	10	11
2	0	0	1	0	8	80	2	68	0	1
2	0	0	1	0	99	85	4	62	0	1
2	0	0	1	0	61	70	2	71	0	1
2	0	0	1	0	25	70	2	70	0	1
2	0	0	1	0	95	70	1	61	0	1
2	0	0	1	0	80	50	17	71	0	1
2	0	0	1	0	51	30	87	59	10	1
2	0	0	1	0	29	40	8	67	0	1
2	0	1	0	0	24	40	2	60	0	1
2	0	1	0	0	18	40	5	69	10	1
2	0	1	0	0	83	99	3	57	0	0
2	0	1	0	0	31	80	3	39	0	1
2	0	1	0	0	51	60	5	62	0	1
2	0	1	0	0	90	60	22	50	10	1
2	0	1	0	0	52	60	3	43	0	1
2	0	1	0	0	73	60	3	70	0	1
2	0	1	0	0	8	50	5	66	0	1
2	0	1	0	0	36	70	8	61	0	1
2	0	1	0	0	48	10	4	81	0	1
2	0	1	0	0	7	40	4	58	0	1
2	0	1	0	0	140	70	3	63	0	1
2	0	1	0	0	186	90	3	60	0	1
2	0	1	0	0	84	80	4	62	10	1
2	0	1	0	0	19	50	10	42	0	1
2	0	1	0	0	45	40	3	69	0	1
2	0	1	0	0	80	40	4	63	0	1
2	1	0	0	0	52	60	4	45	0	1
2	1	0	0	0	164	70	15	68	10	1
2	1	0	0	0	19	30	4	39	10	1
2	1	0	0	0	53	60	12	66	0	1
2	1	0	0	0	15	30	5	63	0	1
2	1	0	0	0	43	60	11	49	10	1
2	1	0	0	0	340	80	10	64	10	1
2	1	0	0	0	133	75	1	65	0	1
2	1	0	0	0	111	60	5	64	0	1
2	1	0	0	0	231	70	18	67	10	1
2	1	0	0	0	378	80	4	65	0	1
2	1	0	0	0	49	30	3	37	0	1

Test

Answers

Chapter 1

True-False Questions:

1. T
2. T
3. T
4. F: step function.
5. F: ranges between 0 and 1.
6. T
7. T
8. T
9. T
10. F: median survival time is longer for group 1 than for group 2.
11. F: six weeks or greater.
12. F: the risk set at 7 weeks contains 15 persons.
13. F: hazard ratio
14. T
15. T

16. $h(t)$ gives the instantaneous potential per unit time for the event to occur given that the individual has survived up to time t; $h(t)$ is greater than or equal to 0; $h(t)$ has no upper bound.

17. Hazard functions
    • give insight about conditional failure rates;
    • help to identify specific model forms (e.g., exponential, Weibull);
    • are used to specify mathematical models for survival analysis.

18. Three goals of survival analysis are the following:
    • to estimate and interpret survivor and/or hazard functions;
    • to compare survivor and/or hazard functions;
    • to assess the relationship of explanatory variables to survival time.

19.

$t_{(j)}$	$m_{(j)}$	$q_{(j)}$	$R(t_{(j)})$
Group 1: 0	0	0	25 persons survive $\geq$ 0 years
1.8	1	0	25 persons survive $\geq$ 1.8 years
2.2	1	0	24 persons survive $\geq$ 2.2 years
2.5	1	0	23 persons survive $\geq$ 2.5 years
2.6	1	0	22 persons survive $\geq$ 2.6 years
3.0	1	0	21 persons survive $\geq$ 3.0 years
3.5	1	0	20 persons survive $\geq$ 3.5 years
3.8	1	0	19 persons survive $\geq$ 3.8 years

$t_{(j)}$	$m_{(j)}$	$q_{(j)}$	$R(t_{(j)})$
5.3	1	0	18 persons survive $\geq$ 5.3 years
5.4	1	0	17 persons survive $\geq$ 5.4 years
5.7	1	0	16 persons survive $\geq$ 5.7 years
6.6	1	0	15 persons survive $\geq$ 6.6 years
8.2	1	0	14 persons survive $\geq$ 8.2 years
8.7	1	0	13 persons survive $\geq$ 8.7 years
9.2	2	0	12 persons survive $\geq$ 9.2 years
9.8	1	0	10 persons survive $\geq$ 9.8 years
10.0	1	0	9 persons survive $\geq$ 10.0 years
10.2	1	0	8 persons survive $\geq$ 10.2 years
10.7	1	0	7 persons survive $\geq$ 10.7 years
11.0	1	0	6 persons survive $\geq$ 11.0 years
11.1	1	0	5 persons survive $\geq$ 11.1 years
11.7	1	3	4 persons survive $\geq$ 11.7 years

20. a. Group 1 has better survival prognosis than group 2 because group 1 has a higher average survival time and a correspondingly lower average hazard rate than group 2.

    b. The average survival time and average hazard rates give overall descriptive statistics. The survivor curves allow one to make comparisons over time.

Chapter 2

1. a. KM plots and log–rank and Peto statistics for the cell type 1 variable in the vets.data dataset are shown below.

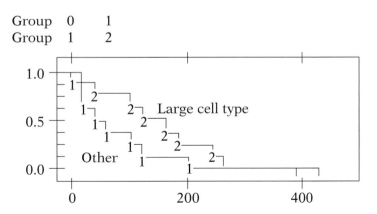

Group	Size	%Cen	LQ	Median	UQ	0.95	Med CI
0	110	7.273	21	56.000	139	44.000	84
1	27	3.704	53	156.000	231	103.000	200

df: 1   Log–rank: 3.021   p-value: 0.082   Peto: 4.906   p-value: 0.027

The KM curves indicate that persons with large cell type have consistently better prognosis than persons with other cell types, although the two curves are essentially the same very early on and after 250 days. The log–rank test is not significant at the .05 level, but the Peto test is significant at the .05 level, which gives somewhat equivocal findings.

b. KM plots and log–rank and Peto statistics for the four categories of cell type are shown below:

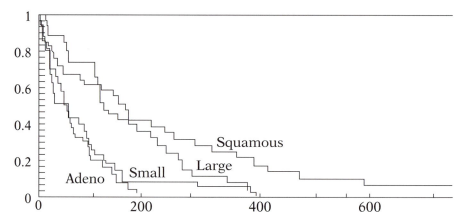

The KM curves suggest that persons with adeno or small cell types have poorer survival prognosis than persons with large or squamous cell types. Moreover, there does not appear to be a meaningful difference between adeno or small cell types. Also, persons with squamous cell type seem to have, on the whole, a better prognosis than persons with large cell type.

Computer results from **SPIDA** giving log–rank and Peto statistics are now shown:

Group	Size	%Cen	LQ	Median	UQ	0.95	Med CI
1	27	3.704	53	156	231	103.000	200
2	27	3.704	19	51	92	31.000	84
3	48	6.250	20	51	99	25.000	59
4	35	11.429	33	118	357	72.000	231

df: 3   Log–rank: 25.404   p-value: 0   Peto: 13.607   p-value: 0.003

Both the log–rank test and the Peto test yield highly significant p-values, indicating that there is some overall difference between all four curves; that is, the null hypothesis that the four curves have a common survival curve is rejected.

2. a. KM plots for the two clinics are shown below. These plots indicate that patients in clinic 2 have consistently better prognosis for remaining under treatment than do patients in clinic 1. Moreover, it appears that the difference between the two clinics is small before one year of follow-up but diverges after one year of follow-up.

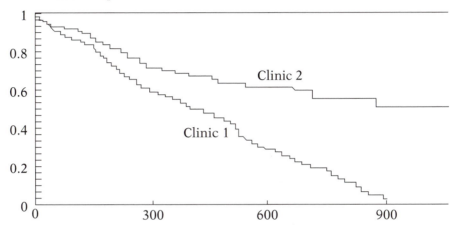

 b. The log–rank statistic (27.893) and Peto statistic (11.078) are both significant well-below the .01 level, indicating that the survival curves for the two clinics are significantly different. The log–rank statistic is nevertheless much larger than the Peto statistic, which makes sense since the log–rank statistic emphasizes the later survival experience, where the two survival curves are far apart, whereas the Peto statistic emphasizes earlier survival experience, where the two survival curves are closer together.

 c. If methadone dose is categorized into high (70+), medium (55–70) and low (<55), we obtain the KM curves shown below.

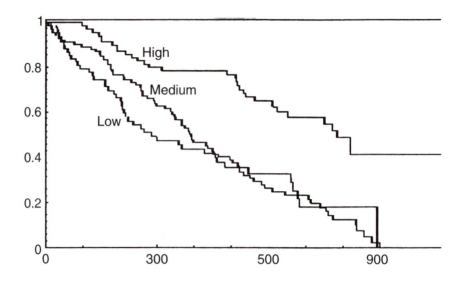

The KM curves indicate that persons with high doses have consistently better survival prognosis (i.e., maintenance) than persons with medium or low doses. The latter two groups are not very different from one another, although the medium dose group has somewhat better prognosis up to the first 400 days of follow-up.

The log–rank and Peto test statistics are shown below for the above categorization scheme:

Group	Size	%Cen	LQ	Median	UQ	0.95	Med CI
1	72	37.500	129	286	679	207.000	480
2	95	22.105	212	393	612	341.000	465
3	71	56.338	514	785		624.000	

df: 2   log–rank: 33.019   p-value: 0   Peto: 19.903   p-value: 0

Both test statistics are highly significant, indicating that these three curves are not equivalent.

Chapter 3

1. a. $h(t, \mathbf{X}) = h_0(t) \exp[\beta_1 T1 + \beta_2 T2 + \beta_3 PS + \beta_4 DC + \beta_5 BF + \beta_6(T1 \times PS) + \beta_7(T2 \times PS) + \beta_8(T1 \times DC) + \beta_9(T2 \times DC) + \beta_{10}(T1 \times BF) + \beta_{11}(T2 \times BF)]$

   b. **Intervention A: $\mathbf{X}^* = (1, 0, PS, DC, BF, PS, 0, DC, 0, BF, 0)$**

   Intervention C: $\mathbf{X} = (-1, -1, PS, DC, BF, -PS, -PS, -DC, -DC, -BF, -BF)$

$$HR = \frac{h(t, \mathbf{X}^*)}{h(t, \mathbf{X})} = \exp\left[2\beta_1 + \beta_2 + 2\beta_6 PS + \beta_7 PS + 2\beta_8 DC + \beta_9 DC + 2\beta_{10} BF + \beta_{11} BF\right]$$

   c. H_0: $\beta_6 = \beta_7 = \beta_8 = \beta_9 = \beta_{10} = \beta_{11} = 0$ in the full model. Likelihood ratio test statistic: $-2 \ln \hat{L}_R - (-2 \ln \hat{L}_F)$, which is approximately χ^2_6 under H_0, where R denotes the reduced model (containing no product terms) under H_0, and F denotes the full model (given in part 1a above)

   d. The two models being compared are:

Full model (F): $h(t, \mathbf{X}) = h_0(t) \exp[\beta_1 T1 + \beta_2 T2 + \beta_3 PS + \beta_4 DC + \beta_5 BF]$

Reduced model (R): $h(t, \mathbf{X}) = h_0(t) \exp[\beta_3 PS + \beta_4 DC + \beta_5 BF]$

H_0: $\beta_1 = \beta_2 = 0$ in the full model

Likelihood ratio test statistic: $-2 \ln \hat{L}_R - (-2 \ln \hat{L}_F)$, which is approximately χ^2_2 under H_0

   e.

Intervention A: $\hat{S}(t, \mathbf{X}) = \left[\hat{S}_0(t)\right]^{\exp\left[\hat{\beta}_1 + \left(\overline{PS}\right)\hat{\beta}_3 + \left(\overline{DC}\right)\hat{\beta}_4 + \left(\overline{BF}\right)\hat{\beta}_5\right]}$

Intervention B: $\hat{S}(t, \mathbf{X}) = \left[\hat{S}_0(t)\right]^{\exp\left[\hat{\beta}_2 + \left(\overline{PS}\right)\hat{\beta}_3 + \left(\overline{DC}\right)\hat{\beta}_4 + \left(\overline{BF}\right)\hat{\beta}_5\right]}$

Intervention C: $\hat{S}(t, \mathbf{X}) = \left[\hat{S}_0(t)\right]^{\exp\left[-\hat{\beta}_1 - \hat{\beta}_2 + \left(\overline{PS}\right)\hat{\beta}_3 + \left(\overline{DC}\right)\hat{\beta}_4 + \left(\overline{BF}\right)\hat{\beta}_5\right]}$

2.   a. $h(t, \mathbf{X}) = h_0(t) \exp[\beta_1 \, CHR + \beta_2 \, AGE + \beta_3 \, (CHR \times AGE)]$

   b. H_0: $\beta_3 = 0$

LR statistic = $264.90 - 264.69 = 0.21$; χ^2 with 1 d.f. under H_0; not significant.

Wald statistic gives a chi-square value of .01, also not significant. Conclusions about interaction: the model should not contain an interaction term.

   c. When AGE is controlled (using the gold standard model 2), the hazard ratio for the effect of CHR is exp(.8051) = 2.24, whereas when AGE is not controlled, the hazard ratio for the effect of CHR (using model 1) is exp(.8595) = 2.36. Thus, the hazard ratios are not appreciably different, so AGE is not a confounder.

Regarding precision, the 95% confidence interval for the effect of CHR in the gold standard model (model 2) is given by exp[.8051 ± 1.96(.3252)] = (1.183, 4.231) whereas the corresponding 95% confidence interval in the model without AGE (model 1) is given by exp[.8595 ± 1.96(.3116)] = (1.282, 4.350). Both confidence intervals have about the same width, with the latter interval being slightly wider. Thus, controlling for AGE has little effect on the final point and interval estimates of interest.

d. If the hazard functions cross for the two levels of the CHR variable, this would mean that none of the models provided are appropriate, because each model assumes that the proportional hazards assumption is met for each predictor in the model. If hazard functions cross for CHR, however, the proportional hazards assumption cannot be satisfied for this variable.

e. For $CHR = 1$: $\hat{S}(t, \mathbf{X}) = [\hat{S}_0(t)]^{\exp[0.8051 + 0.0856(\overline{AGE})]}$

For $CHR = 0$: $\hat{S}(t, \mathbf{X}) = [\hat{S}_0(t)]^{\exp[0.0856(\overline{AGE})]}$

f. Using model 1, which is the best model, there is evidence of a moderate effect of CHR on survival time, because the hazard ratio is about 2.4 with a 95% confidence interval between 1.3 and 4.4, and the Wald test for significance of this variable is significant below the .01 level.

3. a. Full model (F = model 1): $h(t, \mathbf{X}) = h_0(t) \exp [\beta_1 Rx + \beta_3 \text{ Sex} + \beta_4 \log \text{WBC} + \beta_5(Rx \times \text{Sex}) + \beta_7(Rx \times \log \text{WBC})]$

Reduced model (R = model 4): $h(t, \mathbf{X}) = h_0(t) \exp [\beta_1 Rx + \beta_3 \text{ Sex} + \beta_4 \log \text{WBC}]$

$H_0: \beta_4 = \beta_5 = 0$

LR statistic = $144.218 - 139.029 = 5.19$; χ^2 with 2 d.f. under H_0; not significant at 0.05, though significant at 0.10. The chunk test indicates some (though mild) evidence of interaction.

b. Using either a Wald test ($P = .776$) or a LR test, the product term $Rx \times \log$ WBC is clearly not significant, and thus should be dropped from model 1. Thus, model 2 is preferred to model 1.

c. Using model 2, the hazard ratio for the effect of Rx is given by:

$$\text{HR} = \frac{h(t, \mathbf{X}^*)}{h(t, \mathbf{X})} = \exp[0.405 + 2.013 \text{ Sex}]$$

d. Males (Sex = 0): $\widehat{HR} = \exp[0.405] = 1.499$.

Females (Sex = 1): $\widehat{HR} = \exp[0.405 + 2.013(1)] = 11.223$.

e. Model 2 is preferred to model 3 if one decides that the coefficients for the variables Rx and $Rx \times$ Sex are meaningfully different for the two models. It appears that such corresponding coefficients (0.405 vs 0.587 and 2.013 vs. 1.906) are different. The estimated hazard ratios for model 3 are 1.799 (males) and 12.098 (females), which are different, but not very different from the estimates computed in part 3d for model 2. If it is decided that there is a meaningful difference here, then we would conclude that log WBC is a confounder; otherwise log WBC is not a confounder. Note that the log WBC variable is significant in model 2 ($P = .000$), but this addresses precision and not confounding. When in doubt, as in this case, the safest thing to do (for validity reasons) is to control for log WBC.

f. Model 2 appears to be best, because there is significant interaction of $Rx \times$ Sex ($P = .023$) and because log WBC is a likely confounder (from part e).

g. The $P(PH)$ values for the sex variable and for the $Rx \times$ Sex variable are significant, suggesting that the PH assumption is not satisfied for the sex variable. This indicates that the previous conclusions (in 3e and 3f) may be inappropriate, and that it may be necessary to carry out an alternative (e.g., stratified) analysis that does not include the Sex variable in a Cox PH model.

Chapter 4

1. The $P(PH)$ values in the printout provide GOF statistics for each variable adjusted for the other variables in the model. These $P(PH)$ values indicate that the clinic variable does not satisfy the PH assumption ($P \ll .01$), whereas the prison and dose variables satisfy the PH assumption ($P > .10$).

2. The log–log plots shown are parallel. However, the reason why they are parallel is because the clinic variable has been included in the model, because log–log curves for any variable in a PH model must always be parallel. If, instead, the clinic variable had been stratified (i.e., not included in the model), then the log–log plots comparing the two clinics adjusted for the prison and dose variables might not be parallel.

3. The log–log plots obtained when the clinic variable is stratified (i.e., using a stratified Cox PH model) are not parallel. They intersect early on in follow-up and diverge from each other later in follow-up. These plots therefore indicate that the PH assumption is not satisfied for the clinic variable.

4. Both graphs of log–log plots for the prison variable show curves that intersect and then diverge from one another and then intersect again. Thus, the plots on each graph appear to be quite nonparallel, indicating that the PH assumption is not satisfied for the prison variable. Note, however, that on each graph, the plots are quite close to one another, so that one might conclude that, allowing for random variation, the two plots are essentially coincident; with this latter point of view, one would conclude that the PH assumption is satisfied for the prison variable.

5. The conclusion of nonparallel log–log plots in question 4 gives a different result about the PH assumption for the prison variable than determined from the GOF tests provided in question 1. That is, the log–log plots suggest that the prison variable does not satisfy the PH assumption, whereas the GOF test suggests that the prison variable satisfies the assumption. Note, however, if the point of view is taken that the two plots are close enough to suggest coincidence, the graphi-

cal conclusion would be the same as the GOF conclusion. Although the final decision is somewhat equivocal here, we prefer to conclude that the PH assumption is satisfied for the prison variable because this is strongly indicated from the GOF test and questionably counterindicated by the log–log curves.

6. Because maximum methadone dose is a continuous variable, we must categorize this variable into two or more groups in order to graphically evaluate whether it satisfies the PH assumption. Assume that we have categorized this variable into two groups, say low versus high. Then, **observed** survival plots can be obtained as KM curves for low and high groups separately. To obtain **expected** plots, we can fit a Cox model containing the dose variable and then substitute suitably chosen values for dose into the formula for the estimated survival curve. Typically, the values substituted would be either the mean or median (maximum) dose in each group.

After obtaining observed and expected plots for low and high dose groups, we would conclude that the PH assumption is satisfied if corresponding observed and expected plots are not widely discrepant from one another. If a noticeable discrepancy is found for at least one pair of observed versus expected plots, we conclude that the PH assumption is not satisfied.

7. $h(t, \mathbf{X}) = h_0(t) \exp [\beta_1(\text{clinic}) + \beta_2(\text{prison}) + \beta_3(\text{dose}) + \delta_1(\text{clinic}) \times g(t) + \delta_2(\text{prison}) \times g(t) + \delta_3(\text{dose}) \times g(t)]$

where $g(t)$ is some function of time. The null hypothesis is given by $H_0: \delta_1 = \delta_2 = \delta_3 = 0$. The test statistic is a likelihood ratio statistic of the form

$LR = -2 \ln \hat{L}_R - (-2 \ln \hat{L}_F)$

where R denotes the reduced (PH) model obtained when all δ's are 0, and F denotes the full model given above. Under H_0, the LR statistic is approximately chi-square with 3 d.f.

8. Drawbacks of the extended Cox model approach:
    *   not always clear how to specify $g(t)$; different choices may give different conclusions;
    *   different modeling strategies to choose from, e.g., might consider $g(t)$ to be a polynomial in t and do a backward elimination to eliminate nonsignificant higher-order terms; alternatively, might consider $g(t)$ to be linear in t without evaluating higher-order terms. Different strategies may yield different conclusions.

9. $h(t, \mathbf{X}) = h_0(t) \exp [\beta_1(\text{clinic}) + \beta_2(\text{prison}) + \beta_3(\text{dose}) + \delta_1(\text{clinic}) \times g(t)]$

where $g(t)$ is some function of time. The null hypothesis is given by $H_0: \delta_1 = 0$, and the test statistic is either a Wald statistic or a likelihood ratio statistic; either statistic is approximately chi-square with 1 d.f. under the null hypothesis.

10. $t > 365$ days: $HR = \exp[\beta_1 + \delta_1]$

$t \leq 365$ days: $HR = \exp[\beta_1]$

If δ_1 is not equal to zero, then the model does not satisfy the PH assumption for the clinic variable. Thus, a test of H_0: $\delta_1 = 0$ evaluates the PH assumption; a significant result would indicate that the PH assumption is violated. Note that if δ_1 is not equal to zero, then the model assumes that the hazard ratio is not constant over time by giving a different hazard ratio value depending on whether t is greater than 365 days or t is less than or equal to 365 days.

Chapter 5

1. By fitting a stratified Cox (SC) model that stratifies on clinic, we can compare adjusted survival curves for each clinic, adjusted for the prison and dose variables. This will allow us to visually describe the extent of clinic differences on survival over time. However, a drawback to stratifying on clinic is that it will not be possible to obtain an estimate of the hazard ratio for the effect of clinic, because clinic will not be included in the model.

2. The adjusted survival curves indicate that clinic 2 has better survival prognosis than clinic 1 consistently over time. Moreover, it seems that the difference between the effects of clinic 2 and clinic 1 increases over time.

3. $h_g(t, \mathbf{X}) = h_{0g}(t)\exp[\beta_1 \text{prison} + \beta_2 \text{dose}]$, $g = 1, 2$.

This is a no-interaction model because the regression coefficients for prison and dose are the same for each stratum.

4. Effect of prison, adjusted for dose: $\widehat{HR} = 1.475$, 95% CI: (1.059, 2.054). It appears that having a prison record gives a 1.475 increased hazard for failure than does not having a prison record. The p-value is 0.021, which is significant at the 0.05 level.

5. Version 1: $h_g(t, \mathbf{X}) = h_{0g}(t)\exp[\beta_{1g} \text{prison} + \beta_{2g} \text{dose}]$, $g = 1, 2$.

Version 2: $h_g(t, \mathbf{X}) = h_{0g}(t)\exp[\beta_1 \text{prison} + \beta_2 \text{dose} + \beta_3(\text{clinic} \times \text{prison}) + \beta_4(\text{clinic} \times \text{dose})]$, $g = 1, 2$

6. $g = 1$ (clinic 1): $h_1(t, \mathbf{X}) = h_{01}(t)\exp[(0.502)\text{prison} + (-0.036)\text{dose}]$

$g = 2$ (clinic 2): $h_2(t, \mathbf{X}) = h_{02}(t)\exp[-0.083)\text{prison} + (-0.037)\text{dose}]$

7. The adjusted survival curves stratified by clinic are virtually identical for the no-interaction and interaction models. Consequently, both graphs (no-interaction versus interaction) indicate the same conclusion that clinic 2 has consistently larger survival (i.e., retention) probabilities than clinic 1 as time increases.

8. H_0: $\beta_3 = \beta_4 = 0$ in the version 2 model (i.e., the no-interaction assumption is satisfied). $LR = -2 \ln \hat{L}_R - (-2 \ln \hat{L}_F)$ where R denotes the reduced (no-interaction) model and F denotes the full (interaction) model. Under the null hypothesis, LR is approximately a chi-square with 2 degrees of freedom.

Computed $LR = 1195.428 - 1193.558 = 1.87$; $P = 0.395$; thus, the null hypothesis is not rejected and we conclude that the no-interaction model is preferable to the interaction model.

Chapter 6

1. For the chemo data, the -log–log KM curves intersect at around 600 days; thus the curves are not parallel, and this suggests that the treatment variable does not satisfy the PH assumption.

2. The $P(PH)$ value for the Tx variable is 0, indicating that the PH assumption is not satisfied for the treatment variable based on this goodness-of-fit test.

3. $h(t, \mathbf{X}) = h_0(t)\exp[\beta_1(Tx)g_1(t) + \beta_2(Tx)g_2(t) + \beta_3(Tx)g_3(t)]$
   where
   $$g_1(t) = \begin{cases} 1 \text{ if } 0 \leq t < 250 \text{ days} \\ 0 \text{ if otherwise} \end{cases}$$
   $$g_2(t) = \begin{cases} 1 \text{ if } 250 \leq t < 500 \text{ days} \\ 0 \text{ if otherwise} \end{cases}$$
   $$g_3(t) = \begin{cases} 1 \text{ if } t \geq 500 \text{ days} \\ 0 \text{ if otherwise} \end{cases}$$

4. Based on the printout the hazard ratio estimates and corresponding p-values and 95% confidence intervals are given as follows for each time interval:

	HazRatio	p-value	0.95	CI
$0 \leq t < 250$ days:	0.221	0.001	0.089	0.545
$250 \leq t < 500$ days:	1.629	0.278	0.675	3.934
$t \geq 500$ days:	1.441	0.411	0.604	3.440

   The results show a significant effect of treatment below 250 days and a nonsignificant effect of treatment in each of the two intervals after 250 days. Because the coding for treatment was 1 = chemotherapy plus radiation versus 2 = chemotherapy alone, the results indicate that the hazard for chemotherapy plus radiation is $1/0.221 = 4.52$ times the hazard for chemotherapy alone. The hazard ratio inverts to a value less than 1 (in favor of chemotherapy plus radiation after 250 days), but this result is nonsignificant. Note that for the significant effect of $1/0.221 = 4.52$ below 250 days, the 95% confidence interval ranges between $1/0.545 = 1.83$ and $1/0.089 = 11.24$ when inverted, which is a very wide interval.

5. Model with two heavyside functions:
   $h(t, \mathbf{X}) = h_0(t)\exp[\beta_1(Tx)g_1(t) + \beta_2(Tx)g_2(t)]$

where

$$g_1(t) = \begin{cases} 1 & \text{if } 0 \leq t < 250 \text{ days} \\ 0 & \text{if otherwise} \end{cases}$$

$$g_2(t) = \begin{cases} 1 & \text{if } t \geq 250 \text{ days} \\ 0 & \text{if otherwise} \end{cases}$$

Model with one heavyside function:

$$h(t, \mathbf{X}) = h_0(t)\exp[\beta_1(Tx) + \beta_2(Tx)g_1(t)]$$

where $g_1(t)$ is defined above.

6.   The results for two time intervals give hazard ratios that are on the opposite side of the null value (i.e., 1). Below 250 days, the use of chemotherapy plus radiation is, as in the previous analysis, 4.52 times the hazard when chemotherapy is used alone. This result is significant and the same confidence interval is obtained as before. Above 250 days, the use of chemotherapy alone has 1.532 times the hazard of chemotherapy plus radiation, but this result is nonsignificant.

References

*Caplehorn, J., et al., "Methadone dosage and retention of patients in maintenance treatment," *Med. J. Aust.,* 154, 195–199, 1991.

*Crowley, J. and Hu, M., "Covariance analysis of heart transplant data," *J. Amer. Stat. Assoc.* 72, 27–36, 1977.

Dixon, W.J., *BMDP, Statistical Software Manual,* Berkeley, CA, University of California Press, 1990.

*Freireich, E.O. et al., "The effect of 6-mercaptopmine on the duration of steroid induced remission in acute leukemia," *Blood* 21, 699–716, 1963.

Gebski, V., Leung, O., McNeil, D., and Lunn, D., *SPIDA Users Manual, Version 6,* Macquarie University, Sydney, Australia, 1992.

Harris, E., and Albert, A., *Survivorship Analysis for Clinical Studies,* Marcel Dekker, New York, 1991.

*Kalbfleisch, J.D., and Prentice, R.L., *The Statistical Analysis of Failure Time Data,* John Wiley and Sons, New York, 1980.

Kleinbaum, D.G., *Logistic Regression: A Self-Learning Text,* Springer-Verlag, New York, 1994.

Kleinbaum, D.G., Kupper, L.L., and Morgenstern, H., *Epidemiologic Research: Principles and Quantitative Methods,* Van Nostrand Reinhold, New York, 1982.

Kleinbaum, D.G., Kupper, L.L., and Muller, K.A., *Applied Regression Analysis and Other Multivariable Methods,* Second Edition, Wadsworth, Belmont, CA, 1987.

Krall, J.M., Uthoff, V.A., and Harley, J.B., "A step-up procedure for selecting variables associated with survival data." *Biometrics* 31, 49–57, 1975.

Lee, E.T., *Statistical Methods for Survival Data Analysis,* Wadsworth, Belmont, CA, 1980.

SAS Technical Report P-229, *SAS/STAT Software: Changes and Enhancements, Release 6.07,* Cary, NC: SAS Institute, Inc., 1992, 620 pp.

Prentice, R.L., and Marek, "A qualitative discrepancy between censored data rank tests," *Biometrics* 34, 1979.

*Schoenbach, V.J., Kaplan, B.H., Fredman, L., and Kleinbaum, D.G., "Social ties and mortality in Evans County, Georgia," *Amer. J. Epid.* 123:4, 577–591, 1986.

Schoenfeld, D., "Partial residuals for the proportional hazards model," *Biometrika* 69, 51–55, 1982.

*Stablein, D., Carter, W., and Novak, J., "Analysis of survival data with non-proportional hazard functions," *Controlled Clinical Trials* 2, 149–159, 1981.

*These references are sources for practice exercises or test questions presented at the end of chapters.

Index